PENGUIN LIFE

BODY NEUTRAL

Jessi Kneeland (they/them) is a coach, writer, and speaker dedicated to helping people overcome the suffering associated with body anxiety, insecurity, and negativity, and to improve their relationship with their bodies. After working as a personal trainer for a decade in New York City, Kneeland became an iPEC-certified life coach and launched a coaching practice centered around the meaningful work of self-acceptance. Their innovative approach allows them to partner with clients (individually and in groups) to help them find body acceptance, freedom from oppressive beauty and body ideals, and an authentic sense of identity and worth outside of their body or appearance. They are committed to developing and advancing body neutrality—the practice of consciously stripping our bodies of all false or inflated meaning, importance, and moral significance—as a way of combating both individual suffering and systemic, body-based oppression. Their work has been featured in *Women's Health*, *Shape*, *POPSUGAR*, *Refinery29*, *BuzzFeed*, *HelloGiggles*, and more, and their TED talk has been viewed by over fifty thousand people. They live in North Carolina with their partner and cat.

Body Neutral

A Revolutionary Guide to Overcoming Body Image Issues

Jessi Kneeland

life

PENGUIN BOOKS
An imprint of Penguin Random House LLC
penguinrandomhouse.com

A Penguin Life Book

LIBRARY OF CONGRESS CATALOGING-IN-PUBLICATION DATA
Names: Kneeland, Jessi, author.
Title: Body neutral: a revolutionary guide to overcoming
body image issues / Jessi Kneeland.
Description: New York, NY: Penguin Books, an imprint of
Penguin Random House LLC, [2023] | Includes bibliographical references.
Identifiers: LCCN 2022051181 (print) | LCCN 2022051182 (ebook) |
ISBN 9780593491768 (trade paperback) | ISBN 9780593491751 (ebook)
Subjects: LCSH: Body image. | Beauty, Personal—Psychological aspects. |
Self-esteem. | Identity (Psychology)
Classification: LCC BF697.5.B63 K628 2023 (print) |
LCC BF697.5.B63 (ebook) | DDC 306.4/613—dc23/eng/20221031
LC record available at https://lccn.loc.gov/2022051181
LC ebook record available at https://lccn.loc.gov/2022051182

Printed in the United States of America
1 3 5 7 9 10 8 6 4 2

Set in Horley Old Style MT Pro
Designed by Sabrina Bowers

All names and identifying characteristics have been changed
to protect the privacy of the individuals involved.

For my mom

Contents

Part III

THE PATH TO BODY NEUTRALITY

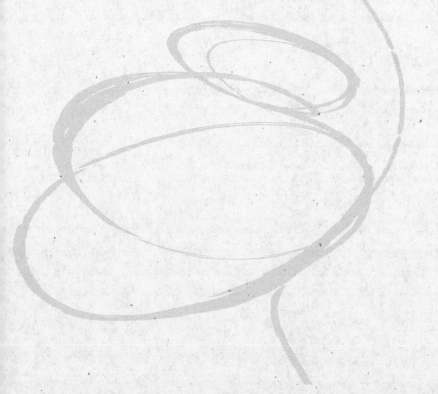

Part I

BODY NEUTRALITY

CHAPTER 1

How I Got Here

OVER A DECADE AGO, I WAS WORKING AS A personal trainer in New York City, overwhelmed by the ubiquity of body image issues. Nearly every single one of my clients (mostly women at the time) came to me with one goal: changing how their body looked. There was a sort of normalized shorthand they all used to talk about their goals. They wanted to work on their "trouble spots," get rid of their "bat wings" and "muffin tops," and "look better" naked. They wanted to tighten this and tone that. Every inch of their bodies was mapped out with specific goals: get bigger, get smaller, get flatter, or change shape completely. They wanted Michelle Obama's arms, Pink's abs, and Gisele's legs. They wanted to attain a thigh gap, but lose their hip dips, and would it be possible to make their boobs a bit perkier? We talked about bodies like Potato Heads; each part considered individually, critiqued without the context of the rest of the body, and given a specific plan for change.

These kinds of conversations happened so often that I barely even recognized them as conversations about body image. It just felt normal. For something to register as a "real" body image issue in my mind, it had to be pretty intense. Like the time a successful model pulled her shorts down to show me a nonexistent flaw that disgusted her so much she felt she couldn't bear it anymore, or the many times clients broke down in tears during sessions because they hated their bodies so much and they were terrified that no matter how hard they worked they were never going to look how they wanted.

I tried to focus on fitness as a tool for building strength and empowerment, and redirect people away from aesthetic goals, but I also understood that the latter was part of the job. People hired me not to get healthier or stronger, but because they felt insecure in their bodies and were absolutely convinced that the key to feeling more peaceful and confident was to change how they looked.

It took me a long time to put into words why this kind of conversation made me uncomfortable, but it didn't take me any time at all to realize that everyone was asking me to help them attain something that simply couldn't be attained through fitness: to stop hating their bodies, and to stop thinking about their bodies all the time. They wanted to feel free, to feel safe, and to find an escape from the endless body-checking* thoughts and behaviors that plagued them.

My clients were desperate to get a "better body," but only because they believed a "better" body would offer them relief from the exhausting and uncomfortable parade of negative body image thoughts, feelings, and behaviors. They believed that with the "right body," they would no longer feel obsessed with food, anxious about people judging them, or self-conscious about their flaws. They believed changing their body meant an escape from suffering; that the "right body" would finally make them feel worthy, confident, good enough, and at peace. But

---

* "Body checking" is the habit of compulsively examining, measuring, monitoring, and assessing the body's weight, shape, size, or appearance in an attempt to gain temporary relief from anxiety. It can refer to behaviors like weighing oneself over and over, always fixating on a specific body part in the mirror, regularly comparing oneself with old photos, repeatedly evaluating the fit of clothing to determine shape or size, and habitually pinching, squeezing, flexing, or handling certain body parts.

I was working with some of the most conventionally beautiful people in the world at the time, including successful actors and models, and they experienced all the same insecurity, guilt, anxiety, and fixation on their bodies as everyone else.

Clearly, having the "right body" wasn't the antidote to suffering my clients were hoping it would be. So while I did help a lot of folks get stronger, build physical competence and athleticism, and tap into power through my work as a personal trainer, I often felt I was failing at the unspoken task my clients had assigned me: to free them from body anxiety, negativity, and preoccupation.

This is what I was dealing with when I first heard the term "body positivity." I immediately loved it, because it sounded like exactly the answer everyone needed—less hating and punishing your body, more celebrating and loving it! At the time, my understanding of body image issues was fairly superficial, and I (like many people) thought body image issues were pretty much just caused by folks comparing themselves with the unrealistic cultural beauty and body ideals being set by exploitative capitalism and the patriarchy. It stood to reason, then, that the answer to body negativity would be a cultural pushback against those ideals (and the systems that drive them), and an embracing of all our supposed "flaws" and "imperfections" as not only normal and acceptable, but beautiful and worthy of celebration too!

In those early days, I considered body positivity to be nothing short of a revolution. We were waging war on the forces that made us feel insecure and hate ourselves, and I had fully bought in. Having struggled with my own body insecurities and shame for so long, I found the concept that we could just "love ourselves, flaws and all" to be wildly exciting and liberating. Conventional beauty ideals be damned, we can reclaim our confidence! The only opinion that matters is our own! Every body is beautiful and worthy!

I dove into the social media #BodyPositivity scene and consumed everything. I reposted photos of women embracing their rolls and dimples and other "imperfections," and shared photos of my own, with captions that said things like "bloating is normal, and all bellies are beautiful," and "this is my cellulite, but I prefer to think of it as fancy fat, because the pattern is so pretty and lacelike!" Messages and comments poured in every time I did this, from people who both admired my courage in showing myself in such an unflattering light, and felt inspired to let go of their *own* body hate.

At the time, my understanding of body image issues was focused entirely on women, so I cheered when Dove and other brands started depicting women in "real" bodies and pledging to ditch Photoshop. It felt like the next wave of feminism, freeing women to cast off the expectations and ideals of the male gaze, and to reclaim our bodies for ourselves. It promised that we could *all* embrace our curves, accept our flaws, love ourselves, and feel equally worthy and confident in the bodies we have right now. Instead of changing our *bodies* to feel better, we could just change our *mindsets*—it was so empowering!

It needs to be stated here that during this time, I looked very close to how a woman is "supposed to look" in our culture. I was young, nondisabled, white, conventionally feminine and pretty, and extremely lean. I was into lifting heavy weights, and through years of dedicated training I had put on enough muscle to look very toned and tight, but not bulky. I had what many of my clients considered the "ideal body," and I sometimes even worked gigs as a fitness model, although in those spaces I was considered to have a very "average" body (compared with physique competitors), and I booked jobs only when the editors wanted someone who was super fit but still "relatable." In short, I had a shit ton of body privilege I was completely unaware of.

I hope by mentioning this, you can see why my message on the internet seemed to empower and inspire some folks, while also coming off as kind of ignorant and disingenuous to others. I hadn't yet heard of concepts like privilege and oppression (because, you know . . . not needing to know about privilege is part of having privilege) and despite everything, I didn't consider myself particularly close to the "ideal" for women at all. I worked with those "ideal" women, and they were all much taller, thinner, younger, and more conventionally feminine than me. At five foot three, I often felt short, stocky, jiggly, and butch next to the models I trained. So when I talked about body confidence online, I focused on the ways *I* was failing society's standard of beauty for women, and how I was choosing to reject those standards, reclaim my body for me, and embrace those imperfections. I genuinely believed it was possible for everyone else to do the same, no matter what their particular "flaws" happened to be.

This ended up being the problem, though. I felt like I had cast off the chains of unrealistic beauty ideals and set myself free from the pressure to meet those ideals, and I seemed to be "inspiring" others into doing the same. But I couldn't quite tell anyone else how to follow suit, especially when society was treating them badly or putting them in danger because of their "flaws"—something I had never had to go through. Maybe you could just . . . try harder to not care what people think of you? Stop letting the patriarchy push you around? Plenty of people resonated with my work (mostly other young, thin/lean, non-disabled, gender conforming, and conventionally attractive white folks), but others wrote me long and painful messages about how desperately they wanted to stop hating their bodies and feel confident, too, but just *couldn't*, and could I please tell them exactly how?

I wanted to be able to break down the systems and paths for how to do the work of addressing and overcoming body image issues, and I wanted it to apply to everyone, not just people who more or less looked like me. I was also getting uncomfortable with the idea that everyone could or even should "love their bodies," because that seemed to put an awful lot of pressure on something that felt completely impossible to so many folks.

From a marketing perspective, as someone running my business online at that point, I knew my job was to figure out what my audience wanted and offer it to them—and my audience unambiguously wanted to fully love their bodies. They wanted to look in the mirror and feel good about what they saw. They imagined how happy and free they would be once they finally achieved body positivity, and how much better life would be when they finally "felt confident" in their bodies. But not only did I not see any reliable or realistic way to get people there, I also felt uneasy about how similar this all felt to the way my personal training clients had approached fitness. *Once I get ____ I'll feel the way I want to feel. Once I have ____ life will be easy.*

I became obsessed with finding the language and concepts required to offer people a clear and repeatable pathway for building body confidence. I consumed everything I could find about mindset, happiness, body positivity, self-worth, trauma, sexuality, mental health, and more. I learned a ton about diet culture, beauty culture, weight stigma, and anti-fat bias, and what all of this has to do with systems of oppression like sexism, racism, ableism, ageism, homophobia, and transphobia. I got my life coaching certification and left the fitness industry to focus on body image. I wrote programs, made content, and taught workshops on self-love and body positivity, encouraging everyone to challenge and heal their relationships with their bodies.

Throughout all of this, I was passionate and proud of the work I was doing, but something still felt off. I would talk publicly about the journey to "body love" and "body confidence," but behind the scenes with clients, I was approaching things differently. I would explain how loving your body isn't what everyone thinks it is—it's not about thinking you look good, it's about believing in your inherent worth as a person, no matter how you look. I was working with men and gender nonconforming clients (who generally seemed to feel less pressure to "love their bodies," and just wanted to stop feeling insecure), and realizing the body image conversation needed to expand far beyond women. And I was honest with my clients about the fact that I wasn't so sure everyone could get to a place of liking how they look, and that actually I didn't think it was such a great idea to try.

Ultimately, my work with clients ended up focused more on relieving the suffering caused by body anxiety, negativity, and obsession than it was about generating feelings of happiness or satisfaction with the body.

After all, body image issues can be unbelievably painful, and feeling better doesn't have to be about feeling *more good*—it can sometimes just be about feeling *less bad*.

It wasn't a very sexy marketing message, all things considered. People wanted promises of body *love*, and all I could promise was a reduction of body *hate*. But that was the work, and the more I saw this play out with clients—the more I saw "success" be defined by less insecurity and suffering, rather than more pride and confidence—the less often I found myself using "body positive"–based language.

It was around this point that I first saw the term "body neutrality" floated as an alternative goal to loving your body. It was presented as a more realistic and attainable goal for people deeply mired in body image issues, and it offered a sort of middle ground for body image, a space in which you neither love your body nor hate it, but instead you just . . . don't think about it much. This concept felt a lot closer to the work I had been doing with clients, and I started folding it into my language around body image, both publicly and behind the scenes.

I also saw that body neutrality had the potential to expose the link between body image issues and self-worth. If you believe your worth and value as a person are based on how you look and what other people think about you, then how you look is always going to feel overly important. This leads to a lot of body image suffering: attachment to the significance and importance of looking a certain way, and a feeling that who you are *as a person* is either too much or not enough. By trying to love how you look, you never have to face that important piece of the puzzle: how you feel about yourself, your value as a person, and your worthiness for respect, connection, and belonging. Body neutrality invites you to examine why you were so attached to your appearance in the first place, asks you to strip away the undue significance you've been placing on your appearance, and encourages you to build a sense of yourself and your worth outside of how you look and what people think of you.

Despite its not having a super-clear definition, the concept of body neutrality felt like instant relief to me, and it seemed to feel like relief for a lot of my audience and clients too. Trying to *change* their bodies had felt impossible and made them feel like failures, but trying to *love* their bodies had felt impossible and made them feel like failures too! Body neutrality offered them a more attainable goal, and the promise of a safe place to rest: a cease-fire in the war against their bodies, and freedom from the endless stream of negative thoughts and feelings about how they look.

As you'll see throughout this book, the concept of body neutrality has taken on a lot more depth, richness, and clarity as I've worked with it over the years in my coaching practice. Combined with the real-life feedback from hundreds of clients of various genders, body sizes, races, ages, and abilities struggling with body image, body neutrality morphed from just an alternative to loving your body to a process and approach for the work of dismantling, healing, and finding relief from the suffering caused by body image. It's not a quick and easy solution, but body neutrality as I now define it offers structure, clarity, and direction so you can heal and improve your relationship with yourself and your body by reducing the pain and suffering associated with it—both in the short term and for the rest of your life.

In my own personal body image journey, body neutrality allowed me to discover that I had subconsciously tied my identity, value, and sense of safety and control in the world to my appearance. I had often thought I was "loving my body" when actually I was just loving the validation, approval, and feeling of power it offered me (and in fact, I was constantly stressing and obsessing over how to maintain it, and what would happen if I lost it). I had to face a lot of dark and painful things that lived inside my subconscious mind as I did the work required to heal and release that attachment, including the impact that childhood sexual abuse had on my self-image, how fundamentally unsafe I felt around men, oppressive biases against certain kinds of bodies, and the fact that there were deep-down hidden parts of myself I absolutely hated.

This insight into the root causes of my body insecurity, anxiety, and obsession set me down a path of self-examination and healing that included a ton of skill building, shame busting, and fear facing. My goal became breaking free from *attachment* to my appearance so I could look at myself without thinking that what I saw was important, rather than loving what I saw. I challenged myself to stop doing all the things I had been doing to maintain a particular appearance, and started examining my relationship to gender, intimacy, emotions, and privilege along the way. I stopped dieting, stopped my intense workouts, stopped wearing makeup, and stopped everything else I'd been doing to fit a standard of femme attractiveness that had, I was realizing, never actually felt like *me*.

What I discovered as I did this was pretty uncomfortable. As I lost my "toned" appearance, buzzed my hair, and wore my face bare, people treated me *very* differently. It was shocking to see how such relatively small changes could so radically shift everyone's perception of me from special and admirable to sort of . . . unremarkable. Without hair, or with a chest binder, I seemed to become almost completely invisible to men, and people automatically made some very different assumptions about my health, lifestyle, relationships, and even competence as my body shape and size changed. It was weird and uncomfortable to see this all play out, but also fascinating, and it gave me space to reprocess my relationship to my appearance, detaching even further from the idea that how I looked (or, more specifically, what other people thought about how I looked) was an important, or even particularly interesting, part of who I am.

It also gave me insight into the discrimination and marginalization facing people in less privileged bodies. If I was being viewed and treated this differently for such relatively small changes—and I still fit a ton of social norms and ideals—what must it be like for folks who don't? This experience drove my commitment to learning everything I could about systems of oppression and privilege, and how they affect a person's lived experience, self-worth, emotional needs, identity, and ultimately body image. It also inspired me to strive to always center the fight for justice and liberation of people in marginalized bodies in both my work and my personal life.

It should be said here that I gave up a certain amount of privilege that I had been "earning" by conforming to certain femme beauty ideals in our culture, but I still had and will always have an extraordinary amount of privilege in this body. I am able-bodied and white, and no matter how I eat or exercise, my body is always relatively thin and small. I identify as queer and nonbinary, but most of the time I'm cis- and straight-passing (which means people just assume I'm a straight woman), and I'm young enough to still have a lot of the privilege afforded to very young women.

I say all this because a person's lived experience of privilege and oppression plays a huge role in their relationship to their body, and I realize it may feel strange to read a book on body image written by someone who has never faced discrimination or marginalization for the way they look. I've even had folks in marginalized bodies ask me how I think I can possibly be qualified to help them find peace in their bodies, when I can't relate to anything they've been through. And my answer to that is, quite simply, that I might not be.

I will never be able to understand or "relate to" the experiences of a person in a marginalized body, and if that turns you off and makes you want to stop reading, I get it. I won't be offended, and in fact I'd like to actively encourage and support you to put this book down and go find resources that resonate with and inspire you. Everyone deserves to feel peace in their bodies, and sometimes you need that message to be delivered by someone who gets your specific lived experience. I wouldn't want to read books about feminism that were written by cisgender men, and I understand if you don't want to read a book on body acceptance written by someone who looks like me.

That said, this is *not* a book about how thin, pretty white women can accept themselves. This is a book about how we can each find the truth underneath our body image suffering. And the truth—once you've stripped away the lies, red herrings, biases, and protective mechanisms that have led to your body image issues—is that your body image issues aren't the *cause* of your suffering, they're a *symptom*. So if your goal is to suffer less over body image, be prepared to dig deep, face fears, challenge beliefs, dismantle biases, and explore the darkest parts of yourself. There is a reason you're in pain, and my approach to body neutrality can help you figure out what that reason is. But don't expect to be able to do it in a vacuum. Because how you look may be the least interesting and important thing about you, but also, as Emma Lazarus once wrote, "Until we are all free, we are none of us free."

I believe the body neutrality concepts and steps you'll read about in this book are aspects of liberation work, and therefore they not only can work for *anyone*, but will also benefit *everyone*. By dismantling the systems of lies and oppression inside ourselves, we collectively move everyone toward social justice and equity. After all, thin, pretty white women learning to "love their bodies" don't do much to help bring justice or equity to people of color, people in fat* bodies, or trans folks. But thin, pretty white women giving up the fantasy that more body privilege will make them happy, facing and healing the darkest parts of themselves, and dismantling the oppressive systems that exist both inside of themselves and in the world? Now that has potential.

---

* You may cringe at my use of the word "fat" in this book, if you've learned to think of fat as an insult, but my use of the word as an unflinchingly neutral descriptor is intentional. "Fat" is the term most often used by the fat justice and liberation communities, and using it this way helps destigmatize fatness. See page 401 for more on why I use the word "fat" rather than "obese" or "overweight."

CHAPTER 2

Body Positivity

WHEN BODY POSITIVITY FIRST started to become popular, I was thrilled. Finally there seemed to be mainstream pushback against the ever-increasingly unrealistic beauty and body ideals causing so many people (women especially) to feel unworthy and insecure.

In my view at the time, the nexus for the movement was on social media, where a growing number of body positivity advocates and influencers were gaining huge followings publicly documenting their own journeys to body love. It all seemed so brave and radical: people showing off their imperfections, reshaping the narrative around what's beautiful, and shining a light on the unconscious biases we're conditioned to believe about which kind of body indicates that a person is worthy of being visible and happy, and which isn't.

As a personal trainer who had recently gained a small following on Instagram, I loved being a part of it. It was exciting to make posts challenging my audience to think more deeply about their desires and assumptions with regard to fitness and bodies, and to encourage them to question everything. A picture of me naked with my belly relaxed and bloated instead of sucked in, and a caption about why we need to destigmatize round bellies. A "before" and "after" showing how easy it was to fake a "perfect body" for social media, and exposing how even those supposedly "perfect inspo" bodies have cellulite, rolls, and unflattering angles when they're not posed and edited. A side-by-side of me covering my nipples, one with my breasts pushed way up into perfect bubbly spheres where society says they "should" be, and the other with my breasts sagging down where they are naturally. People loved these posts, and I was inundated with messages about how brave and inspiring I was and how the fitness industry needed more voices like mine.

Looking back, I find this all very cringy for a lot of reasons, the least being that my naked body is now all over the internet, and the most being that I contributed to the soon-to-be-popular trope of a thin, able-bodied white girl in her twenties being celebrated in a movement that was founded to uplift and center the rights and dignity of folks in marginalized bodies. Because as it turns out, that's what body positivity actually was. I didn't know it at the time because the mainstream perception of the movement was that it was all about individuals embracing their bodies, flaws and all, but body positivity wasn't ever actually intended to be a movement for individuals—it was intended to be a political movement.

Chelsea Kronengold, the former manager of communications at the National Eating Disorders Association, puts it this way: "The body positive movement was created by and for people in marginalized bodies, particularly fat, Black, queer, and disabled bodies." And she's right; body positivity was based on the work of fat-acceptance activists from the 1960s. According to journalist and *Refinery29* senior staff writer Elizabeth Gulino, "This movement was rooted in social justice; it birthed organizations like The National Association to Advance Fat Acceptance, a non-profit fat rights organization that fought and continues to fight against societal anti-fat bias, fatphobia, and systemic fat oppression."[1]

So the body positive movement was focused entirely on fighting for the socioeconomic equality of opportunities, treatment, representation, safety, and dignity of all people living in marginalized bodies, and was never intended to affect self-love or body confidence at all. The two concepts are unrelated; in fact, you could totally hate your body while pushing for greater accessibility and antidiscrimination policies, and you could also totally embrace your body while *in no way* participating in the movement for justice or equality.

Let's take a moment here to define what I mean when I refer to a person in a "marginalized body." A person in a marginalized body is someone with a statistically higher chance of facing discrimination, exclusion from social, political, or economic activities, and being kept in powerless positions in society, due to society's biases about and response to something about the person's *body*. It doesn't define the person in any way, other than to say the person is at a statistically higher risk of facing these inequalities in their lifetime.

When people think about body positivity, they often think about people in fat bodies, and people in fat bodies are certainly marginalized in our society. But that's only a small part of it. People in disabled bodies, people in bodies of color, people in older bodies, and people in transgender or gender nonconforming bodies are all marginalized in our society to different degrees as well, and a person's intersecting identities of race, age, gender, weight, and ability inform how marginalized a person is likely to be. As such, someone we can say is unlikely to be facing marginalization for how they look would be a thin, white, young, able-bodied femme. Unfortunately, that category not only includes *me,* but it also includes the vast majority of the people who ended up becoming the faces of mainstream body positivity. Predictably, then, because marginalization is built into the systems of who is most visible and powerful, a movement centered on the social inequity facing the most marginalized folks became centered on the individual insecurities of the most privileged.

This is important to understand, because the shift from centering marginalized people to privileged people was only able to come about because of the shift from inequity to insecurity: the political to the personal, the social to the individual. Fighting for antidiscrimination legislation keeps the focus automatically on the people being discriminated against, but fighting to "feel confident in your skin" can apply to anyone. And anything that can apply to everyone will always end up centering privileged bodies, because that's how social hierarchies, unconscious biases, and systems of power and oppression work. A fat trans woman of color accepting her body won't get the same kind of traction on social media—or, thus, in her modeling career—as a thin, cisgender white woman accepting her body, both because of the biases built into the algorithms and company leadership, and the biases built into consumer behavior and the user base. For example, the nonprofit news organization the Intercept reported that TikTok intentionally "filtered out users they viewed as 'unattractive, poor, or disabled.'"[2]

With body positivity's move into the social media mainstream, more and more people across different parts of society participated in the collective reinterpreting and recrafting of it, making it less extreme and more palatable, focusing it on individual feelings rather than on systems of oppression, and downshifting it from progressive to center. As the message of body positivity was watered down and corrupted, it became something else entirely: a movement for everyone to reject society's idea of how they "should" look, and embrace their (beautiful) bodies exactly as they are. Instead of talking about the legislation needed to protect marginalized people, we were talking about loving ourselves no matter how society treats us. Instead of talking about ways to *change* the system, we were talking about ways to cast off and rise above the system. And the people succeeding at this new goal most fabulously were folks already pretty close to the top of the body hierarchies. Thin, pretty white girls with cellulite and belly rolls when they leaned over. Fat women with perfect hourglass shapes. Conventionally attractive folks with one notable disability or difference, like being in a wheelchair or having visible scars or vitiligo.

The fact that body positivity started as a political movement can be understood as the reason it functioned so beautifully as a social movement raising awareness and inspiration—but failed to adequately provide the body image relief so many individuals were looking for. Because that's where we are; despite the extraordinary popularity of the idea that we should all feel good about our bodies, here we are over a decade after body positivity's mainstream rise, and body image issues haven't become any less frequent, intense, or destructive to people's lives. (In fact, quite the opposite!)[3]

Mainstream body positivity moved the dial against body oppression by bringing awareness to the widespread problem of body negativity, cultivating a movement of social values based on self-acceptance and self-love, and pressuring brands to be more inclusive and representative of body diversity. But as we look to the future and consider the question of individual body image relief, we have to consider and appreciate some of the reasons body positivity wasn't effective.

I once had a client who had been doing "body positivity work" for many years (and actually taught and coached others to feel better in their bodies!), but still struggled with a lot of body hatred. By "body positivity work," she of course meant "trying to achieve a feeling of warmth, approval, pleasure, and love when seeing or thinking about my body," because that is the colloquial definition most often used in the mainstream. She told me that she tried really, really hard to feel differently, to "let things go" and "care less what people think," and to "not take things so personally," but she just couldn't seem to do it. She couldn't understand what was wrong with her that it hadn't worked yet, because she understood the issue so well, knew all the tips and tricks, and did everything "right." But no matter how many times she repeated mantras like "I am beautiful" and "I am worthy," she still looked in the mirror and felt disgusted, anxious, and unhappy. No matter how many books she read about how diets don't work[4] and the BMI doesn't mean anything,[5] she still desperately wanted to lose some weight. All this work, all this time and effort trying to love and accept herself, and she didn't feel *any* closer to her goal.

This kind of story is unfortunately so common that I often spend my first few sessions with new clients unpacking why their approach to body positivity hasn't worked yet so they can release the shame and anger at themselves they've been carrying for not being able to "get it right." I explain the political origins of the movement, and the fact that it was never designed to help individual people feel differently about their individual bodies, and we unpack some of the ways in which mainstream body positivity was simply not equipped to effectively tackle the issue of how a single person can feel more positively toward their own body and appearance.

If you're reading this book, I have to assume that you didn't get what you were looking for out of body positivity either. Maybe you found it inspiring and healing and helpful, or maybe it never quite resonated with you. Either way it probably didn't provide you with everything you needed to overcome your personal body image issues, and before we dive into body neutrality, I think it's important to unpack some of the reasons why that is.

There's no shade being thrown on body positivity here—both the original political activists and mainstream social advocates have done some amazing and necessary work in the world. They've raised awareness, built communities, and slowly moved legislation forward. They've changed the popular conversation about bodies entirely, influenced clothing brands to be more inclusive and realistic in their portrayal of bodies, and successfully pressured social media platforms to protect people from scammy diet culture bullshit. They've given folks the tools, resources, and courage to fight back against diet culture and the objectification of women when they see it, and they've given *so* many people hope, relief, and a sense of belonging.

The way I see it, I am standing on the shoulders of giants. Political activism and liberation workers made the mainstream body positivity movement possible, and the mainstream movement made it possible for this book to be written. This chapter is not here to belittle body positivity. It is, however, here to offer a critical exploration of why and how body positivity wasn't able to ultimately offer what we were all hoping it would: a way to break free from our individual body image issues, and to access a feeling of peace, confidence, and worthiness in our own skin.

My hope for you is that in reading this chapter, you're able to find some relief and self-compassion in the knowledge that if body positivity didn't "work for you," it's not because there's anything wrong with you. You are not "crazy," broken, weak, or stupid for still struggling with body image. You are not too vain, or too self-absorbed, or "too emotional" to overcome these issues. The structure of body positivity was just simply never designed or equipped to help you look at what was really going on with your body image issues, or to deal with them effectively.

Let's take a look at a few reasons body positivity couldn't provide the individual body image relief we were all hoping it would, and why body neutrality *can*.

BODY IMAGE ISSUES ARE ALWAYS ABOUT SOMETHING DEEPER

A tipsy woman in the bathroom of a bar once remarked offhand, more to her reflection in the mirror than to me, "oh my god I look like shit." Perhaps she expected me to respond that she looked great, or maybe she just assumed I would ignore her altogether. I responded by asking, "What do you think would be different tonight if you looked the way you wanted?" Stunned, she paused for a moment and then responded in a quiet voice, "I would feel like I belong here."

Boom. There is *always* something deeper going on when you're suffering over your appearance. We know this because not liking how you look, or preferring to look different, is one thing. But it's never just that, is it? You might not like how your kitchen looks either, but it's unlikely that you stress and obsess about it all day, or feel gutted, panicky, or like a failure every time you catch sight of it. And you might wish you lived near the ocean, or had a nice new car, but you probably don't feel incapacitated by hatred and resentment every time you come home, or a sickening shame and grief every time you get in your car.

I'll be honest, I don't always *prefer* to look the way I look. Many mornings I would prefer for my curly hair to cooperate differently, I would prefer my belly didn't swell up to make me look pregnant after I eat certain foods, and as I'm writing this, I have a big old zit on my chin I would definitely prefer weren't there. But none of that causes me any suffering, because while I have my preferences, I still see them with neutral vision, meaning, I don't assign any meaning, significance, or moral judgment to them. I know that my hair is always going to be a bit wild and doesn't mean anything about me; bloating is sort of annoying but doesn't have any impact on my identity, life, or worth; and this zit isn't a sign of failure or shame. It's just a zit; it's neutral.

This is body neutrality: this is seeing ourselves with clear and neutral vision, without layering stories, interpretations, meaning, or moral significance on top of our bodies.

To be honest, if you kinda wish you looked different but it hardly takes up any mental space or makes you feel bad, this book isn't for you. This book isn't here to help you prefer to look the way you look, it's here to address the pain, stress, distress, anxiety, and dysphoria created by your relationship with your body and appearance. Because that suffering is the real problem, isn't it?

Thinking about your body, picking it apart, trying to "fix" it, and berating yourself for failing becomes an all-consuming obsession for many people, cannibalizing their ability to feel worthy, be present, connect with others, build a life in which they can thrive, and like themselves. I can't tell you how many clients have shared stories of full-blown mental and emotional breakdowns—sometimes lasting days, weeks, or months—brought on by discovering a pair of jeans didn't fit, catching sight of themselves in a bathing suit, or seeing an unflattering photo. And it's that completely out-of-proportion and out-of-control reaction that tells us something else—something deeper—is going on. Something that repeating mantras, giving up dieting, and trying to feel attractive just can't touch.

There is always a deeper reason, a deeper need, a deeper wound, or a deeper level to body image suffering. And while body positivity moved us in the right direction (inward and downward from the superficial layer of conventional beauty ideals), it stopped a bit short. Committing to seeing yourself neutrally (which is to say without interpretation, moral judgment, or undue significance) requires that you find, name, and deal with that deeper wound or reason directly. For example:

♦ If you feel like you need to lose weight so people will think you have your shit together, then what you're really seeking isn't weight loss. Instead, it might be respect, dignity, social status, belonging, or a feeling of being "good enough."

♦ If you hate your flabby belly because you want the validation of having a "perfect" body, then what you're really seeking might be more like attention or connection . . . or *maybe* you're hoping that enough external validation will convince *you* that you have value and are worthy of love and belonging.

♦ If you feel panicky when you think about "losing your looks" as you get older, you might have been subconsciously using your looks to get one or more of your emotional needs met, and you're actually terrified of those needs going unmet as you age.

The work of body neutrality is about getting radically honest: acknowledging the lies you've been telling yourself (like the lie that your body image suffering just comes down to a preference, for example), dealing with your deeper truth, and learning to see yourself and your body with clear, neutral, and objective vision. This requires us to go much deeper into knowing ourselves than most people have learned how to do or are comfortable with! It asks us to prioritize courage over comfort and to be wildly vulnerable with ourselves about how we really feel, what hurts, what we crave, what feels intolerable, what we're avoiding, and what we need protection from.

In this way, body neutrality *can't* stop at the surface; it requires that we dig deeeep into who we are, and learn to see ourselves, others, and the world through different eyes. It pushes us to get curious and honest about the root cause of our suffering, and what's blocking our ability to see ourselves and our bodies clearly, neutrally, and objectively. It invites us to explore and examine everything—to keep digging until we get to the root of our suffering, to understand how that suffering has been serving us, and to come up with a plan that puts our suffering out of business.

BODY IMAGE ISSUES ARE UNIQUE TO THE INDIVIDUAL

Looking back on the early body positivity messages on social media, I can see why individuals sharing their personal stories gained massive followings. There was so little information available on how to actually overcome *our own* body image issues, everyone just tried to copy the people who seemed to have figured it out already!

But body image issues aren't a monolith. Each individual person's body image suffering has its own unique root cause and purpose, having developed to try to help them solve a specific and unique problem, so copying someone else's path rarely works. Body neutrality, on the other hand, requires you to get super specific about *why your relationship to your body isn't neutral in the first place.* After all, the terminology and concept of body neutrality may be relatively new, but the experience itself has been around forever.

Body neutrality isn't some newfangled invention, after all. It's just . . . our natural state. It's the way we all came into this world. It's our birthright.

Kind of like how nobody is born racist or sexist, nobody is born thinking some bodies are better than others, or that how we look determines what we deserve and what kind of life we'll have. Babies don't have an innate disgust for fatness, a fear of balding, or a preference for women with perfectly hairless, poreless skin. I sometimes think of body neutrality as the "intuitive eating" of body image for this reason: we were all born with it, but living in a society full of messages that interrupt, corrupt, and deny it can make it feel completely inaccessible.

I encourage you to think of your journey to body neutrality not as a journey to something new, but as a *return* to your natural state: the state of seeing yourself without moral judgment, meaning, interpretation, or significance. The state of recognizing that there are *so* many more interesting and important things about a person than their body or appearance. The state of being able to look in the mirror, and—*even if you would prefer to look different*—not being too attached to or affected by what you see.

To get there, you'll need to figure out what exactly is blocking that experience for you in the first place; what problems your body image issues have been trying to solve, how your suffering has been trying to protect you, or what lies you've been telling yourself about your body that get in the way of your ability to see yourself with clear and neutral vision. The rest of this book will offer you concepts and tools to help you look inward, get radically honest with yourself about why your body image issues exist, and then create a plan to make them unnecessary. And while the general steps of body neutrality can apply to anyone, each individual's specific journey will be unique!

LOVING YOUR BODY JUST ISN'T ALWAYS REALISTIC

There is a popular idea out there that a person should be able to love and celebrate themselves and their bodies, unequivocally and unconditionally. This idea is lovely, of course. *You are already worthy of unconditional acceptance and love, exactly as you are! Don't let society make you feel bad about yourself!* But unfortunately, given the world we live in, trying to actually feel that way can be difficult, even downright impossible, for some folks.

Many of my clients feel like complete failures by the time they come to me, because they've been trying and trying (and *trying*) to love their bodies, and they *just freakin' can't*. It's often a source of added distress, because they feel like loving and celebrating their bodies should be *easy*, and they can't figure out why they can't do it. But then at the same time, it sounds completely unfathomable to them, to go from hating their bodies to loving them. I once had a client tell me that she felt the same way about loving her body as she did about going to Hogwarts—she *desperately* wanted to but felt absolutely heartbroken, because she knew it could never happen.

Now, listen, I'm all for loving your body if that's available to you. I even love mine! But I love my body the same way I love my friends, my family, and my partner, which is to say I believe my body is fundamentally worthy of respect, kindness, and care. But I don't love my body in an unconditional state of euphoria and gratitude and bliss, nor do I feel I should, because frankly that's just not how love works.

Surely you don't feel a constant stream of euphoric affection and gratitude toward your partner, your best friend, your child, or your dog? Why then do we think we should feel that way toward our bodies in order to properly "love" them? Sometimes the people we love are annoying, wrong, and disappointing. That doesn't mean we love them any less! And we certainly don't always love the way they *look*, right? Do you love your partner less when they look sick and disgusting? I doubt it! Do you love your child less when they get a terrible haircut? Good gracious, I hope not.

I say all this to make clear that there is nothing wrong with *actually* loving ourselves or our bodies, if we're being realistic about what "love" means. But I *do* take issue with the notion that we should be able to feel a constant flow of celebratory happiness and affectionate gratitude toward our bodies, or that we have to love every dimple, every jiggle, and every inch of our bodies. As far as I'm concerned, that's neither a necessary nor a realistic goal, and its absurd loftiness is more likely to make you feel *worse* about yourself than it is to make you feel *better*.

Body neutrality, on the other hand, takes the pressure way off, and tends to feel like a *much* more realistic, approachable, and achievable goal for many people. I can often literally see my clients' bodies relax when I describe it, because it offers them a glimmer of hope and possibility, like: "Oh, thank goodness, I could do *that*." Instead of asking you to become some one-dimensional saint who feels "good vibes only" toward your body, body neutrality allows you to be your whole self, and feel all your feelings. Don't like what you see in the mirror today? That's okay. Through a body neutrality lens, both how you look *and how you feel about it* are morally neutral. Your thighs don't mean anything good or bad about you, but neither does the fact that you wish they were smaller. Your belly fat doesn't increase or decrease your worthiness for love, connection, respect, or happiness . . . but neither does the fact that in this moment, you hate your belly fat.

Neutrality gives you space for everything that previously felt like a huge problem to kind of just be . . . whatever. Not good, but not bad. Not something to freak out about. Not even a problem to solve. Sort of an annoying thing maybe, worthy of an eye roll or a shrug before you move on with your day, but ultimately pretty powerless.

If you've been trying to love your body without success for a while, try this: say to yourself, in your head or out loud, your big complaints about your body (or yourself!), and follow each one up with the phrase "and that's not a problem" (alternatively: "and that makes sense and is okay" or "and that doesn't mean anything bad about me").

For example:

- ◆ I wish I were smaller, and that's not a problem.

- ◆ I hate my stretch marks, and that makes sense and is okay.

- ◆ I'm constantly worried about how I look, and that doesn't mean anything bad about me.

- ◆ I hate the way my _____ looks, and that's not a problem.

- I desperately want to lose weight, and that makes sense and is okay.

- I'm so embarrassed by _____, and that doesn't mean anything bad about me.

Whew! Can you feel the difference in your body when you add that second part to neutralize the first part?

I sometimes wish I would never get another pimple as long as I live, and when I think about just that fact, it's easy to tumble down a negative spiral about how gross pimples are, and how much it sucks that I can't do anything to stop them, because they're hormonal. So frustrating! But if I tried to *love* my pimples—to suddenly think they're beautiful and perfect just the way they are—I would fail miserably.

That said, if I adopt a body neutral lens, I can just acknowledge that two things are true and neither of them is a problem. One true thing is that I get pimples, and the other is that I don't *like* when I get pimples. Neither of these facts means anything about me, neither of them affects my self-worth, identity, or life, and neither has any moral value, significance, or power over me. And because neither of them is likely to change anytime soon, this neutral perspective offers a huge relief.

This is the power of body neutrality: it offers a safe place to rest as you exit body hatred, without putting pressure on you to somehow magically love every iota of your body and self. It gives you the ability to see yourself and the world clearly, which means you can take your emotional power back from the places that don't deserve it, and de-escalate a lot of your triggers and spirals.

TRYING TO OUTTHINK BODY IMAGE ISSUES JUST MAKES US FEEL WORSE

With the meteoric rise of the body positivity movement online in the early 2010s, a handful of body positivity advocates and influencers skyrocketed into visibility and fame. There was a lot of pressure on these individuals to come up with a solution, formula, or plan to teach other people how to get the same body positive results they had gotten . . . *even if* they couldn't yet put into words what they had done, and had no way of knowing whether it would work for anyone else.

So what happened is that—because it's damn near impossible to persuade anyone to *feel* differently—the vast majority of mainstream body positive messaging started to focus on how to *think* differently.

All flowers look different, but we still find them beautiful, right? Companies are manipulating us into feeling insecure, and everyone is unique, so we shouldn't compare ourselves! You wouldn't talk to your best friend the way you talk to yourself, and nobody notices or cares about your belly rolls. Diets don't work anyway, and you just need to be confident!

These messages were trying to appeal to our logical side, from a place of assuming that body image issues are *illogical* and the person suffering from them needs to simply be *set straight.*

This doesn't work for two reasons. The first is that you can't outthink body image issues any more than you can outthink grief, depression, trauma, or shame, meaning: not at all. Body image issues are rooted deeply in the murky and emotional subconscious mind, not the conscious mind. Think about someone who got viciously attacked by a dog as a child and now struggles with an "irrational" fear of dogs as an adult. Saying, "Don't be afraid, this dog is friendly!" to them isn't going to make them feel any less afraid. That's because logic (or at least, logic *alone*) doesn't have much of an impact on the subconscious mind or emotional landscape.

Not to mention how trying to change the way we feel through logic and willpower has a way of making us feel stupid, weak, irrational, invalid, and out of control . . . which means appealing to logic not only doesn't help people overcome their body image issues, but also tends to cause more issues in the form of shame, guilt, self-criticism, and low self-worth.

The second reason these messages don't work is that, even though they seem illogical on the surface, body image issues actually are extremely logical.

Your negative feelings toward your body make sense, given everything you've learned and experienced in your life, and given what problems you've needed solutions to. Body neutrality gives you the opportunity to explore your beliefs, fears, and feelings without judgment, shame, or criticism so that the unique logic of your body image issues can become clear. And this is important, because when we recognize how reasonable, rational, and useful our body image issues are, we have the power to invite compassion for ourselves and our suffering, instead of judgment. This compassion can help decrease the tension and disconnect between our minds and our bodies, restoring a feeling of wholeness, and moving us in the direction of healing.

You are not unintelligent, irrational, unreasonable, feeble, or misinformed just because you're struggling with body image. And frankly, rejecting our body image issues isn't all that different from rejecting our bodies. If the goal is peace and acceptance, we have to work *with* ourselves, not *against* ourselves, and that means letting go of the idea that body image issues are illogical. Approaching our body image issues with kindness, curiosity, and understanding is key if we're going to stand any chance of dismantling them. And kindness, curiosity, and compassion are the natural result of body neutrality.

WE DON'T NEED TO FIND EVERYONE BEAUTIFUL

I understand the appeal of messages that help people, especially women, reframe their idea of what's beautiful. Beauty standards have been unrealistically narrow and homogenous for so long, it can be a huge relief to hear things like "you're beautiful just the way you are!" and "curvy is the new skinny," and other seemingly more inclusive messages about beauty.

But messages like this can also keep our attention focused on attractiveness, and reinforce the idea that beauty is *important*. So while I appreciate the invitation to reexamine our definition of beauty (there's actually a lot of interesting work that can come out of self-inquiry around what you find attractive and what you don't!), these messages can actually have a counterproductive effect on body image. After all, as coauthor of *More Than a Body* Lindsay Kite said during her TED talk, "Girls and women aren't only suffering because of the unattainable ways beauty is being defined; they are suffering because they are being defined by beauty. They are bodies first and people second."[6]

How could you *ever* be able to see yourself (or anyone else, for that matter) with clear and neutral vision if you still believe beauty (either having it or feeling it) determines a person's worth, value, character, identity, or what they deserve in life?

Body neutrality invites us to understand ourselves and others as whole human beings first, and to form our concept of worth, value, and identity around a person's internal self instead of their external self. It helps us strip away the many layers of complex social conditioning telling us what different bodies mean about a person, so that we can see this clear and objective truth: beauty and attractiveness can be pleasant and nice, but they can't tell you anything about a person's character, personality, value, lifestyle, or the kind of life and treatment they deserve.

By taking the focus off aesthetics and beauty altogether, body neutrality frees us up to see that we are innately and inherently worthy of love, respect, connection, belonging, and happiness no matter how we look, and that how we look is the least interesting and important part of who we are.

SOCIAL CONTEXT MATTERS

When body positivity stepped into the mainstream spotlight in the early 2010s, it came with the same kind of rugged individualism approach as most things in Western culture. That is to say, it assumed that any individual should be able to overcome any social context, with enough hard work, determination, and strength of character. This makes sense, because it had become a movement about how individual people felt about their individual body image issues, and also because there was very little mainstream awareness at the time of how a person's identity and social context create different levels of privilege or oppression.

The problem with this idea of course is that we actually live in an inequitable and unjust system, in which some people have much *less* to overcome and are praised and celebrated when they succeed, while other people have much *more* to overcome, and are shamed and belittled when they can't succeed in the same way.

No matter what we *want* to believe, a person's race, age, ability, gender identity and expression, sexuality, and body size all carry *enormous* significance in our society, bestowing a person with either a lot of unearned social privilege and power, or a lot of unearned marginalization, trauma, erasure, exclusion, and oppression.[7] And while the fantasy that any person can overcome any obstacle if they try hard enough is uplifting and tempting, it's just that: a fantasy.

Body neutrality is about getting to the objective truth; it's about seeing *clearly,* without moral judgment, interpretation, lies, stories, added meaning, or undue significance. That means stripping away everything society taught us about what different bodies *mean.* It's also about stripping away fantasies—like the fantasy that we live in a fair and equal meritocracy, and everyone can pull themselves up by their bootstraps and overcome their own oppression if they try hard enough. There are very real consequences to looking a certain way in our society, and we must acknowledge those consequences, both as a means to understanding and healing our own individual body image issues, *and* as a means to building a more equitable and just society so that future generations don't have to fight the same battles.

After all, it's all very well and good for a fat person to love their body, but their body is still going to *statistically inhibit* them from getting into college, getting a job, or getting a loan—because they live in a fatphobic (that is, discriminatory toward and negatively biased against folks with fat bodies[8]) and ableist society.[9] A transgender person can try to "be confident," but transgender people are still four times more likely to be the victim of violent crimes than cisgender people.[10] And a Black woman can "embrace her imperfections" until the cows come home; it still won't change the fact that Black women face significantly higher rates of domestic violence, rape, and homicide than white women.[11]

There are people facing a society that is systematically abusive toward people who look like them, and focusing on body image issues as an "individual problem" in the face of that truth is nothing less than violence. We simply cannot ignore or deny social context when we talk about our relationships with our bodies, whether on a global *or* an individual scale.

A person's social context is an *objectively true story*, and therefore it's an important part of body neutrality. It may be a false interpretation to say, "People with fat bodies are lazy," but it's *not* a false interpretation to say, "It's been statistically proven that most people carry a negative bias toward people with fat bodies, seeing them as lazier than people with thin bodies."[12] Do you see the difference? The first one is a lie that we have to strip away in order to arrive at neutrality, but the second one is a fact we'll need to acknowledge in order to arrive at neutrality.

A person's relationship with their own body is individual and personal, of course. But we can't pretend that it exists in a vacuum and is untouched by the influence of their family culture, community culture, media intake, social conditioning, religion, traumas, social status, or privilege. We can't pretend it's untouched by popular beliefs about, and treatment of, both people who *look like them* and people who *don't*. We can't pretend a person's body could *ever* be completely divorced from their experience in the world, their wounds and fears, their identities, their relationships, or their emotional needs.

Do you think women would ever have felt insecure about having hairy armpits if advertisers in *Harper's Bazaar* hadn't taken advantage of the new sleeveless dress trend to start hawking depilatory creams in 1915?[13] No. Do you think you ever would have wanted six-pack abs if the only people who sported them were low-status losers? Unlikely.

Bodies of all genders have represented a person's status, social position, class, and more for a long time, with the specific meaning of each body changing over time and location. In some eras, wealthy women were more likely to have fatter bodies because food was abundant and they didn't need to perform manual labor—which showed off the fact that their fathers or husbands were wealthy. Poor women were more likely to have thin, toned bodies because they were more likely to be out working in the fields, and more likely had dealt with food scarcity from the time they were children. Due to the context of who had social and economic power during these eras, women with soft, curvy bodies were considered more desirable and of higher status, and women with thin, toned bodies were considered less desirable and of lower status.[14] Today, of course, the exact opposite is true.

All of this is to say that we develop our body image issues in a social context, and we must heal our body image issues in a social context as well. This starts by *acknowledging* a person's social context, and recognizing that it has a real and valid impact on their life experience, social conditioning, and relationship both to their own body and to everyone else's. Instead of asking people to "rise above" and "cast off" their social context, body neutrality asks us to accept, acknowledge, consider, and explore it with open eyes and a clear mind. Only by doing so can we fully recognize the truth that an individual's body is *never* the actual problem. The real problems—the evil core of their body image issues—are the biases, bigotry, stereotypes, and systems of body-based oppression our culture upholds.

Body neutrality requires unflinching honesty about the existence, violence, and untruthfulness of those biases and systems, as well as a deep personal commitment to anti-oppression and liberation work. (I won't be going into anti-oppression work or liberation work here, because I am not the most qualified leader, teacher, or educator in those areas, but I will include a list of book recommendations at the end of the book for you to explore.) In this way, body neutrality goes beyond an attempt to clean up our own individual messes and heal our own individual wounds; it offers us an opportunity to also work together to create a more equitable and just world for everyone.

Acknowledging social context allows us to clearly see and fight against social systems and policies that need changing, and to keep those of us with privilege from gaslighting, erasing, or harming the most marginalized. And while these two things should be a priority for all of us anyway, it also helps each individual to understand the deeper issues and root causes for their body image suffering, and therefore to see and understand what they actually need to heal. What helps you will help everyone, and what helps everyone will help you.

CHAPTER 3

What *Is* Body Neutrality?

I DEFINE BODY NEUTRALITY AS **THE PRAC**-
tice of approaching your body through a clear, unbiased, and
impartial lens, attempting to see and deal only with what's
objectively true in the moment, without moral judgment, interpretation, projection, added meaning, or undue significance.

More similar to a mindfulness practice than to a self-love practice,
body neutrality is about striving to see the truth of every moment, and
resisting the urge to judge, assess, or interpret that truth as good or
bad. It's the practice of seeing and accepting your body's truth from
moment to moment, and recognizing that the truth of that moment is
morally neutral and doesn't require you to have an opinion about it. Put
another way, body neutrality is the practice of receiving the information we get about our bodies without resistance or judgment. That's not
to say we have to like what we see, but we sort of . . . give our consent for
it to be true. Because whether or not we consent, our bodies in that moment are *always* going to be our bodies in that moment. Even if we decide to change something (totally fine), trying to fight the truth of the
moment doesn't do anything but make us feel frustrated, violated,
helpless, and miserable.

As anyone who has tried meditation knows, accepting the truth of the moment without resistance or judgment is often very difficult, especially when the truth of the moment is uncomfortable, scary, or painful. That's why it's important to remember not to judge discomfort, fear, and pain as inherently bad or wrong in and of themselves. They're unpleasant, yes, but when we notice the unpleasantness without adding a layer of meaning, significance, or interpretation on top of that unpleasantness, then the experience stops there and passes quickly. When it comes to body image issues (and, frankly, most other areas of life!), however, we never seem to stop there, and it never seems to pass quickly.

Here's the deal: Through a clear and neutral lens, things that suck will still suck. Stubbing our toes will still hurt, skydiving will still feel scary, and we'll still feel the pain of grief when we lose someone we love. But when we're able to avoid interpreting that unpleasantness as bad or wrong, or adding layers of meaning or judgment on top of it, then there's only one layer of unpleasantness to deal with. Unfortunately, interpreting and adding meaning to things is exactly what we tend to do: we judge an unpleasant experience as a Huge Terrible Problem, invent a story about what it means, and tell ourselves it shouldn't be happening. In this way, we send ourselves into far bigger spirals of unpleasantness.

Our suffering skyrockets when we stub our toe on an otherwise bad day, and we tell ourselves a story about how we have chronically bad luck, we're stupid and clumsy and deserve to be in pain, or we seem destined to suffer more than everyone else and it's just not fair. Our distress increases when we interpret our heartbreak or fear as a shameful sign of weakness. Our pain is compounded exponentially when we lose someone we believe was "supposed to" be in our lives longer (or in a different way), or if we blame ourselves for their leaving.

I personally know very little about Buddhism, but I do have to point out that for anyone who is familiar with its Four Noble Truths, body neutrality will probably feel pretty intuitive. (I won't be diving into all four Noble Truths, but the first two are particularly applicable here).

The first Noble Truth, as I understand it, is the existence of suffering. Basically, it's the acknowledgment that unpleasant stuff is going to happen in life, and we can't stop it. (Accurate.)

The second Noble Truth, however, says that the source of all suffering is twofold: ignorance—defined as an inability to see ourselves as we are, or the world as it is—and "attachment" to our desires.[1] The definition of that second bit is a very complex topic that's been thoroughly unpacked and debated by scholars, and frankly I have no business trying to summarize it here. But I think it can provide a helpful context for body neutrality, so I'll share how I understand it.

To me, "attachment to our desires" just means wanting things to be different than they are, wanting reality itself to be different moment to moment, and getting upset when reality doesn't cooperate with our idea of what it *should* be. We suffer, then, because we're attached to the story that things should be how we want them to be.

That makes sense, right? A while back, I tried to fix a structural issue with my website myself instead of hiring someone, and I ended up accidentally deleting the page I had spent so long building, *and* completely screwing up the formatting of the rest of my website. This was, as I'm sure you'll agree, an undeniably frustrating situation. But I didn't respond with frustration; I responded with red-hot fury. I became practically unhinged with rage, crying to my partner about how I don't know how to do *anything* and should never have tried to build a business online, and maybe I should quit this whole thing and go live in the woods without a computer for the rest of my life because clearly I can't do anything right!

A tad dramatic, I know. My feelings were valid, and my reaction was real, but I hope you'll agree I was causing myself a lot of extra suffering by adding layers of subjective interpretation, meaning, significance, and stories on top of the already-frustrating situation. I escalated my distress by telling myself that I was doltish and incompetent, my brain was bad and wrong, I'm not equipped to run a business online, and if I keep trying, I'm going to fail.

Had I applied a clear and neutral lens to the situation, I probably wouldn't have gone into a rage. More likely, I would have just felt irritated or annoyed for a while, maybe taken a break to clear my head, and then tracked down a good solution to my problem. But that's easier said than done. We're so accustomed to adding interpretations, judgment, or meaning to the story of the moment that we often aren't even aware we're doing it. I would have had to strip away a bunch of thoughts that felt like facts to me in that moment, to say, "I don't like what's happening right now, and that's okay. Because it *is* happening, I'll consider my options for moving forward from here, and make a decision that suits me best."

Rejecting reality is a silly thing to do, really. It's almost like we think disapproving of reality will influence it to change; that putting up a fight will convince the very fabric of the universe to be different. And yet we do it all the time, especially when it comes to our bodies. We decide the truth of our bodies in the current moment is unacceptable, and then we rail against the injustice of it, get emotional, bombard ourselves with terrible stories about what it *means*, and find ourselves unable to let it go or to make clearheaded decisions about what to do next.

When we stand in front of the mirror and say, "I hate the way my body looks, I'm so gross!" we're fundamentally rejecting the truth of the moment, saying, "It shouldn't be like this; the truth of my body in this moment is bad and wrong." We make such audacious assessments as if *we* are the existential or moral authority on how reality should be, and our disapproval has the power to do anything other than hurt ourselves. **We believe there should be no contrast between how things *are*, and how we *want* them to be,** and then we suffer when there is.

This is where body neutrality offers us a tool for instant relief—not relief from the actual source of pain, fear, or discomfort, but relief from the suffering caused by deciding that the truth of the moment is a Huge

Terrible Problem, and therefore also from the exhausting labor of fighting, rejecting, and adding meaning to it. Essentially, body neutrality frees us from the need to form an opinion on the truth of the moment at all. Despite what you may believe, you don't actually even need to ever have an opinion about your body! You don't need to decide whether it's good or bad, or to interpret what it means, or to like it or dislike it.

Once you adopt a neutral lens, you can approach the original source of unpleasantness from a calm, present, grounded, and curious place, without suffering. That is to say, once you relinquish the need to assess and control the very fabric of reality, you can focus on the things you *can* influence (i.e., what you do next), instead of the things you *can't* (i.e., the fact that this moment is happening). And that shift alone has a way of completely changing your internal experience, turning passivity into self-determination, impotence into empowerment, and hatred into disinterest.

This kind of neutrality means you might look in the mirror, see a huge zit on your face, decide that you don't like how it looks, and put some concealer on it—all without getting upset. Maybe you notice your clothes are too tight, feel uncomfortable for a while, and then go buy new clothes. Or you could see a photo of yourself that makes you feel uncomfortable, say to yourself, "Huh, I don't like that photo of me," and then just move on.

Having a zit isn't inherently bad, after all, nor is weight gain, or having an unflattering photo of you taken. But it's *also* not inherently bad to cover up a zit, to take action to feel more comfortable, or to dislike a photo of yourself. All of these are neutral bits of information, and none of them are problems. Through a neutral lens, you might get curious about these bits of information, but not upset. You'll allow them to each exist without interpretation or moral judgment, along with anything you decide to do about them, because you're not trying to fight reality in any way.

To be clear, you don't have to be Buddhist to practice body neutrality—you're still welcome (and even expected!) to have opinions and preferences about how you look, even through a neutral lens. But when those preferences and opinions exist on a foundation of acknowledging and accepting your body's truth in the current moment, you're likely to feel a lot less distressed. In order to do that, however, we must give up the ridiculous notions that reality needs our permission to be itself, that by fighting or rejecting reality we stand a chance of getting our way, and that unpleasantness is inherently bad or wrong.

While the majority of this book is focused on your relationship with your physical body, it also has to be said that neutrality applies to *everything* about you! It applies to your feelings, thoughts, behaviors, opinions, needs, desires, impulses, patterns, character traits, skills, and preferences, including the uncomfortable stuff. Those are *all* morally neutral bits of information; they may be worth considering and getting curious about, but it serves you best to accept them exactly as they are in each moment, without the audacity of judgment, interpretation, rejection, or resistance.

With that in mind, I want to encourage you from here on to view your body image *issues* through a neutral lens too. I know they're unpleasant, but instead of rejecting them, judging them, or fighting against them, try just acknowledging that they exist, exactly as they are, in this moment. It may sound counterintuitive, but the more you give yourself permission for your body image suffering to exist when it shows up, the less suffering you'll experience in the long term, because nonjudgmental awareness (sometimes called mindfulness) opens the door to both healing and appropriate action. According to Bessel van der Kolk in his book *The Body Keeps the Score*, "Awareness puts us in touch with our inner world. . . . Simply noticing our [emotion] helps us shift our perspective and opens up new options."[2]

Giving yourself permission for your body image issues to exist is an important part of the practice, because body neutrality is all about allowing the truth of the moment to exist without adding interpretation, judgment, or meaning to it. And if you're reading this book, the truth of *your* moment is very likely to include body image issues. Better to meet yourself wherever you are, in each moment, and allow your body image suffering to be just one more neutral bit of information to notice, get curious about, and allow to exist without judgment. *Allowing* something doesn't mean you have to give up on changing it, however. Quite the opposite! Noticing and allowing something to exist without judgment or interpretation gives you space to consider it more clearly, calmly, and rationally—including the impact it's having on you, and your options for dealing with it. For this reason, noticing and allowing your negative body image thoughts and feelings without judgment makes it *more* likely that you'll find a way to overcome them. (And yes, I know it's weird that a body image coach is telling you to accept your body image issues, but trust me: this is an all-important first step for many of my clients!)

However, before we dive any further into body neutrality and the role it can play in healing body image issues, I'd like to back it up for a moment to understand what body image issues are in the first place.

This might seem pretty obvious to anyone who has experienced them, but body image issues are actually not as easy to define as you might think. Body image is the way a person perceives their body in their own head—the picture they hold in their mind of their own body—and the sum total of all their thoughts and feelings about it. So body image *issues*, then, can be anything negative, unrealistic, or concerning to a person about the picture they hold of their body, their thoughts about their body, or their feelings toward their body. These issues often focus on specific aesthetic details such as body size, facial features, hair, skin, or the shape and size of specific body parts, and often refer to the negative feelings a person feels toward their body when they perceive themselves as unattractive.

Because a person's relationship to their body includes their *whole* body, however—including face, hair, genitals, reproductive and immune systems, various aspects of performance and function, and even internal organs!—*any* distorted or negative thoughts or feelings that come up in your perception of your own body can be considered a body image issue. I say this because while the mainstream portrayal of body image issues tends to focus on people—usually young women—who want to lose weight, get more toned, or look more attractive, body image issues can span a hugely diverse array of complex and underrepresented issues!

I once worked with a woman with hirsutism who felt fine about the shape and size of her body, but suffered from enormous anxiety about the thick dark hair on her face, chest, and back. This may not be a part of the mainstream narrative around body image issues, but it absolutely qualifies! So does a distress caused by insecurity, dysphoria, or anxiety about anything else body related, like facial features, genital shape and size, height, body odor, or even bad breath. And even *less* talked about in the mainstream are the body image issues caused by negative thoughts or feelings toward an internal or systemic issue in a person's body, like chronic illness, injury, pain and fatigue disorders, sexual dysfunction, fertility issues, or disability.

With all this in mind, it's clear that the experience of body image issues will vary dramatically from individual to individual, but there are two things all body image issues have in common.

DISTRESS

The first thing all body image issues have in common is that they cause the person distress.

This usually means a level of distress that interferes with day-to-day life and functioning, but it can also be any amount of distress that is out of proportion to the situation. For example, it might be appropriate for someone to be upset about their weight gain if it means needing to buy a whole new wardrobe, and that requires expending a lot of time, energy, and money that they don't have available. It's probably not, on the other hand, appropriate for someone to be upset because they gained three pounds on vacation. A transgender person might have an appropriate amount of body anxiety due to their increased chances of being a victim of a hate crime, but their insecurity about their abs not being flat enough might be totally out of proportion. It's all about what amount of distress is appropriate and proportional for the context. And even if a person rarely feels insecure about something small, like having an outie belly button, it could be argued that the presence of *any* distress ever over such a harmless detail is disproportionate to the situation, and therefore in need of some neutrality work.

It's hard to quantify what counts as an "inappropriate" or "out-of-proportion" amount of distress for someone else, just like it's hard to quantify what "interfering with daily life" means, so I can't define that for you. It could be a constant impulse like wanting to check your appearance in a mirror or your phone all day, a daily habit like weighing yourself or criticizing yourself in the mirror every morning, a yearly situation like not swimming in the summer because you're not comfortable in a swimsuit, or even just the presence of a negative feeling that keeps you from living your best life. So while I can't tell you where the line is, I can tell you that if you're reading this book, odds are good your body image issues are causing you distress and interfering with your life enough to count, and you deserve to heal and find neutrality.

Back when I was a personal trainer, one of my peers would spend a lot of time looking in the mirror and talking about what he wanted to change about his body. But despite these behaviors, he didn't seem to be suffering from body image issues, because there was no distress present. Assuming he was telling the truth, this guy just saw changing the body as a sort of fascinating project, a curiosity and a hobby. He thought it would be *so cool* to look like the Hulk, but it didn't seem to bother him whatsoever that he looked more like Bruce Banner. He liked the idea of challenging himself to change his appearance, but he felt good about himself and didn't attach any meaning to his body either way. Without the presence of distress, then, I would argue he didn't have body image issues.

MORAL OR SOCIAL HIERARCHIES

The second thing all body image issues have in common is they were created within a moral or social hierarchy.

All body image issues suppose that there are better bodies and worse bodies, and there is always a body-ranking system of some kind. This is why my trainer friend didn't struggle with his body image: because even though he loved the aesthetic of hugely muscular bodies, he didn't presume one size or shape of body to be any *better* than another, or attach any interpretation or moral significance to a person with either kind of body. And without a hierarchy of some kind, body preferences and opinions just don't have the power to create distress or suffering. Even my client who suffered from hirsutism was distressed and affected by her face and body hair because she believed women "should" have hairless faces, and that a hairy woman was fundamentally less desirable and acceptable.

Interestingly, we often don't agree with each other on which hierarchies are real, which ones matter, who is at the top and bottom of each one, or where we (and everyone else) are on each one. Think of the classic conundrum of those with curly hair versus those with straight hair—each often thinks the *other* is at the top of the hair hierarchy, holding a place of superiority that causes them to dislike their *own* hair and wish for the other.

I have a friend with very straight, very blond hair and small breasts, and she and I often compare the exact opposite things we learned to believe about women's bodies growing up and laugh-slash-cry about it. *She* learned that everyone (read: men) preferred wild, curly-haired brunettes with big boobs (read: me), and that women who looked like *her* came off as too little girlish, and weren't "sexy enough." I, on the other hand, grew up believing that everyone (read: men) preferred delicate, straight-haired blonds with small perky breasts (read: her), and that *I* came across as intimidating, sloppy, or "too much."

This is why other people's body image issues can seem totally confusing and invalid to us! We each hold hundreds if not thousands of individual opinions and hierarchies in our heads when it comes to bodies. They each play out on a bigger "stage" of structurally enforced and socially "agreed-upon" body hierarchies that determine a person's levels of social privilege or oppression, but often even our best friends won't understand how we ended up with the specific preferences and hierarchies we use to torture ourselves with.

While we don't always agree on the specifics of each individual body hierarchy, the fact remains that all body image issues are built upon the belief that one kind of body can be (and is) *inherently better and more worthy* than another. **Body image issues then can be understood as the result of a person considering where they are in any particular body-related hierarchy they hold, as well as where they *want* to be on that hierarchy, and then feeling distressed about the difference.**

From this simplistic definition of body image issues, we can see that in order to stop the suffering of body image issues, we have only a few options.

1. We could try to claw our way up the hierarchy.

One way to stop ourselves from suffering over body image is to improve our standing on the body hierarchy in question, to claw our way up a bit higher by trying to change our appearance and conform to whatever we believe would make us have a "better" body. This can often be accomplished in our culture by losing weight, building muscle, getting surgeries or procedures, or making over your hair, makeup, or wardrobe.

This kind of aesthetically driven hierarchy climbing is considered common wisdom for how a person can "feel more confident" about how they look. Feeling unattractive? Go on a diet, hit the gym, buy some lingerie, get Botox, or try some new makeup! This kind of advice is such a default in the mainstream conversation about body image that we're rarely even aware of what we're doing, or that there are other options to reach the same goal.

Unfortunately, this solution doesn't work, though, because the top of the hierarchy can only ever be occupied by a small percentage of the population at any given time, so the harder people work to get there, the more intensely competitive the requirements for getting there become. Put another way, we don't end up with more people at the top, we just end up making the top even more inaccessible. Plus, a lot of what determines a person's position in the hierarchy is beyond our control. After all, certain things are pretty unchangeable, like our height and our race, and we'll all get older and wrinklier if we live long enough.

2. We could convince ourselves we're already at the top of the hierarchy.

Because body image issues come from not liking where we are on a particular body hierarchy in our minds, another thing we could do to overcome them is to convince ourselves that *we already are* higher up on the hierarchy. This is a tactic often employed interpersonally when someone expresses that they feel insecure about how they look. Whoever is listening will automatically say something like "No, you look *great!*" in an effort to convince that person that they are further up on the hierarchy than they feel.

In the body positivity space, you might also see people trying to reimagine the hierarchies so that *everyone* is at the top! But of course everyone *can't* all be at the top, or the hierarchy wouldn't be a hierarchy anymore . . . so sometimes this approach just seems like gaslighting people who aren't at the top, or asking people to lie to themselves. For these reasons, this approach is ineffective for most people, like trying to believe you're rich when you're poor. It also maintains the (false) notion that social hierarchies give us important and accurate information about a person's worth, by upholding the idea that it's important to be at the top of them!

3. We could stop wanting to be higher up on the hierarchies.

As a third option for how to handle the problem of not liking where we are on the body hierarchy in our minds, we could try to simply *stop wanting* to be at a different place!

This is a common bit of "wisdom" often given to my female clients by their male partners: *You're never going to look how you want, so let it go.* Understandable, certainly, as from their perspective, she would be able to stop suffering if only she could stop wanting to look different. But not particularly helpful.

This approach asks us to notice that we're *not* at the top of some kind of body hierarchy, and just, like . . . be okay with that. And of course, that *is* the direction this book is going, so I support this idea in theory. But for most people, trying to stop wanting something they want is about as effective as asking a five-year-old to stop wanting candy, or a cigarette smoker to stop wanting a cigarette. We want things for a reason, and until that reason is dismantled and neutralized, no amount of trying to "let it go" is going to be effective.

Think about how badly you wanted that one item in high school (Abercrombie & Fitch jeans, anyone?), because it was the Cool Thing. Maybe your mom told you it wasn't worth it, because you could get something almost identical, or of better quality for less money, in another store. And maybe that's what you ended up doing. But that did not stop you from still wanting the Cool Thing. Why? Because the Cool Thing had power in your peer group. It had the power to make *you* cool. The Cool Thing was not neutral to you. Even though it was neutral to your mom, *you* were not able to see it neutrally or stop wanting it.

Trying to stop wanting to lose weight when you believe your weight has the power to "make you cool" will ultimately be as effective as my mom telling me to stop drooling over low-rise Abercrombie flares, because Walmart jeans are "just as good." (In other words, not effective at all.) We have to strip away the power and significance we've assigned to the Cool Thing to be okay without it, and likewise we have to strip away the layers of power, meaning, and significance we've assigned to our bodies in order to be okay with them.

To be perfectly honest, however, even when you've learned to strip away the power and significance, you *still* might just want a body that looks or acts a certain way, and that's okay! That's neutral information too! After all, we live in a capitalist society, and sometimes you might just wish you had more money, right? Even if you don't think of money as the Cool Thing you need to become worthy of belonging, the desire to have a lot of it might still be there, and that makes sense. We're influenced by what we see and the world we live in, and it's normal to want the things that offer a person real social power and privilege, and we know that certain bodies *do* offer those things.

Plus, wanting to look a certain way is sometimes about wanting to *express ourselves* a certain way, which may or may not be possible, but *is* normal and healthy. I occasionally wear hair extensions, for example, because I like the sensation of ultra-long hair swirling around me when I'm feeling particularly femme, but I don't assign any moral significance to my hair, so wearing it naturally doesn't cause me any distress or insecurity, either.

So not only is this approach pretty damned impossible for most people, it's also kind of missing the point. You might always *want* to have green eyes, a six-pack, clear skin, or longer legs, and that desire does not have to completely disappear for you to escape from body image suffering.

4. We could just get over it.

Similarly, a fourth option is the idea that we can "cure" our suffering over where we are on a body hierarchy by just "letting it go" and "not letting it bother us." This is the gist of the popular "stop caring what people think of you" advice, which is generally well-intentioned, but still infuriating. After all, has anyone *ever* stopped being upset about something just because they were told to?

Like the previous option, this advice gets *close* to body neutrality, insofar as it suggests a person could notice that they're not where they want to be on a body hierarchy without it bothering them. And if this is an option for you, great! Put this book down and go do it! But for most people, this is like telling a depressed person to cheer up, or an anxious person to relax—not helpful in the slightest, and actually rather rude and counterproductive.

The truth is that trying to change how you feel using logic and will-power doesn't work. As trauma researcher and expert Bessel van der Kolk explains, "The rational brain cannot *abolish* emotions, sensations, or thoughts." That means we can't just decide to stop being upset about something. We can numb, repress, ignore, or run from such feelings, but we can't just *stop* them from happening. And van der Kolk goes on to say "the neuroscientist Joseph LeDoux and his colleagues have shown that the only way we can consciously access the emotional brain is through self-awareness. . . . Neuroscience research shows that the only way we can change the way we feel is by becoming aware of our *inner* experience and learning to befriend what is going on inside ourselves."[3]

Put another way, we can't forcibly stop ourselves from being upset about or caring about the way our bodies are, but by learning to notice, accept, and welcome those feelings without judgment, they *can* shift over time. So the best chance we have of changing how we feel is approaching our feelings with nonjudgmental self-awareness—i.e., body neutrality.

5. We could dismantle all the hierarchies.

The fifth and final way to ease the suffering caused by hating where you are on a body hierarchy is the body neutrality approach, which is to completely dismantle the hierarchy's existence inside yourself altogether.

If you don't believe that some bodies are better than others, then there will be no need to be distressed about yours not being good enough. Social and moral hierarchies are, after all, *just made up*. They're subjective, erratic, and ever evolving, and they're designed to both reflect and uphold a world in which certain people have power and certain people don't. Fat people used to be considered more attractive than thin people, and now thin people are considered more attractive.[4] In a matriarchal society, women are at the top of the social hierarchy and men are at the bottom, while in a patriarchal society it's the opposite. Social hierarchies are all entirely subjective from place to place and time period to time period, and dependent on who is powerful.

In *The Sneetches*, my favorite story by Dr. Seuss as a kid, we see how fickle and arbitrary our body hierarchies and beauty ideals are, by following the actions of a sly capitalist named Sylvester McMonkey McBean as he manipulates the status-conscious Sneetches to make himself rich. At first, the Sneetches with stars on their bellies occupied a higher social status, which made the Sneetches *without* belly stars feel inferior, so McBean builds a machine to sell belly stars to those with "no stars upon thars," and business booms. But when all the Sneetches have belly stars, those who had previously enjoyed a higher social status no longer feel special or superior, so McBean tells them belly stars have gone out of style, and starts offering belly star removals. McBean's plan is possible both because the Sneetches place so much (false and inflated) meaning onto belly stars, and because those who had been enjoying a high social status are invested in upholding a hierarchical social system. But this ends up costing *all* Sneetches a lot of money, and the only one who benefits is the businessman with a machine selling both belly stars and belly star removals.

Body neutrality in the world of the Sneetches, then, wouldn't just be about everyone deciding it's equally beautiful to have a belly with or without stars, deciding to simply stop wanting the "right" kind of belly du jour, or to "get over" their feelings of inferiority when their bellies are out of vogue. It would be about the Sneetches acknowledging that they'd been functioning in a false reality where a body even *could* be better or worse based on something as trivial as belly stars, and exploring and challenging this concept within themselves (and in their social, political, and economic systems) until their concept of worthiness was based on something more equitable and meaningful than belly aesthetics. Then, a scammer trying to exploit their hierarchical system would just be laughed out of town.

This is the kind of body neutrality I believe in: a neutrality that comes from having knocked down the whole system of ranking people's bodies relative to each other as good or bad in the first place, and acknowledging that despite how our society is set up, there actually *aren't* any objectively better or worse bodies! Just like how the truth of the current moment can't actually be right or wrong—it just *is*—a body can't be right or wrong either.

I believe in a neutrality that comes from having stripped away all the false and inflated meaning, significance, and importance we learned to assign to bodies in the first place. Of course, dismantling these hierarchies inside ourselves isn't easy. We've all learned that it's our right, and even our *responsibility*, to have an opinion about absolutely everything, bodies included; we've learned that everything both *can* and *should* be assessed and ranked. Dismantling long-held associations, bias, interpretations, meaning, and ideas about moral significance inside our own minds, therefore, requires radical honesty, courage, dedication, humility, patience, and plenty of practice.

To share a personal example of a body hierarchy *I* grew up with: in my rural, conservative hometown in upstate New York, I learned that cisgender people (i.e., those whose gender identity aligns with the sex they were assigned at birth) were *good and right*, and transgender people (i.e., everyone else) were *bad and wrong*. Nobody outright said this to me exactly, but I absorbed the message from thousands of tiny moments, exchanges, and bits of negative representation on TV and in the media that a transgender body was a *wrong* body, signaling that the person was morally corrupt, sick, broken, or disgusting. I learned that such bodies were shameful, and this specific hierarchy lived in my head for decades. In 2015, however, when Caitlyn Jenner came out and joined Chelsea Manning and Laverne Cox in pushing the conversation around transgender folks into the mainstream,[5] I—like so many of us at the time—started dismantling this hierarchy inside my own mind.

What I discovered was that this hierarchy had been nothing more than the result of bigotry, bias, stereotypes, misinformation, moral judgment, fear, and violence. And as it turns out, every single major body hierarchy is exactly the same.

Not all hierarchies are quite as overtly bigoted and explicitly oppressive as that one, but think about all the layers of interpretation and significance you've learned throughout your life about what it means to be Black, white, Indigenous, Latinx, East Asian, or South Asian. What nuanced layers of "better" or "worse" are in your mind about each race, their character, and their appearance? How about what it means to be able-bodied versus disabled—including every specific variation of what "disabled" can mean? What kinds of bodies did you learn were right or wrong when it comes to age, weight, fitness, gender, sexuality, and gender expression? What does the hierarchy in your mind look like when it comes to beauty ideals and attractiveness for each kind of person? How is it different for men? Women? Black folks? White folks? Fat people? Thin people? Straight folks? Gay folks? Trans people? Nonbinary folks? Who did you learn was better than whom, and which bodies did you learn to associate with being *more* or *less* worthy of respect, belonging, autonomy, and happiness because of something about their bodies?

And to take it even further, what happens when we zoom in and look at the micro-hierarchies underneath each category? What did you learn about blonds versus brunettes, long versus short hair, or curly versus straight hair? Who is at the top in your mind, and who is at the bottom? And what hierarchy do you hold in your mind about acne, stretch marks, eyelash length, fertility, neurodivergence, wrinkles, cellulite, and freckles? Which versions of skin, lashes, brains, and faces did you learn meant something good about the person, and which ones did you learn meant something bad? What about breast size, penis size, body hair, teeth color, and butt shape and size?

Think about how different each layer of interpretation, meaning, and significance changes when you consider different kinds of people and bodies. It's right for women to get breast implants, but not men. It's wrong for boys to wear dresses and high heels, but not women. The nuanced layers of what's *more right* and *more wrong* inform the body hierarchies in our minds depending on whom we're applying it to, which means they, too, were created by, and continue to enforce and uphold, the systemic oppression of certain people based on their bodies.

Because body image issues uphold body hierarchies, they are also almost always upholding systemic oppression too. This wouldn't be the case if the changes you wanted to make to your body were completely outside any social hierarchy, of course, like if you hated the skin you were born with and preferred to dye it green instead. But most of the changes we want to make to our bodies are about trying to climb the social body hierarchies; they're about trying to "improve" our bodies enough that we earn ourselves more social privilege and power. And this individual act helps uphold the entire social hierarchy, because in order for some people to have bodies that are worthy of respect, some people must have bodies worthy of disrespect; in order for some people's bodies to be *good*, some have to be *bad*. Body image issues are built on a hierarchical comparison of some kind, which means that (often without meaning to) they automatically uplift some people (i.e., those with a lot of privilege) and oppress others (i.e., those who are marginalized).

There is literally no way to uphold the idea that some bodies are better without upholding the idea that some bodies are worse, which is why teachers, activists, and leaders in the most marginalized bodies— Black, Brown, Indigenous, disabled, transgender, very fat, and particularly those with multiple marginalized identities—are in a unique position to teach us how to identify and dismantle these hierarchies. Body neutrality is born out of and functions to *supplement* rather than stand in for the work of the extraordinary Black, Brown, trans, fat, and disabled activists who have been fighting to dismantle the body hierarchies inside the minds of individuals, and society at large, for generations. Again, because I have multiple privileged identities (white, thin, able-bodied), I am simply not the right person to teach you how to dismantle body hierarchies and systems of oppression. Luckily, there are many wonderful authors, coaches, speakers, teachers, and leaders who *are*, and I've compiled a list of liberation-focused books and authors for you to use as a jumping-off point in the back of the book.

I encourage you to seek out the body liberation and anti-oppression leaders in multi-marginalized bodies to guide you on that journey, as they are best suited to the role, and to pay them extremely well for their insight, wisdom, skill, energy, and time. For the purposes of this book, I will give you as much information as you need to move through the individual body neutrality process as I've outlined it, but dismantling an entire society's worth of oppressive body hierarchies in your own mind *will* require you to seek out and learn from the people whose life experiences best qualify them for that work.

For now, just know that a nonnegotiable aspect of body neutrality is to recognize the body hierarchies in your mind for what they are (subjective and false interpretations) and dismantle them inside yourself until they no longer cloud your vision when you look at a body—yours, or anyone else's.

Yes, this is a tall order. Dismantling what you've learned about bodies will be a journey that takes you the rest of your life, and even so you'll never completely strip away everything, because this stuff has been taught to us since the moment we were born. But luckily, you don't have to be perfect at this, you just have to be present, curious, brave, and self-aware enough to recognize in the moment when you're coming up against your false interpretations about bodies at first, and to be willing to interact with those thoughts differently.

When I started dismantling my internalized transphobia, for example, I discovered some nasty, cruel, shameful stuff in there. It was painful and embarrassing to acknowledge the prejudiced, oppressive, and vicious beliefs I'd been holding about trans people, and the inexcusable amount of harm to trans people I had been unconsciously causing by believing them. It was even *more* mortifying when I realized that I don't identify as a cisgender woman . . . so I had actually been holding on to a lot of those nasty beliefs toward trans people as a way of hiding from and burying my own truth. I was ashamed of who I was, so I tried to separate myself from it by being anti-trans. Unfortunately, this is a very common experience: we tend to reserve our most violent biases and judgments for the things we're most ashamed of within ourselves.

Dismantling this particular body hierarchy inside myself has been deep, painful, and slow. I'm still working on it, and I'll probably be working on it forever. I went through a similarly personal experience around being queer, and struggling with mental health, and have also spent a huge amount of time and energy identifying and dismantling the hierarchies that lived in my subconscious mind around race, weight, and ability. I can tell you from experience that facing your own conscious and subconscious biases, bigotry, and prejudices in this way is wildly uncomfortable. But ultimately even those thoughts are neutral, insofar as they don't mean anything bad about *you*. They just mean you grew up with prejudiced and bigoted conditioning. We all did.

Try to apply the clear and neutral lens of body neutrality to this part of the work too. No need to start spinning out a story about what it means about you that you have a mind full of body hierarchies. Just notice and acknowledge the hierarchical thoughts and feelings wherever and whenever you find them, accept the fact that they exist, stay curious, and hold yourself accountable to the continual dismantling of the idea that one kind of body is (or frankly even *could be*) better and more right than another.

While the body neutrality process can mitigate a lot of body image suffering, ultimately the only way to completely free yourself from it is to free yourself from the body hierarchies they're based on. And while I know you probably didn't mean to pick up a book on how to make the world more just, fair, and equitable, it's important to point out that doing this work inside ourselves is actually a critical first step to dismantling it in our society. Because once you've committed to dismantling these hierarchies wherever and whenever you find them . . . and you've done a lot of that work inside yourself (by learning from marginalized activists and leaders), the next natural step is to help the people around you do the same. In this way, pushing back against body image issues is a way of pushing back against injustice and oppression, and moving our society forward toward justice, fairness, and true equality.

Or dare I say . . . *human* neutrality?

CHAPTER *4*

The One Big, Crucial Lie

MY CLIENT BEX, AN EX-FIREFIGHTER in her midthirties, told me in our first session together that she understood that most people who struggle with body image issues are chasing an unrealistic fantasy, but that *she* was different. The first year she trained to fight fires, she got into incredible shape and lost a significant amount of weight. During this period of her life, she told me she was the happiest she had ever been—full of energy and brimming with confidence, friends, and joy.

When we met, however, Bex had regained all that weight and felt isolated, insecure, and unhappy. "So you see," Bex said to me, "it's not all in my head. I actually *know* that being thin makes me feel happy and confident. I have *proof* that my body is the only thing standing in the way of the life I want."

Each person's individual journey to seeing themselves with clear and neutral vision will be different, because body image issues are based on a plethora of different beliefs, interpretations, experiences, biases and prejudices, identities, and moral associations. This can make it difficult to talk about (or write about) body image healing more generally, because each person has to explore which specific blocks to body neutrality they're dealing with, in order to dismantle them and strip them away.

There is, however, one fundamental and universal lie that every single person who is suffering from body image issues believes—one lie to rule them all, as it were.

That lie is that *their body is the problem*— *their body* is the source of their pain or suffering, or their body is the thing standing between them and what they want. Bex thought she was a unique case, but actually *all* my clients believe their body is the problem on some level. Body image issues simply couldn't exist if a person didn't believe their body was the source of their pain and suffering, because then, well, the ruse would be up, and they'd already be dealing with the deeper issues.

If you've been paying attention, you might already have guessed that dismantling this one crucial lie is at the heart of body neutrality work. In fairness, body neutrality is about dismantling *all* the layers that get in the way of seeing yourself and your body clearly, but this particular lie is extremely important, because it's the one that gives your body image issues so much power and influence over you. It's the *first* lie we have to expose and tackle on the body neutrality journey, and also the most important one. Frankly, the rest of this book won't even be able to help you much, if you refuse to acknowledge that this lie is a lie. (That said, if right now you're reading this and thinking, "Actually, Jessi, I *am* the exception . . . ," don't worry. You're normal, and in excellent company. Just keep reading!)

After Bex made her declaration to me, I asked her to reflect on that time of her life and why *else* she might have felt so confident and happy during her "thin year." We quickly discovered that it had been a wonderful year for multiple reasons: she was finally doing meaningful work that she loved, she had come out to her friends and family and started dating women, and then she met her first serious girlfriend. Most important, I think, Bex was living with two of her best friends in a house together, where she felt abundantly connected, supported, and taken care of. She felt good in her life, her heart was full, and she had just thrown off a layer of inauthenticity and secrecy she'd been carrying for years. But, yes, she was also thinner than ever, and people gave her a lot of positive feedback on how she looked, which felt great. All these feelings sort of melded together and made Bex feel liberated, empowered, sexy, and happy.

Given all this information, I asked Bex if she still thought it was truly her body that had made her so happy and confident during that time. It sounded to me like there were many other reasons she had felt so good about herself that had nothing to do with her body at all, and that getting positive feedback on her appearance had made it possible to give herself permission to be her most dazzling self, and to live her most dazzling life. That permission made her bolder and more authentic so that people were drawn to her—her energy, her joy, and her full, interesting life—and a positive feedback loop was created.

When I asked Bex about life now, she talked about feeling isolated, living in the suburbs with her girlfriend, and rarely seeing friends. She missed firefighting, all the adventures she used to go on, and all the people she used to connect with, but she felt like none of that was "realistic" anymore, given her age, responsibilities, and stressful new job. It was very clear to me that losing weight wouldn't actually have helped Bex feel how she wanted to feel at this point, because the things that were actually hurting her had nothing to do with her body at all—other than the fact that in Bex's mind, thinness was strongly associated with boldness, joy, and confidence, and she seemed unable to give herself permission to live fully in a bigger body.

I share this story because despite how sure she was, Bex wasn't an exception to the rule, and neither are you: the presence of body image suffering indicates the presence of this one big, crucial lie. But because I can't be there to convince you that your body isn't the problem *even in your particular case*, I just want to validate that sometimes this lie can be *very* difficult to see, and that's okay. It's hard to see because your brain has been searching for and storing moments of "evidence" and proof on its behalf for a long time, and because society at large has been encouraging and supporting the lie for your entire life.

The human mind loves a good narrative; stories are how we make sense of the world, so it makes sense that we would naturally try to come up with stories to understand our lives, our experiences, and ourselves. But the thing is, despite our believing that we're intelligent enough to interpret everything correctly, and despite those stories *feeling* true, they generally just . . . aren't. We tell ourselves a story about how the guy who cut us off in traffic is a selfish asshole, even though he might have just had a moment of thoughtlessness or distraction. We tell ourselves a story about how our crush doesn't like us because they always take hours to respond to texts, and how our coworker is mad at us because they signed their email kind of weird. We tell ourselves a story about how our partner only cheated on us because we weren't attractive enough; how everyone will judge us for gaining weight; how if we were thinner, it wouldn't be so hard for us to make friends. And it all *feels* real; it *feels* provable. But it's not.

The experiences you've had—the ones that convinced you that your body really *is* your problem—are real and valid. But the stories, interpretations, meaning, and significance you've assigned to them probably aren't. A lot of the conclusions we draw about our own lives are actually just wildly imaginative storytelling; we tend to create false narratives about which factors caused which outcomes, we confuse correlation with causation, we extrapolate based on cherry-picked data points to prove a point we want to prove, and we unconsciously absorb only the information that supports whatever story we're invested in telling ourselves, thanks to our brain's confirmation bias.[1]

This is often how we end up convinced that our bodies are the source of our suffering—by using true experiences to create a false narrative. After being teased for being fat, we think, "If I get thin, everyone will always be nice to me." After seeing other people succeed in the areas we crave, we think, "If I looked like that, I would be confident enough to get what I want." After attaching our self-worth to our appearance, we think, "If I fix this one flaw, I'll finally feel good enough." After facing marginalization, prejudice, or violence, we think something about our bodies was to blame.

It's important to understand that this internalization and self-blaming isn't about a lack of intelligence. The false narratives we weave aren't random accidents; they exist to help us make sense of the world, and they are always trying to serve, protect, or help us in some way. This is important because the big lie about your body is trying to solve a problem for you, and you need to know *what problem* in order to know what to do next.

Counterintuitively, because this big lie is the source of our body image suffering, instantly erasing it from our minds probably wouldn't actually make us feel happy and free, even if we could! Or, at least, not at first. That's because the *lie itself* often offers us something we want and need, such as hope, certainty, structure, or a feeling of control in our lives. Taking it away actually tends to make us extra miserable for a while, because we have to face the fact that something else is causing our suffering, and the real problem might not be so easy to understand or fix, and might mean the loss of hope or certainty.

This is why body neutrality work is so complex, deep, and slow; your mind is deeply invested in its stories, interpretations, and lies. For any number of reasons, it wants to believe them, and often at some point it may have even needed to believe them to survive—so it will often go to some pretty impressive lengths to keep you from dismantling them!

Have you ever reached one of your "body goals," but still not felt the way you wanted to? Maybe you felt great about the work you put in, or the way you actually looked, but did it give you what you really wanted? Did you feel as worthy, connected, happy, whole, confident, secure, or free as you were hoping? Probably not, because your body wasn't really the problem, so it *couldn't* be the solution. But the mind can still send us on a wild-goose chase in these moments, to protect the lie it's invested in. We might find ourselves thinking that maybe the problem wasn't our weight after all, but that it's actually this little pouch of fat where it shouldn't be! And if we get rid of the fat pouch and still don't feel happy, maybe the problem is our wrinkles and "old-looking" skin! After we get Botox and fillers to change that, suddenly the problem is that our thighs just aren't in proportion to our torso. Surely *that* is what stands between us and the confidence and happiness we seek, right? Plus, if we never actually "succeed" at making the body changes we're sure would solve our problems, that might make us miserable, but it also protects us from needing to notice or face the real problem underneath! In fact, spending your entire life trying to solve an unsolvable problem (i.e., weight loss) is an extremely efficient way to avoid ever challenging the reality you've built for yourself about *what the problem is.*

So let us recognize the one big crucial lie for what it is, and acknowledge that your body isn't actually your problem or the cause of your suffering. It's just the lie that allows you to buy into your own body image issues . . . and there is *always* a reason your brain wants you to buy into them. To help you understand why, let me return your attention to that Cool Thing you really, really wanted in high school.

If you were anything like me, you were completely, totally, and unwaveringly sure that the Cool Thing would solve all your problems. I imagined myself walking into homeroom smelling like that iconic Abercrombie body spray, with my midriff perfectly exposed and my butt perfectly flat (don't judge me, it was the early aughts), and everyone wondering if I had become a model like the store employees were rumored to be. I imagined the cool kids recognizing me as one of their own by the prominent label on my butt, and suddenly becoming superconfident and popular. But this fantasy had a flip side too. I felt like if I *didn't* get those jeans, I would *never* become confident and popular, and I would instead be destined for—not to be too dramatic here—a life of awkward loserdom.

I was positive that my problem—the source of my pain—was the *lack* of those dark blue low-rise jeans. It wasn't my debilitating self-objectification, chronic low-level depression and anxiety, deeply buried shame about my queerness, or the fact that I never felt like I quite belonged anywhere in my hometown. No, no. The problem was that I was wearing the wrong jeans. Can you relate to this at all? Most people can think of an item or experience they projected an inappropriate amount of power, meaning, and significance onto, and deluded themselves into thinking could solve all their problems.

Luckily, I was eventually able to see through this particular lie, but why did my mind come up with it in the first place?

This is the question we need to be investigating when it comes to body image issues—the lie that your body is your problem and the source of your suffering. Why has your mind come up with this lie, and why does it want you to buy into it so badly? What purpose is it trying to serve? What might you really be seeking, or avoiding, by focusing on your body? In what ways might you be benefiting from this lie? And what is the real cause of your suffering—the *actual* problem—if not your body?

No matter who you are, what body hierarchies you hold in your mind, and how your body image suffering looks, everyone must start their body neutrality journey the same way.

1. Acknowledge that your body isn't actually your problem.

2. Get curious: investigate why you're telling yourself the lie that it is, and the purpose of this false narrative.

As with everything else, I encourage you to adopt a neutral lens as you explore this part of yourself, and understand that we only ever lie to ourselves for a good reason. It's normal and it makes sense to lie to ourselves, as you'll see in the next chapter, and sometimes it's even the best and healthiest thing we can do, because it helps us survive.[2] So no criticism or judgment as we unpack the reasons we lie to ourselves, please. After all, those criticisms and judgments are just more false interpretations and narratives.

CHAPTER 5

Why Am I Lying to Myself?

I N UNDERSTANDING THE PHENOMENON OF why we sometimes lie to ourselves, it can be useful to imagine a person who has recently lost a loved one, and for one reason or another hasn't been able to properly grieve for them. Then one morning they can't find their keys, get increasingly upset, and end up sobbing uncontrollably in the kitchen because *where the fuck are their keys?!*

Obviously, in that moment, there is something else going on below the surface, causing something fairly insignificant (the loss of the person's keys) to come with a significant emotional reaction. Sometimes the real source of our suffering feels too big, or too painful, to face and acknowledge. As that suffering pops up, or gets projected onto various unrelated sources, we might be aware only that we're suffering, and not aware that there is something underneath it.

All of this is to say that, sometimes, hiding things from ourselves is an act of mercy or self-preservation. We don't lie to ourselves because we are stupid, weak, or irrational, and it's not usually a conscious decision. We do it because we need to do it, or at least some part of our mind *believes* we need to do it, to function and survive. Being a human can be scary, painful, and overwhelming; sometimes we just don't have the capacity, skills, or support to face it head-on. Hiding the real source of our suffering is sometimes the kindest thing our minds can do.

Plus, we tend to project our suffering onto things we think we can fix, so buying into the lie can help us reclaim a feeling of control, power, or self-determination. If the problem—the source of our suffering—is the *body*, then all we have to do to escape suffering is fix the body! It's a tangible, manageable problem we can solve (or, at least, spend our lives *trying* to solve), whereas the deeper problem might not be.

If, at some point in your life, you had to face something you didn't have the tools or capacity to face at the time, your mind might have protected you by creating a fantasy world for you to live in[1]—a world in which you could get thin enough to be lovable, look perfect enough to be safe, be pretty enough to get your needs met, stay pure enough to avoid pain, or get so lean that nobody would ever abandon you.

It's genius, really; our minds hide things and make things up to make life feel more doable, and help us survive.

Don't get me wrong, body image issues are far from the only place we create fantasy worlds or project our feelings. Plenty of people project their suffering onto their financial life, career, partnership status, sex life, or ability to have children. We imagine our lives would be so much better if only we made more money, found a partner, had kids, got married, or got a promotion. And while some of these types of changes do provide a temporary mood boost, they rarely lead to long-term satisfaction or happiness, because they're not actually addressing the real source of dissatisfaction or unhappiness.

What's interesting is that while the details of the lies we invent are informed to a great extent by the trends of our culture, social conditioning, and environment, the deeper pain driving them is pretty universal and ubiquitous throughout time and location. People have been having problems and suffering—and finding ways of solving those problems and coping with their suffering—for as long as we have written history. There's nothing new about feeling lonely or wishing you had a different lot in life, but there are constantly evolving trends surrounding the stories, expressions, and interpretations our minds assign to that suffering, and how we deal with it.

A thousand years ago, for example, a European woman who was struggling to land a husband wouldn't have thought to feel insecure about her cellulite or armpit hair. That's not to say she wouldn't have felt anxious or insecure, though. Worrying you won't find the love and intimacy you crave (or, more realistically for the time, the social and financial security that marriage could offer) and feeling the pain of isolation and rejection are universal. A woman today worrying about the same issue might find herself mired in body insecurities, whereas a European woman from the Middle Ages might have found herself stressed out and insecure about something more relevant to *her* environment and culture instead, like, say, how well she could sew or how many goats her father had.

Similarly, the painful thing underneath *your* body image issues probably would have found a different narrative, expression, or interpretation, even if you never encountered a single message about weight, bodies, or beauty ideals in your whole life. The details of *how* you understood your unmet needs and how you numbed, coped, or distracted yourself from the pain of them would be different, but the suffering itself would be the same. If nobody in your world cared about body shape or size, you might not find yourself dieting or worrying about belly rolls, but you *might* find yourself measuring your worth by something else, like how clean your house is, how pious you are, or whatever else you were taught makes a person important, worthy, and happy.

The lie that something superficial is our problem is a beautifully flexible and resilient one. It can change shape to fit any situation, society, or person, but the structure more or less always stays the same: that the problem is ____.

Cultural and social context inform how we understand ourselves and our suffering, and given the current body- and appearance-obsessed culture, our suffering often gets organized into body image issues.

We're bombarded with messages and images everywhere we look, reinforcing the lie that our bodies are the problem, and supporting the fantasy that the key to getting everything we need is *changing our bodies*.[2] But no matter how real that fantasy feels, body image issues are only ever a red herring.

"Look over here at your weight, your thighs, your scars, your cellulite!" your mind says urgently. "Don't look over there at your oppression, emotions, unmet needs, desires, or pain!" It may not feel good, but like a parent jangling a toy in front of a crying child, your body image issues *are* genuinely just trying to help.

The brutal irony of this whole thing, however, is that the lie itself still causes suffering.

The big lie that our body is the source of our suffering exists to protect us, but we still go through an immense amount of suffering to uphold it. Projecting your pain onto your body might be more tangible and manageable than facing the fact that you feel fundamentally unworthy of love . . . but it still really freakin' sucks. You still spend years in pain, wondering what's wrong with you that you can't lose weight, hating yourself, and raging against how unfair it is that some people just look perfect, while you have to suffer. Ultimately, it's probably not any more pleasant to exist within this lie than it would be to face the deeper truth of feeling unworthy. It just offers more of a sort of contained, tangible, manageable, and understandable form of suffering.

This is true for most of our body image suffering. Believing that you feel unworthy or insecure only because of the size, shape, or function of your body might provide you with a somewhat contained and manageable form of suffering, but it doesn't necessarily offer any *less* suffering in the long run.

Struggling with body image issues can be unbelievably painful, and it has the power to take over and ruin a person's entire life. But on some level, your mind believes obsessively worrying about people seeing your flaws or endlessly striving to lose weight is a better alternative to, say, facing the depth of your feelings, needs, or pain. And this is an important point about the purpose of our body image suffering: sometimes we are in immense pain deep down, and our body image suffering functions simply as a form of suffering that *we think we can survive.*

Ika, an office manager who uses a wheelchair, went through a body image healing program with me. She did brilliant work during that time to dismantle internalized sexism, ableism, and beauty ideals that had made her feel unworthy of belonging, love, and intimacy. By the end of the program, Ika reported feeling hardly any attachment to her appearance at all anymore, but something strange had started happening. Ika had started drinking, a *lot.* Where previously she might have a glass of wine with dinner, she was now drinking a bottle of wine nightly. She didn't think to mention this change in her drinking until the very end of her work with me, because she didn't see it as connected to the work we were doing, but I saw the connection immediately.

Ika was in a tremendous amount of emotional pain. Due to childhood abuse and a lifetime of inaccessibility as a person who uses a wheelchair, she had a lot of trauma that hadn't yet been dealt with. Obsessing over her body had provided Ika with a distraction and sort of "cover story" for her pain, so once we blew her cover story, she needed another way to cope with the pain. Acknowledging that her body wasn't the problem meant the lie no longer "worked" to protect her— but she wasn't yet ready or well resourced enough to deal with her pain directly, so she turned to alcohol to numb it.

Sometimes an individual, like Bex the ex-firefighter, will insist that surely *some people's* body image issues aren't actually covering anything up, or solving a deeper issue. And she's right, in a way, because certainly a person could suffer from a body image issue that came exclusively from a bit of misinformation, misunderstanding, or cultural conditioning that can be set straight, and erase the issue altogether. For example, I once worked with a nineteen-year-old girl who struggled with intense dysphoria around the shape and size of her vulva. After our second session, we realized she was pretty much "cured," and I refunded the rest of her coaching package. Why? Because I had sent her some information and resources on the vast diversity of normal vulval shapes and sizes—something she'd had *no* idea about, and had therefore been assuming that something about hers was gross and shameful—and all her insecurities pretty much just went up in smoke.

I have very occasionally worked with clients like this who didn't have any deep-down problems or pain driving their body image issues, but it's *extraordinarily rare.* This girl had been suffering exclusively from a misunderstanding! Her body shame and negativity hadn't existed to protect her from anything else, or solve any deeper problem, so once she learned the truth, there was no more reason for that suffering to stick around. So while this is possible, it's also fairly unusual. Ninety-nine point nine percent of body image suffering is the result of something deeper, and each person's body neutrality journey will require them to identify their own personal "something deeper."

To be clear, sometimes acknowledging the existence of a deeper issue makes things get worse before they get better, because looking at what our minds have been hiding from us can be incredibly scary and painful. Facing the stuff we've been avoiding for a long time is *not* a fun or easy process. I've even worked with a few people who straight up refused to do it.

Beth, a stay-at-home mom in her forties, figured out that her body image issues were covering up for an unhappy marriage, and because she wasn't willing to get divorced until the kids were older, she didn't want to keep digging. She told me point blank that she preferred to hate her body for another decade rather than let herself see what her body image issues were helping her avoid about her marriage, and have to split up the family. So we stopped working together, and Beth went back to a life of constant dieting and obsessing over her appearance, fully aware of the choice she was making.

For most people, though, pulling back the curtain on the big lie is liberating, as it's the only path with the potential to decrease suffering in the long term. It can be phenomenally uncomfortable and scary to face your deeper issues, but doing so paves the path to peace, acceptance, confidence, self-trust, and relief. It feels *good* to stop running, to get your actual needs met, to live in the present moment instead of a fantasy, and to know you've faced your scariest demons and survived! The journey may be difficult and even painful, but the destination is worth it. It's a bit like coming in from the cold after your hands have gone numb: it might hurt before it gets better, but all that burning and tingling in your hands as you warm up is a *good* sign, because it means blood flow is increasing again. If you were too scared of that pain to ever come inside and warm up your hands, you would end up with permanent damage in your hands, possibly even losing them to severe frostbite.

That example might sound a bit silly, but it's what a lot of us do when we suffer from body image issues: we suffer a *lot* to avoid suffering a *little*; we spend a lifetime hurting ourselves to avoid feeling pain. We're so scared to face the truth that we torture ourselves endlessly with a lie. Body neutrality is the process of noticing this pattern, pulling back the curtain on the lie, and facing that deeper truth directly. This helps us reclaim the power we've given to our bodies, *and* it gives us the information we need to understand the next steps of our unique, specific body neutrality journey.

Remember Bex? Well, during our work together, she was eventually able to recognize that her intense desire to look different wasn't just about "preferring" a certain kind of body—it was about chasing the feelings and experiences she *associated* with that body: freedom, purpose, community support, permission to take up space, and confidence. By identifying and acknowledging these underlying needs and problems, she was able to separate her body from her actual needs and desires and start going after those things more directly and effectively. Over time, as more of her needs were getting met and she was feeling happier overall, the false significance, meaning, and power Bex had attached to her body fell away, until her body was just a body, not the key to her confidence and happiness.

In the next part of this book you'll learn about the four body image avatars, which I use to help my clients start understanding the deeper issues and root causes leading to body image suffering, so that you, too, can pull back the curtain on your body image issues, expose the big, crucial lie for what it is, and face whatever it is *your* brain has been hiding behind it.

Part II

THE AVATARS

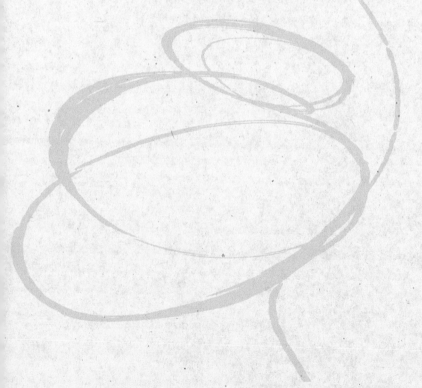

CHAPTER 6

Meet the Body Image Avatars

OR YEARS, I HELPED MY COACHING clients recognize that their bodies weren't the actual problem, and then individually and organically discover what problems lurked behind their body image issues. What were they subconsciously seeking, or avoiding? What problem were they trying to solve? What emotional needs were they trying to get met? How did they help the person cope or survive? Everyone's journey was so different though, I couldn't imagine ever creating content that applied to *everyone*. One woman hates her breasts because they're too small and she doesn't feel sexy, while another hates her breasts because they're too big and attract unwanted attention. One person hates their belly fat because they believe visible abs are a sign of hard work and discipline, and another hates their belly fat because an abusive partner once pinched it and told them nobody would ever love them unless they lost weight.

A person comes into their body image issues through a lifetime of unique experiences, influences, social conditioning, and their own individual makeup, so there's no telling what will cause a person to feel one way or another about their bodies—not by looking at them, and not even by hearing them talk about their insecurities. It's entirely possible for two people to go through the same exact experiences and come out with completely different body image issues, *and* it's totally possible for two people who went through completely opposite life experiences to struggle with the same exact body insecurities.

What I discovered over time, however, was that while the details of a person's body image journey were personal and individual, there were some overarching patterns, based on the underlying root cause and hidden purpose of a person's body image issues. As it turned out, by discovering how a person's body image issues were attempting to help them, I could start to make more accurate predictions. By paying attention to these patterns, I was able to determine which kind of body image healing work a person needed much more quickly.

Based on what I've seen in my coaching practice, people suffering from body image issues tend to fall into four major categories: those focused on *looking attractive*, those trying to earn *external validation* for being "good" (i.e., better than others; special), those seeking *connection and social safety*, and those just trying to *cope*. These categories are still broad, of course, but by helping a client figure out which umbrella category most fit them, I found that our work together was significantly expedited. Instead of spending months trying to figure out where to even get started, we could more quickly and easily identify what kind of healing work had the best chance of helping them and then just dive right into the deep end. A person whose body image issues exist in the hopes of attracting a potential partner, for example, might have absolutely *nothing* in common with a person whose body image issues exist to help them cope with a deep fear of abandonment, so even if both people end up hating their thighs, the solution to their underlying problems would look completely different.

By introducing these four categories, I could help my clients more easily identify their subconscious body image "purpose," i.e., how their body image issues had been attempting to help them. This gave us all the information we needed, as you'll see later in the book, to create an individualized plan for *them*, to strip away the layers of moral judgment, false meaning, significance, and blame that had been blocking *their* ability to access body neutrality.

Presenting the four categories this way also made my clients immediately feel seen, which turned out to be extraordinarily healing and helpful. So many people struggle with body image issues in isolation, feeling misunderstood by the people around them and wondering why they're so weird and broken. Learning about these patterns helped them see how normal, common, and valid their experiences are; that they're not alone, and they're not weird—in fact, quite the opposite! This immediately started to strip away layers of shame for some folks, and allowed them to take their first step toward self-acceptance and self-compassion.

For others, learning about these patterns gave them *hope*, because it meant maybe they weren't too broken to heal after all, and that maybe their experience wasn't actually "the exception." This hope that things could get better for them (something so many people sadly don't have, when it comes to body image issues) seemed to fuel their journey from then on, motivating them and helping them persevere through the scary, difficult, and painful parts so they could get to the other side.

Eventually, I found myself thinking in terms of these four categories when I met with new clients, asking questions to figure out which were driving their body image issues, and then shocking them by making a few educated guesses about who they are, how they experience life, and what they struggle with. Once, on a Zoom call with a potential client, I had been talking to a woman for only about five minutes when I accurately guessed a few very specific details about her sex and dating life. She got so flustered about how I could know something like that that we had to spend the next five minutes backtracking so I could share how I made those leaps and convince her that no, really, I didn't have any inside information.

This is how the four body image avatars emerged. Through years and years of experience talking to people about their body image issues, and paying attention to the patterns, I saw that the root causes generally fell into four categories. Then, to make the four categories easier for people to connect with and understand, I fleshed each one out to create a sort of symbolic representation of each category, which is what I call the **avatar**. I wanted to organize the patterns into a system that could help people more quickly and easily understand their suffering, recognize that they're not alone, and start figuring out the unique and specific reason why their body image issues exist.

This specific reason why a person's body image issues exist is something I call their **hidden body image purpose**, and every single person suffering from body image issues has at least one hidden body image purpose lurking below the surface and fueling their suffering. A person's hidden body image purpose is basically a summary of which problems their body image issues are trying to help them solve, what need or desire they're trying to meet, or what they're trying to help protect the person from. And while each person's hidden body image purpose will be as personal and unique as they themselves are, each of the four body image avatars represents a distinct way in which a person's body image issues tend to function, operate, or try to help them. Each avatar expresses a broad category of characteristics of, and probabilities about, the root cause and purpose of their body image suffering. This allows people to locate themselves quickly and easily so they can cut through all the confusion, and more effectively and expeditiously start digging into their own story, to discover their own specific hidden body image purpose. By learning about the four body image avatars, then, a person can immediately feel less alone, access a sense of hope, and (most important) start to gain the insight they need about *why* their body image issues exist so they can begin the process of letting them go.

Before I introduce the four avatars, I ask that you try not to take the descriptions of each too literally, or worry that you're not a perfect match for any of them. Of course you won't be a perfect match for any of them, you're a three-dimensional human, full of nuance, complexity, and individual lived experiences! Each avatar is just a two-dimensional stand-in: a personified depiction of an underlying pattern. Like personality quizzes, or astrology, the avatars are just a set of containers; *nobody* will fit into them perfectly, and they're not supposed to. But if you use them as a jumping-off point for understanding your own hidden purpose, the body image avatars can offer you a powerful source of insight and information about the path that will best help *you* overcome your body image suffering.

With all that in mind, allow me to introduce the four body image avatars!

THE SELF-OBJECTIFIER

The self-objectifier is the body image avatar who is focused on looking attractive as a way of motivating other people to meet their needs. They see their appearance as deeply connected to their identity and worth, they tend to spend a lot of time imagining themselves from a third-party perspective in their minds (often a version of the "male gaze" that reduces them to the status of a sexual object), or feel like they need *everyone* to find them attractive. Often focused on conforming to conventional beauty ideals, sometimes the self-objectifier's hidden purpose is to earn or secure something in the realm of sex, intimacy, and partnership, but other times they see attractiveness as the key to something else entirely, like power, status, or money.

THE HIGH ACHIEVER

The high achiever is the body image avatar focused on getting what they want and need by "proving their worth," which is to say they try to rack up socially sanctioned accomplishments, achievements, and accolades to make people see how good and impressive they are, in the hopes of finally feeling good enough. To the high achiever, the body is just a place to demonstrate the excellent quality of their character, climb the social ladder, and give themselves a feeling of being special, different, or better than other people. They need to be perfect all the time, hate making mistakes or being bad at things, feel guilty a lot, and revere discipline, hard work, and self-control. For all of these reasons (and more), the feeling of superiority, righteousness, structure, organization, and sense of purpose provided by controlling one's body is incredibly appealing to the high achiever.

THE OUTSIDER

The outsider is the body image avatar focused on fitting in, being accepted, and avoiding rejection and humiliation. They tend to be people pleasers who focus so much on other people's needs, desires, thoughts, and feelings that they don't make any space for their own, and struggle to express their authentic selves because they worry so much about what other people think and feel about them. Terrified of being judged, some outsiders believe looking a certain way will earn them the feeling of belonging, acceptance, and connection they crave, while others believe looking a certain way will protect them from the rejection, abandonment, and humiliation they live in fear of.

THE RUNNER

The runner is the body image avatar focused on surviving. Their hidden body image purpose is often to help them cope with, avoid, or stay distracted from pain, and they are primarily focused on protecting themselves and feeling safe. They tend to be drawn to *control* (over their bodies and other areas) in the hopes that it will keep them safe, and they struggle with vulnerability and intimacy. They're often disconnected from their bodies and emotions, they struggle with self-sabotaging behaviors, and they engage in many different forms of numbing, not just ones related to body image. This is because the runner is always running from, hiding from, or coping with something—and more often than not, that *something* lives deep down inside them.

We'll be going into much more depth about each avatar later, so for now just think of the body image avatars as a place to start organizing your understanding of your body image issues. Each individual's journey will be unique, but placing yourself within the landscape of the avatars will offer you two important bits of insight right away. The first one is how multifaceted and complex your body image issues are, which will help you create a realistic view of how long this journey might take, and the second one is where to start digging.

Each of the four body image avatars represents a distinct reason for body image issues to exist, a person's primary motivation for being so attached to their body or appearance. So more than one avatar might resonate with a person (in fact, individual qualities and aspects of all four resonate with most people!), but when it comes right down to it, there is usually only one or two that best fit them. That said, some people will find all four strongly resonate with them because their body image issues actually have *four separate reasons* for existing, and the person has *four separate motivations* for being so attached to their body or appearance.

In such cases, I encourage people to set realistic expectations for themselves about how long this journey will take, how much work it will require, and what kind of outcome to expect. The work will be the same whether one body image avatar or four resonate with you, but the increased complexity has to be taken into account. If your body image issues exist to solve four huge problems, for example, you might be looking at a journey that's four times longer and harder than someone whose body image issues exist only to solve one huge problem. Each avatar is likely to require a big chunk of dedicated time, and heaps of practice, patience, courage, and processing to overcome—so it wouldn't be reasonable for a person in that situation to expect to feel neutrally about their bodies in, say, six to twelve months. The more reasons a person's body image issues exist, the longer they've existed, and the deeper they go, the more time and energy the body neutrality journey will take.

I say all this because it's very trendy to present self-development work with ridiculously exaggerated timelines, and I don't want anyone thinking they're just a few months away from body neutrality when it actually might be more like a few years. Placing yourself on the body image avatar map should give you an idea of how complex your body image issues are, and how time-consuming and complex your body neutrality journey is likely to be, so that you can set realistic expectations.

In the next chapter you'll be given a self-assessment—a multiple-choice quiz—to help you discover which of the four body image avatars resonates most strongly with you. Then, in the chapters following the self-assessment, you'll be taken on a deep dive into each individual body image avatar, including some common characteristics, struggles, and patterns for each, so that you can deepen your understanding of where you fit in the avatar landscape.

As you move through the rest of this book, remember that the body image avatars are a tool for understanding yourself, not a tool to pathologize, pigeonhole, or judge yourself—and they're *definitely* not a tool to replace your inner wisdom. You are the ultimate expert on yourself, not me, and this system is designed to guide you back to that wisdom, not to take its place. So be careful about letting the avatars become another box, hindrance, or limitation. If at any point the avatars feel more oppressive than liberating, the system may have crossed over from tool to dogma, which is the exact opposite of its intent.

To that end, I need to include a standard disclaimer here too. This book is intended for informational use only, in service of your personal growth and self-development. It should not be used to diagnose, or as a substitute for evaluation or treatment by a trained and licensed medical or mental health-care provider. And if the work outlined in this book becomes too triggering, upsetting, scary, or painful for you to do alone, please stop doing it immediately, and seek out the support of a qualified medical or mental health professional.

Lastly, try not to get too hung up on whether every specific detail, quality, characteristic, or experience of an avatar perfectly fits you. Take the quiz and read the chapters describing each one, but then look inward to see what feels right and true for you as you read through the rest of the book. Remember that *you* are the expert on you; take what applies to you, and let go of the rest!

CHAPTER 7

The Self-Assessment

NSWER THE QUESTIONS IN THE ASSESS-ment as truthfully as you can, choosing the answers that resonate with you most.

You can circle as many of the answers as apply to you for each question—that means you might be circling two, three, or even all four answers at times! That's okay. If you're not sure, go with the answer that feels the closest to your experience, and if absolutely *none* of the answers resonate with you, just leave it blank.

At the end, simply tally up how many of each letter you circled. Your "score" will indicate which body image avatar or avatars are likely to be dominant, based on which has the highest number. The key at the end will help you decipher which letter corresponds to which avatar.

For example, let's say you tally up your score and it looks like this:

A: 7

B: 19

C: 3

D: 16

That would mean that your dominant body image avatars are the ones that correspond to B and D, with B being your primary avatar and

D being your secondary avatar. And while you might learn a lot by perusing the material for the avatar that corresponds with A (or even C!), you will likely find that you connect most with the characteristics, struggles, fears, and common paths to healing laid out for B and D.

Be brave, and push yourself to be totally honest in your answers. This assessment is about how you show up in the world now, as opposed to the way you used to show up, wish you showed up, try to show up, or want other people to *think* you show up.

THE AVATARS SELF-ASSESSMENT

1. When you're getting ready to go somewhere, you're mostly thinking about:

    A. Looking attractive.

    B. Looking impressive, or like you have your shit together.

    C. Being accepted, or not being judged.

    D. Steeling yourself for whatever happens.

2. When you see parts of your body you perceive as "flaws," you mostly feel:

    A. Disgust

    B. Shame

    C. Anxiety

    D. Hate

3. When you think about your "perfect body," it's mostly focused on:

    A. Wanting to meet conventional beauty and body ideals.

    B. Wanting people to know you're special and "good," just by looking at you.

    C. Making people like you, or avoiding judgment.

    D. Whatever it would take to feel like you can finally relax.

4. One of your biggest body image fears is:

    A. Someone thinking you're ugly or gross.

    B. Someone thinking you're lazy or out of control.

    C. Being humiliated, because people were making fun of your appearance behind your back.

    D. That if you let your guard down for even one second, your body will betray you or put you in harm's way.

5. Something you spend a lot of time craving or wishing for is:

A. Attention, intimacy, or power.

B. People's respect or admiration.

C. Belonging, community, or nourishing friendships.

D. A feeling that you can trust yourself, your body, or other people.

6. You most closely identify as striving to be:

A. Hot, sexy, or desirable.

B. Good, special, or exceptional.

C. Normal, likable, or acceptable.

D. Logical, independent, or in control.

7. During sex you are often:

A. Focused on your partner's experience and pleasure, how your body looks to them, and what they might be wanting, thinking, or feeling.

B. Focused on your own body shape or size, and worried that your partner will see something "unflattering" and think less of you.

C. The giver of pleasure, but rarely the receiver.

D. Pretty numb and disconnected.

8. You often find yourself thinking:

A. That in order to find a partner (or keep your partner interested and loyal), you have to maintain a high aesthetic standard.

B. That it's important to excel at something, to be in the top percentile of things, or to be better than "average."

C. That other people are judging you, mad at you, or disappointed in you.

D. That your needs or emotions are embarrassing, shameful, bad, or dangerous.

9. Deep down you really believe:

A. That being attractive gives a person a sort of "free pass" through life—that when you look good enough, people are motivated to just give you what you want and need.

B. That there is a sort of organized justice to the universe—that if you do things right and are good, you'll be rewarded, and if you don't do them right or are bad, you'll be punished.

C. Something about you is different, bad, or broken—and if you want to be accepted or loved, you have to hide that part of yourself from people.

D. The world is a scary place, and you can't trust anyone—it's every person for themselves, and you have to protect yourself, because no one else will.

10. In your ultimate body image fantasy, you imagine:

A. That if you looked good enough, you'd never again feel lonely, jealous, insecure, anxious, needy, or vulnerable. You'd have a great partner who would worship you, and you'd always feel beautiful, appreciated, and loved.

B. That if you were thin, lean, or fit enough, nobody would ever be able to question your discipline, self-control, or willpower. Everyone would admire you and wish they could be like you, and you would feel special and worthy.

C. That achieving the body you want would make you feel socially confident and secure, and you'd never worry about being judged, rejected, or excluded again. Everyone would like you, and you'd be able to easily make friends and freely express yourself without worry.

D. That if you finally got your body under control, you'd feel safe. You would feel less vulnerable and more capable of handling pain, but life would also feel a lot easier, and you wouldn't feel as anxious or afraid all the time.

11. Other people would describe you as:

A. Caring a lot about how you look, or someone who loves attention.

B. Goal oriented, disciplined, hardworking, or perfectionist.

C. Conflict avoidant or a people pleaser.

D. Guarded, or fiercely independent.

12. If someone were to say something negative about you, they might say you come off as:

A. Vain, self-absorbed, "slutty," or manipulative.

B. Snooty, boring, overly rigid, or a buzzkill.

C. Fake, weird, anxious, or socially awkward.

D. Cold, awkward, mean, or bitchy.

13. You worry a lot about:

A. Someone feeling disgusted by you.

B. Other people thinking you've "let yourself go."

C. People secretly judging you.

D. Being self-destructive or self-sabotaging.

14. You feel most insecure about body and appearance:

A. In a context around sex, dating, or partnership.

B. When you're surrounded by other people who are higher in status, or excel at body control.

C. All the time.

D. When you feel vulnerable or sad.

15. You've spent a lot of your free time learning to perfect:

A. Your appearance, via makeup, hair, fitness, skin care, or other beauty work.

B. How to eat and exercise to get results (at least in the short term).

C. Your ability to pick up on what other people are thinking and feeling.

D. Your ability to disconnect from, numb, or suppress your emotions.

16. Sometimes you wonder why you:

    A. Care so much what men (or potential romantic or sexual partners) think, want, and like.

    B. Can never seem to relax or let things go.

    C. Struggle with boundaries and self-advocacy.

    D. Often can't stop scrolling, eating, drinking, shopping, procrastinating, or numbing out with Netflix.

17. You tend to compare yourself with others in order to:

    A. Determine which one of you is better looking.

    B. Determine which one of you is thinner or leaner, or more impressive.

    C. See whether or not you'll "fit in" with them.

    D. Be prepared for whatever worst-case scenario you're most worried about.

18. You're sometimes very afraid that:

    A. You're too much (too emotional, too sensitive, too sad, too opinionated, too needy, too overwhelming, etc.).

    B. You don't have anything else special or valuable to offer the world outside of diet, fitness, and controlling your physique. If you gave that up, you'd be doomed to a life of mediocrity.

    C. There's something wrong with you deep down, something that makes you fundamentally unworthy of love and belonging.

    D. You'll let someone in, only to have your heart completely broken, and you won't be able to survive it.

19. You feel most jealous of:

    A. Conventionally attractive folks: the bombshells and hotties you think everyone wants to be with, people who you think compete with you in your "category" of attractiveness.

B. People who have accomplished things that are objectively *impressive*; who demonstrate extraordinary discipline and self-control; and whom people admire, gush about, and see as high status.

C. People who seem to be effortlessly and authentically *themselves*, oozing confidence, expressing their weirdness, taking up space, and connecting with people easily wherever they go; those rare compelling, magnetic souls whom everyone immediately wants to get to know.

D. People who seem to have an easy, comfortable, connected relationship to their bodies; the ones who talk about "listening to their bodies" as if it's easy, who seem to effortlessly identify and express their emotions, and who can eat a bowl of ice cream without even giving a second thought to the rest of the pint.

20. **When you walk into a party or event, you're mostly focused on:**

   A. Imagining who might be checking you out, and hoping that they like what they see.

   B. Scanning the crowd for your competition—who is a threat to your social niche or status here?

   C. Imagining how other people might be judging or criticizing you.

   D. Judging, criticizing, or nitpicking the people, or the details of the event.

KEY FOR SCORING:

A: Self-Objectifier

B: High Achiever

C: Outsider

D: Runner

Once you've taken the quiz and gotten your score, move on to the next chapters to learn more about each body image avatar! If you prefer, you can skip directly to the avatar or avatars you scored highest on, but I recommend reading through all of them. Most of my clients report learning valuable insights from *all* the avatars, including the ones they scored low on, or not at all. After reading through all four, you might even make a new connection or gain a new insight into yourself that makes you adjust your understanding of your primary avatar!

Reading them all can also help you understand where you came from (or where you might go in the future!). For example, many of my clients report things like "I'm definitely a self-objectifier *now*, but I used to be a high achiever, too, before I got into therapy" or "I think I'm an outsider with my family, but a self-objectifier everywhere else." One person can move between avatars over time, or in different contexts, because body image issues can step in to "solve" different problems for them. So it can be helpful to know about them all.

Learning about all the different avatars can also help you identify and understand other people who might be struggling with body image issues, whose experiences are completely different from your own. One of my clients identified strongly as a runner, so she almost didn't even read the self-objectifier or outsider parts. When I encouraged her to anyway, she realized that her husband was a self-objectifier, and her teenage daughter was an outsider, and she would have never been able to understand or support them properly without that insight.

Reading about all four avatars will give you the fullest possible picture, and I encourage you to do so. After all, the better we each truly understand the various reasons and patterns that lead to body image suffering, the better we can heal ourselves, support each other, avoid causing harm, and move toward building a culture where body neutrality is the default.

CHAPTER **8**

The Self-Objectifier

HE SELF-OBJECTIFIER PLACES AN INAP-
propriate amount of importance on attractiveness, and
believes attractiveness (or sexual desirability) is the key
to having value, being worthy as a person, or motivating
other people to give them what they want and need.

PATTERNS OFTEN SEEN AMONG SELF-OBJECTIFIERS:

- They have a history of being sexualized, objectified, or fetishized (for any reason), or a history of sexual abuse, sexual
assault, sexual trauma, sexual harassment, rape, or other unwanted sexual attention.

- The way they've been treated at times has taught them that
people don't see or respect them as fully autonomous humans,
but rather as sexual objects, sources of labor, or a resource to
be exploited, consumed, and enjoyed. (And they often come to
see themselves that way too.)

- They measure their own value, power, or safety by how attractive other people find them, or how desirable they are to others.

- They care a lot about meeting conventional beauty and body ideals, so they engage in a variety of beauty work behaviors (i.e., exercise, diet, makeup, skin care, hair care, clothing, injections, surgery, and so on) to get closer to them.

- On some level, they believe their job on earth is to give other people a pleasant or pleasurable experience.

- They frequently develop body dysmorphia: by constantly zooming in on certain body parts and assigning them huge mental and emotional significance—to the extent that they ultimately see a distorted and unrealistic version of their bodies in the mirror, like a fun house image—they become preoccupied with "flaws" that are tiny, insignificant, or even invisible to others.

- They tend to feel a lot of body anxiety, which leads them to constantly check on, monitor, worry about, or try to change their appearance throughout the day.

- On a bad body image day, they will often say they "feel disgusting" or "feel gross."

- They often imagine themselves through other people's eyes, and imagine what other people's experience of them might be.

- They tend to feel like they "owe" other people (usually men) sexual arousal, pleasure, and gratification—but consider their *own* arousal, pleasure, and gratification to be optional, secondary, or even off-limits.

- They tend to report feeling like "too much" for other people: too emotional, too needy, too complicated, etc.

- Though many are women or femmes who see themselves through the male gaze and are focused on being attractive to men, they may be any gender, any sexuality, and focused on being attractive to anyone.[1]

While these are common characteristics of the self-objectifier, don't forget that each individual will have their own experience. Even if most of the points in the list above (or even any of them!) don't resonate with you, you could still be a self-objectifier, because the unifying factor for each body image avatar is the hidden body image purpose.

THE SELF-OBJECTIFIER'S HIDDEN BODY IMAGE PURPOSE

The self-objectifier's hidden body image purpose is to be attractive or desirable enough that they have value, and that other people are *automatically motivated to offer them what they want and need.* The specifics of what an individual is wanting or needing (aka what they're seeking through attractiveness) can vary dramatically from person to person, but all self-objectifiers believe on some level that attractiveness and desirability are the key to getting it, and that unless they are attractive and desirable enough, they will have to go without.

Wanting to be attractive or desirable is commonly associated with a person seeking out sex, intimacy, romance, or partnership, and sometimes that's true for the self-objectifier too. Some self-objectifiers want to be attractive enough to get (or keep) the kind of sex, romance, or relationship they desire, and feel insecure about anything they imagine could threaten their ability to do so. People who have been encouraged to think of themselves through the perspective of a potential sexual or romantic partner often end up developing a self-objectifying mindset, taking offhand statements like "men don't like body hair," "women don't like skinny guys," or "nobody will date you unless you ___," to be mandatory prerequisites for getting what they want, or veiled threats that they'll end up alone if they don't make themselves attractive enough.

In this way, many people become self-objectifiers because they've learned that their worth or value as a person is directly linked to their attractiveness, or that they have to achieve or maintain a certain aesthetic standard in order to have sex, access intimacy, land a partner, or keep a partner interested. This kind of conditioning leads to a very high importance placed on a person's appearance, and a lot of meaning and significance attached to their bodies, which immediately clouds body neutrality and can easily turn into body anxiety, a hyper-fixation on appearance, body dysphoria, disordered eating, and an obsession with achieving or maintaining a certain aesthetic. After all, how could a person ever feel neutral about a body that they believe to be their only pathway to sex, intimacy, or partnership, or that they believe could block or threaten their access to those things?

That said, not all people wanting to capture the eye of a potential lover are self-objectifiers. A man showing his abs on Grindr or Tinder may be doing a little casual self-objectification in the hopes of catching the attention of his desired sexual or romantic partner, but if he doesn't experience any body image *distress*, then he's not really a self-objectifier. A man who struggles with chronic shame and insecurity about his belly, however, because he believes defined abs are critical for getting laid or being considered a worthy partner, may indeed be a self-objectifier.

Also, while some self-objectifiers are focused on looking good enough to get what they crave in terms of sex and intimacy, many are seeking something else entirely. I've known self-objectifiers who, consciously or subconsciously, viewed attractiveness as their main (or only) path to motivate people to meet their needs for attention, respect, kindness, connection, safety, money, power, or even opportunities. Sometimes they were even right! Thanks to growing up in a white supremacist, ableist, fatphobic patriarchy, many self-objectifiers have learned that their full humanity is either invisible or undesirable, and that their *only* source of value comes from their ability to give other people visual or sexual pleasure and gratification.

Lindsay Kite and Lexie Kite explain how this gets internalized in their book *More Than a Body*:

> When we are self-objectifying, our identities are split in two: the one living her life and the one watching and judging her. We become our very own self-conscious identical twin, an onlooker to ourselves, monitoring how we look rather than how we are feeling or what we are doing. We live, and we imagine how we look as we live, adjusting and contorting ourselves accordingly. We watch from afar as our bodies become our primary means of identity and value. Our feelings about and perceptions of our bodies—our body image—become warped into our feelings about how we appear to ourselves and others. We learn that the most important thing about women is their bodies, and the most important thing about women's bodies is how they look.[2]

This is especially true for women, of course, but anyone can become a self-objectifier in this way, shifting from thinking about themselves through their own eyes to assessing how they look to others, and tying their very sense of identity and worth to that assessment. Many self-objectifiers even come to feel like they owe it to other people to be attractive because they think of themselves as existing for this purpose, and this purpose only: to be a source of pleasure for other people to enjoy and consume. With this purpose so entwined with their sense of identity and self-worth, there is a lot of pressure on the self-objectifier to fulfill their assigned role and be adequately attractive, or else see themselves as a completely worthless failure of a person. And this isn't some defect in the self-objectifier's mind, it's the natural result of growing up in a culture that regularly dehumanizes, objectifies, and exploits people based on what kind of body they have. When a person is consistently treated like a sexual object for other people to enjoy, or a resource for other people to consume, it's natural for them to assume that their value comes exclusively from their ability to provide pleasure, labor, or gratification to others.[3]

And when a person's identity and value is consistently coupled with and dependent on their appearance, it's natural for them to assume that they themselves must not have any inherent worth.

Because of this conditioning, the self-objectifier's sense of self, and confidence as a person, tends to go through rapidly cycling highs and lows based on their appearance: on a day they feel good about how they look, they're likely to feel good about themselves as a person, and on a day they feel bad about how they look, they're likely to feel worthless and struggle with a lot of shame and self-loathing. And because they're focused on being attractive to others, how they feel about their own appearance tends to be heavily informed by how other people respond to them. Getting a lot of positive attention, praise, validation, or compliments on their appearance can make them feel incredibly "confident," while criticism or insults about their appearance (or even just a lack of attention and validation) can quickly make them feel like garbage about themselves again.

While the self-objectifier tends to see attractiveness as the key to getting what they want and need, they're just as likely to be focused on using their appearance to avoid or protect themselves from something as they are to gain or earn something. In my own personal body image journey for example, I identified most strongly with two body image avatars: the self-objectifier and the runner. So at first, I thought being attractive was the key to getting what I wanted in life: men's attention, approval, care, kindness, respect, and love. But as I learned more about myself through the body neutrality process, it became clear that I had also been using attractiveness to avoid the things I was afraid of: men's rejection, indifference, abandonment, cruelty, and even violence. On a subconscious level, I believed I could avoid the apathy, anger, and brutality of entitled men who dehumanize and objectify women by meeting conventional beauty ideals and giving them what they wanted. My body image issues existed, therefore, both to help me "earn" the attention, care, and love I craved, and also to keep men from feeling disappointed, getting angry, and wanting to hurt me.

There are plenty of things a self-objectifier might be wanting to avoid, from uncomfortable feelings (like rejection, heartbreak, or grief) to painful experiences like being cheated on, abandoned, or attacked. Sometimes they're trying to "skip" doing or learning hard or scary things, like being vulnerable, advocating for themselves, building a career, setting boundaries, working hard, communicating, or figuring out who they are. And they may just imagine that being attractive enough means they get to bypass all the hard work, and gives them a free pass to an easy life, which is what their body image issues are trying to secure for them.

No matter what specific and unique hidden body image purpose a self-objectifier has, they believe that being attractive and desirable is the way to get there, which places an extraordinary amount of pressure and significance on their body and appearance. The self-objectifier isn't usually consciously aware that this is happening, though, or that their desire to be hot has any deeper meaning at all. They often have no idea that they're trying to earn or avoid anything, that their full humanity has been stripped away, or even that they measure their value by their ability to give other people pleasure and gratification. All they know is that they want to look as attractive as possible, and that they feel extremely upset when they don't.

A SELF-OBJECTIFIER CASE STUDY: MARIE

Marie was a married woman in her late thirties who started coaching with me in the hopes that she might finally stop hating her body and feel more confident. She spent a lot of time picking her body apart in the mirror, berating herself for "letting herself go," feeling "disgusting," shopping online for clothes to feel sexier, and going on and off diets to try to lose weight.

Marie told me she had been the ugly duckling of her family, never quite delicate or cute enough to catch the attention of the boys who *drooled* over her thinner, prettier sisters. When she met her now husband, she had only ever been with one other person sexually, and considered herself unbelievably lucky that this wonderful, handsome man wanted to marry her. Marie had always struggled to feel confident in her body, imagining that her husband would be happier if she were thinner or prettier, feeling jealous of more conventionally attractive women she imagined he'd prefer to be with, and imagining he was bothered by her physical flaws. When these thoughts and feelings came up, though, she could always kind of ease them by reminding herself how undeniably *into* Marie (and Marie's body) her husband was.

Since the beginning of their relationship, Marie's sex life with her husband had been abundant and enthusiastic. He expressed effusive desire and appreciation for her body, and backed it up with hard erections and eagerness for sex so that even though she sometimes felt insecure about her body, she always felt secure about her *marriage.*

Since Marie had gotten pregnant and given birth to their son, however, things were different. She had gained weight, her skin was sagging, and now her husband rarely complimented her body or initiated sex anymore. Plus, when they *did* have sex, he sometimes couldn't keep his erection the whole time.

When Marie told me all this, she said it with absolute certainty that her husband no longer found her attractive, because she was fat and disgusting now. When I asked if her husband had ever actually indicated that he found her less attractive now, she responded, "No, of course not, he would never say that. He says I'm beautiful, but I clearly just don't turn him on anymore."

I asked Marie how she came to believe it was the changes to her appearance that were at the root of the changes to her marriage, and she said it was just obvious. She had gotten fat and ugly, so he had stopped wanting her, end of story. After a lifetime of thinking *all* men preferred a different kind of woman, a thinner and prettier kind of woman, she had finally proven it. There was no other possibility, so every day when

Marie looked in the mirror and saw her sagging breasts, stretch marks, and fat rolls, she saw the end of her marriage. It was only a matter of time, Marie was sure, before her husband left her for someone younger, thinner, and better looking.

Can you see how Marie was objectifying herself, essentially boiling down her worth and value to her ability to arouse and sexually gratify her husband? Because of the messages she had learned growing up, she had come to believe that men's loyalty and commitment are based on their sexual desire and satisfaction, and that finding her sexy was the main reason her husband had fallen in love with her, and therefore the only reason he would stick around. She had been objectifying herself and worrying about her appearance for a long time, but her negative thoughts and feelings were always alleviated by her husband's obvious desire for her. When his desire for her seemed to lessen, her body image suffering was suddenly standing front and center, and her body anxiety, hatred, insecurity, and resentment exploded.

Marie's body image issues made sense, given her situation, beliefs, and worldview. She had subconsciously assigned her body the job of keeping her husband happy and loyal, and then measured her relationship's safety and her own worth by how often and how eagerly he expressed desire for sex. She viewed her body as a threat to his desire, and therefore to her marriage; her hidden body image purpose was to keep her husband from abandoning her. I would hate my body, too, if I thought it was going to make someone abandon me!

During our work together, Marie decided to finally try asking her husband about their sex life, and she was shocked by his answer. As it turned out, Marie had been completely wrong about what was going on . . . but her lifelong habit of self-objectification had led to a whole bunch of false assumptions that not only made her hate her body, but also kept her from talking to her partner about it.

Marie's husband had had no idea she was feeling that way, and he couldn't even fathom her theory that he wanted her less because her body looked different. He explained that he still desired her just as much as before, but that he hadn't gotten the impression she was ready or interested in sex yet.

Apparently, Marie's pregnancy had been physically and emotionally difficult, with various medical issues and several months of her on bedrest. Then the birth itself had been very scary, ending in an emergency C-section, and during the newborn stage, Marie struggled with postpartum depression. It had been nearly two years since their son was born, and Marie had been stable for a while, but the experience had been incredibly stressful and difficult. Her husband had seen how much pain she had been in, both physically and emotionally, for a long time, and had just been trying to give her the space she needed to heal and recover. He was amazed by how strong she had been, and said he felt more in love with her than ever before as they raised this incredible little being together, but he was still very anxious about her well-being. The *last* thing he wanted was for her to feel any pressure from him about sex until she was ready.

Marie's husband said he had just hoped and assumed that *she* would start initiating regular sex again when she was ready and interested. In the meantime, however, he sometimes got so anxious about accidentally hurting her that when they did have sex, he ended up totally in his head, and lost his erection. Marie's husband even showed her his browser history, where he had been masturbating most nights to porn featuring women whose bodies looked a lot like hers. He wanted her to understand that he wasn't interested in thin young supermodels—he watched videos featuring full-figured women in their thirties or forties, whose bodies jiggled and sagged, and had a real, lived-in look, because they reminded him of Marie, and it was Marie whom he desired.

While this insight was eye-opening and healing for Marie, she still had to do a significant amount of work to uproot and release the many false beliefs that had led her to draw such false conclusions in the first place. This included a lot of the beliefs underlying her lifelong habit of self-objectification, like:

- Men are superficial and only want sex, not a deep emotional connection or a partner they respect as an equal.

- All men would prefer to be with women more conventionally attractive than their wives, if they could.

- Men are naturally cheaters and liars, so it's a woman's job to "keep him interested" so he doesn't stray.

- A woman's value is based on her appearance, and she doesn't have anything else to "keep a man interested" if she loses those looks.

- A woman is responsible for her husband's sexual desire, pleasure, and satisfaction.

- A good sex life is one that never needs to be talked about, because it's just effortless.

Over time, as Marie challenged these beliefs, exposed herself to new perspectives, and engaged in a sort of "reeducation" on these topics, she started showing up differently both in her marriage and in her life. She started having more transparent conversations with her husband, which led to better understanding and more intimacy and connection between them, as well as much more sex. She also started to build a more three-dimensional sense of her own identity and self-worth outside of her appearance—and even outside of her marriage—which made her feel more secure, less anxious, and more confident overall.

COMMON CHARACTERISTICS AND EXPERIENCES OF THE SELF-OBJECTIFIER

Now that you understand how the self-objectifier's body image issues tend to show up and why, let's take a look at a few experiences and characteristics that many self-objectifiers share. (Just remember: these are *patterns*, not *requirements*. You can still be a self-objectifier without having any of these experiences or characteristics.)

Spectatoring, Body Checking, and Hypervigilance

Before sharing their body image struggles, self-objectifiers will often say things like "I don't know why I even care so much about this stuff" or "I know nobody else cares, but . . ." or "I know I'm being ridiculous, but . . ." They often report feeling stupid, silly, or embarrassed about how much time, money, and energy they actually spend managing, working on, picking apart, or trying to change their appearance, because they recognize that not everyone seems to be playing by the same rules they are, and they don't know why they care so much. But self-objectifiers don't just wake up one day and *decide* to measure their worth by their attractiveness. Typically, they have a history of being objectified, sexualized, or fetishized by others (or by seeing things like that happen to people like them) first.[4]

Maybe a self-objectifier had their appearance scrutinized, assessed, or commented on throughout their entire lives without their permission, for example. Maybe they've been regularly treated as less than fully human, or they've discovered that other people seem to see and value them *only* as a source of labor or pleasure, to consume or exploit. And maybe, given the world they live in, they've discovered that leaning into, encouraging, or participating in their own objectification is just easier, and gets them further, than trying to fight or reject it.

This is usually happening below the level of consciousness, though, so a lot of self-objectifiers are completely unaware of what they're doing, and live with a frustrating amount of conflict between what they consciously think and how they actually feel and behave.

One of the most common behaviors displayed by the self-objectifier is called "body checking," in which they compulsively seek out information about their body or appearance in the hopes that this information will reassure them and reduce their body anxiety.[5] Body checking

behaviors include picking oneself apart in the mirror; grabbing, pinching, or squeezing certain body parts over and over; weighing or measuring one's body regularly; or frequently trying on a specific item of
clothing to see how it fits. In my personal trainer days, for example, I
used to examine my abs in the mirror every single morning, to see if
they were more or less defined than the day before, and I kept one pair
of my smallest-size jeans to try on every once in a while, even though
they weren't comfortable and I never wore them out, just to see if they
still fit.

Obviously, there's nothing *innately* wrong with wanting to know
how you look. You might check your teeth in the mirror after eating a
spinach salad, or want to see how your hair looks after getting caught in
a sudden downpour without an umbrella, and those behaviors are unlikely to cause you much distress. But the kind of body checking seen
among self-objectifiers tends to be far more frequent, intense, urgent,
and born out of the constant anxiety they feel about how they look.
One client sheepishly told me that since working from home, he probably stepped on the scale to see how much he weighed twenty or thirty
times a day. It's not that he actually thought his weight was likely to
have changed much in the forty-five minutes since he last weighed
himself, but he *did* find himself feeling anxious and having the irre-
sistible urge to check again, just to be sure. Another client told me that
she checked her appearance in her phone camera or bathroom mirror
every half hour or so (if not more), all day every day. She described the
habit as a response to the anxiety that would build up about how she
looked since the last time she checked, until she eventually gave in and
checked once more, reassured herself that she looked fine, and started
the cycle over again. (Note that body-checking behaviors like these are
sometimes caused by or related to mental disorders like obsessive compulsive disorder or eating disorders, so be sure to consult a medical or
mental health professional if these behaviors interfere with your daily
functioning.)

These kinds of body-checking habits might seem bizarre to someone who hasn't experienced them, but the self-objectifier believes their value, worth, and ability to get their needs met are based on their attractiveness and ability to give other people a positive experience, so it actually makes a lot of sense. It's a safety check, a ritual to reassure and calm themselves, and a preventive measure to stay aware of any issues that might pose a threat. *How do I look? Am I okay? Do I still have worth? Is there anything I should be worried about?* But the temporary relief a person feels by seeking out this information doesn't last very long, so they have to seek it out again soon after.

Another habit seen among many self-objectifiers is called spectatoring, which is a term coined by William Masters and Virginia Johnson in 1970 to describe how some people focus on themselves from a third-person perspective (as though through the eyes of a spectator) during sex, instead of focusing on their own feelings and experience.[6] Emily Nagoski, sex educator and author of the book *Come As You Are*, puts it this way:

> "Spectatoring" is the art of worrying about sex while you're having it. Rather than paying attention to the pleasant and tingly things your body is experiencing, it's like you're floating above the bed watching, noticing how your breasts fall or the squish of cottage cheese on the back of your thigh or the roll at your belly, or you're worried about the sex you're having instead of enjoying the sex you're having.[7]

While the term "spectatoring" was intended only to describe a person's experience during sex, I've found that many self-objectifiers do this *all the time.* They often imagine themselves through the perspective of someone who is looking at them, and consider how that person would think or feel about them, instead of thinking about how they themselves think or feel.

And while spectatoring has only been shown to have a negative impact on a person's sexual experience, the same seems to be true in every other area of life. Focusing on someone else's experience of you all the time means you never get to be fully and wholly present with your *own* experience. A friend of mine once said that at least 25 percent of her brain was constantly focused on how she would look to anyone who might be looking at her. This was true when she was working, when she was hanging out with friends, and even when she was home alone. She was *always* mentally scanning her body for any signs of ugliness, un-flattering angles, or potential turnoffs, even when nobody else was around. She just couldn't turn this part of her mind off.

Unfortunately, this is very common for self-objectifiers, and be-cause a person has only so much time and energy, every minute they spend connecting to someone else's experience of them is a minute spent disconnecting from their own experience. That's why the self-objectifier often struggles to know what they themselves think, feel, and want, or to connect to their own authentic self; their entire aware-ness of themselves comes through the imagined lens of someone else experiencing them. This leads to a variety of issues for the self-objectifier, who tends to have a hard time setting boundaries, saying no, and advo-cating for their own needs and desires. They're too used to thinking about what other people want from them to know what they themselves want, and their self-worth is too wrapped up in other people's approval to assert themselves.

What's interesting about the habit of spectatoring is that it can easily shift from an effort to look good into an effort to more broadly manage or manipulate other people's thoughts, feelings, and overall ex-perience. Constant spectatoring tends to get confused with empathy, emotional intelligence, or sensitivity in this way, because spending so much time thinking about the perspective of other people makes it easy for a person to believe they actually know what everyone else thinks, feels, likes, and wants. And because the self-objectifier often feels obli-gated to make other people feel good, they will often try to use this in-formation to do exactly that. Often disguised as an act of kindness or generosity, this kind of "for the greater good" manipulation tactic is just the self-objectifier's way of trying to secure their "value" in the other person's mind, and thereby ensure they'll get their needs met.

Because they see attractiveness as the key to motivating other people to give them what they want and need, the self-objectifier often ends up living in a state of nonstop hypervigilance around their appearance, anxiously checking how they look to themselves, and imagining how they look to others. They think about how they look, worry about how they look, and spend a lot of time and energy managing, safeguarding, and trying to look "better," by which I mean, trying to conform more closely to conventional beauty ideals. This will sometimes make the self-objectifier seem chronically anxious, preoccupied, and unable to relax, be present, or just be themselves. Sometimes it even looks to other people like vanity, self-absorption, narcissism, distraction, dissatisfaction, fakeness, or even disinterest, which makes people feel uneasy, and makes it difficult for them to connect with the self-objectifier.

This is the ironic and unfortunate side effect of the self-objectifier's obsession with how they look and attempts to be desirable: it often pushes people away, turns people off, and makes the self-objectifier less pleasant to be around in the long run.

They Struggle with Low Self-Worth

Amelia, a thirty-two-year-old doctor, is hilarious, kind, driven, involved in activism, and just an all-around impressive human. But because she *isn't* conventionally attractive (and doesn't have a partner), Amelia feels worthless, and like a total failure as a person. She learned from her family that women are supposed to be thin and hot so they can attract a great partner, get married, and have kids, so sometimes it feels like none of her accomplishments will "count" until she is also fulfilling those roles.

Becca, on the other hand, is a part-time dance teacher who, at twenty-four, has spent the majority of her adult life investing in—and succeeding at—the project of being "hot." She has put thousands of hours of learning and practice into her hair and makeup skills, is obsessed with beauty products and treatments of all kinds, spends most of her free time at the gym, and got a boob job when she was twenty-one. Becca's hotness is integral to her identity, and it makes her feel good to know men want her and women are envious of her. But because she's spent so much time, money, and energy on her appearance, Becca doesn't feel like she has anything to offer the world *other* than being hot and, deep down, also feels worthless.

I'm sharing these two client stories to illustrate the paradox facing the self-objectifier: whether or not they meet conventional beauty ideals, most self-objectifiers seem to have a very low sense of self-worth, because the game is rigged. When you're sexualized or objectified on a regular basis (or see other people you relate to being sexualized or objectified on a regular basis), you learn that *you*—the real, whole, three-dimensional person that you are on the inside—have no value whatsoever. When you learn that your value comes exclusively from your ability to look hot and give other people a pleasurable experience, you come to understand your worth not as intrinsic or innate, but as conditional, transactional, and ephemeral; something to be earned (or lost) moment to moment, based on what kind of experience you're giving someone else. If you fail to meet these ideals and be valued in this way, then you have to face the uncomfortable experience of simply not being valued. And if you "succeed" at being valued in this way, it's for something superficial, impersonal, and manufactured, so your deep human need to be seen, enjoyed, and valued for who you are still goes completely unmet.

It has to be said here that some conventionally attractive self-objectifiers report feeling "confident" because they get a lot of positive feedback for how they look, and that makes them feel good. But these are often the same people who live in constant fear of gaining weight, or losing their looks as they age, because they don't believe they have any intrinsic value *as people*. So even if they do feel (temporarily) good about themselves when they get compliments or attention for how they look, their sense of self-worth is conditional, transactional, and easily lost. That tends to make them incredibly insecure and anxious, because their worth is based on their desirability, and their desirability is based on how closely they conform to conventional beauty ideals, and that means that at best, their worth will slowly disappear as they age. This leads to a lot of supposedly "confident" people who stress and obsess over their appearance, meticulously monitoring and managing it, and living with the constant fear of "losing their looks."

Also, when a person believes their worth comes from looking hot and giving other people what they want, they automatically learn that they're not allowed to be a whole three-dimensional person with needs, desires, emotions, boundaries, or opinions of their own. A lot of women in particular have learned that the "ideal woman" in a man's eyes is one who meets his needs both sexually and emotionally, while demanding absolutely nothing of him in return. It stands to reason that someone in that situation would consider the very fact that they are a whole person with their own feelings and needs to be a source of shame, self-disgust, and even lower self-worth. *Who am I to have feelings or needs, when my job is to give other people a pleasurable experience? How selfish and greedy must I be that I secretly want to be so much more than pretty, pleasant, and nice? Why am I so messy and complicated inside, and why do I have to work so hard to be desirable, when other people can do it effortlessly?*

Low self-worth among conventionally attractive self-objectifiers often leads to an intense obsession with and management of their appearance, a feeling of constant pressure and obligation to look a certain way, panic about people seeing how they really look (without all the work they put into looking good), impostor syndrome, dread and terror about aging, and wild swings between feeling "superconfident" and feeling completely worthless, depending on other people's reactions to them.

But what about when you learn to think of yourself as having value only if you give other people a pleasurable experience of looking at you, but then you also know you just *don't*? When you're so far from the conventional beauty ideals that you seem to have no value to others at all? Self-objectifiers in this situation often experience a lifetime of invisibility, rejection, criticism, unsolicited advice, and harassment for their appearance, leading again to feelings of shame, failure, insignificance, and worthlessness.

Something many people don't realize is that *negative* attention and harassment for how a person looks is often still objectification. A stranger on the street telling a woman to smile is objectifying her, because the stranger thinks of her face as existing for his pleasure, and so he feels entitled to give her an instruction about how to make it more pleasing to him. The same is true for someone who writes, "Lose weight, fatty," on a fat woman's Instagram picture, a mom who tells her daughter she needs to wear makeup to look prettier, or a teen boy who tells a teen girl her hairy arms are disgusting. Objectification and sexualization aren't just compliments and desire, they can also be insults and disgust, because they're fundamentally about stripping a person of their full humanity, believing a person has no innate value, worth, or purpose of their own, and reducing a person to nothing more than a resource to be mined and enjoyed by others.

This is, unfortunately, how many men are taught to see women: not as full humans, but as sexual objects and emotional laborers for them to exploit and enjoy.[8] Through that lens, it's pretty rude for an objectified person to go around being unattractive or displeasing, isn't it? A man who sees women this way is more likely to give a woman patronizing and inappropriate advice on how she can better please him, whether by smiling more, losing weight, or dressing differently, because he thinks of her as existing for his pleasure, not her own. He's also more likely to respond with anger, vitriol, or violence when a woman's appearance doesn't meet his standards, because he feels like she *owes* him a pleasurable experience of looking at her; that he's *entitled* to such an experience, and she deserves to be punished if she doesn't provide it. In this way, the harassment and insults faced by people whose appearance diverges from conventional beauty and body ideals is often just as much the result of objectification as catcalls and compliments. And all of it comes from the systems of oppression conditioning us to believe that some people, in some bodies, simply don't have any innate value or worth.

Low self-worth among self-objectifiers who are marginalized or not conventionally attractive often leads to extreme body hatred and shame, a feeling that they will be alone forever and never find someone to love or desire them, an inability to treat themselves or their bodies with respect or kindness, acts of self-harm and punishment toward the body and self, and a roller coaster of extreme hope and despair as they come up with plans to "fix" themselves and then crash back into reality when the plan doesn't work.

Self-objectification blocks a person's ability to cultivate a resilient, authentic, and three-dimensional sense of their intrinsic value and innate worth, which is why so few (if any) self-objectifiers seem to have that. Plus, that kind of self-worth isn't based on what other people think of you, it's based on what *you* think of *yourself*, which is a very difficult thing to connect with when you've spent a lifetime imagining yourself through the eyes of others. True self-worth is an evaluation that comes from within, the result of a well-developed connection to your inner self, and the ability to see yourself clearly and objectively.

After all, both self-objectification and low self-worth are just false interpretations and significance created and reinforced by the systems of oppression, power, and privilege that form the basis of our society. The truth is that there is no such thing as a person who deserves to be dehumanized, objectified, or exploited, just as there's no such thing as a person who exists to give other people pleasure, or a person who has no worth or value at all. These lies exist because they benefit the people in power, who feel entitled to dehumanize, objectify, and exploit people in certain kinds of bodies, but that doesn't make them true. By learning to dismantle these lies, a person can see themselves with clear and neutral vision, and connect to the *truth*: that they are a gloriously three-dimensional human being with innate worth and inherent value, who was born for something other than to be consumed or give other people pleasure, and whose appearance is the least interesting and important thing about them.

They Often Feel "Gross" and "Disgusting"

The vast majority of self-objectifiers I've worked with use the words "gross" and "disgusting" a lot when talking about their bodies. Sometimes these words are used as an intellectual assessment or criticism, as in "ugh, I look disgusting today," and other times they're used to describe a feeling, as in "I've been feeling so gross all week."

These words tend to be the worst insults a self-objectifier can think of, and the most intense expression of their contempt. Someone who says, "I don't mind my legs, but my belly is just absolutely disgusting," for example, is likely to do so in a voice dripping with revulsion and hatred. Invoking the skin-crawling feeling of *disgust* like this allows the person to express and share the intensely visceral experience they have whenever they think of their belly. They could have said their belly was "ugly" or "unattractive," or said something like "I don't like how big it is" or "I wish it were more toned." But instead, they chose to call it absolutely disgusting, because it wasn't really an expression of their thoughts, but rather an expression of their powerful, visceral, full-body experience of revulsion, repugnance, and abhorrence toward this body part.

Think about what we describe as absolutely disgusting, outside of bodies. Puddles of chunky dog vomit on the carpet. Poop-clogged, overflowing toilets. Discovering your kid playing with some roadkill. Waking up to your kitchen being overrun by rats. These images might provoke a visceral disgust reaction in your body (as they did for me when I wrote them), and maybe you even made the universal "disgust face," with your nose scrunched up, eyebrows knitted low, and your upper lip lifted. If so, you had this reaction because the feeling of disgust is hardwired into us as an evolutionarily clever form of protection.[9] Disgust, or at least "pathogen disgust," which I'm referring to here, exists to keep us from going near things that carry pathogens and will make us sick, like vomit, poop, rats, and corpses. Disgust makes us want to get away from the toxic source immediately!

But there's another kind of disgust that we develop within our environment and culture, called moral disgust. Moral disgust is what we feel when we see a moral violation, which of course means it's extremely subjective, biased, and dependent on what an individual learned to see as a moral violation. A person might feel moral disgust if they found out their friend had been cheating on their spouse, for example, but not feel disgust if they found out their friend was in two separate, consensual, and ethical polyamorous relationships, because the disgust isn't in response to having multiple partners, but rather to the perceived moral violation of cheating.

Disgust serves an important purpose: to get us the hell away from stuff that's toxic or bad for us. But what we consider "morally toxic" is highly influenced by our biases and social conditioning, so it varies from culture to culture, and person to person, and even changes over time. In the early 1970s, for example, a large majority of people polled in the United States—70 percent—considered homosexuality to be morally "wrong," so many would have experienced a visceral disgust reaction to the thought of two gay men being together.[10] But as of 2022, thanks to decades of LGBTQIA+ activism, the figures have swapped; about 70 percent of people in the United States now see being gay as morally neutral—indeed, "acceptable," so most of us won't feel any disgust at the sight of, say, two men kissing.[11]

This is important to understand about disgust, for two reasons. The first is that, due to its visceral nature, most people misunderstand their feelings of disgust to be *proof* that something is a moral violation, instead of recognizing that it's their *perception* of something as morally wrong that creates the feeling of disgust. And the second is that most people are unaware that moral disgust can be dismantled and eliminated if they dismantle their bias and perception of something as a moral violation.[12]

With that in mind, let's get back to the self-objectifier, who feels so much disgust toward their body. It's unlikely to be pathogen disgust they feel, because their body isn't actually toxic, which means it must be moral disgust. But what is the moral violation they're perceiving? To understand that, we have to recognize that the self-objectifier often feels their role, job, or existential purpose on earth to be making other people feel good, letting themselves be consumed, or fulfilling other people's needs and desires. More specifically, especially when the self-objectifier is someone who partners or sleeps with men, it's to make *men* feel good, give *men* pleasure and gratification, and fulfill *men's* needs and desires—which means it's a moral imperative that they be attractive and desirable so men may enjoy them. In this way, the self-objectifier's body has committed the moral violation, by failing to provide men (or whomever) with the pleasurable experience that it owes them.

Writing this out makes my stomach turn, both because it shows us the horrifying depths of brainwashing so many self-objectifiers have been exposed to, and also because, as a self-objectifier myself, I remember feeling this way. When I was younger, I felt like I *owed all men* a pleasurable experience when they looked at me, even though I couldn't have told you why at the time. All I knew was that "gross" and "disgusting" were the absolute worst things I could be called, because they represented some kind of catastrophic failure on my part. And that brings us to another reason the self-objectifier struggles so much with feelings of disgust, which is that desire and disgust are antithetical, and mutually exclusive.[13]

Sexual attraction, desire, and arousal are all about feeling drawn *to* something or someone, and feeling a desire to get closer. Disgust, on the other hand, is the exact opposite. Disgust is about feeling repelled by something or someone, and feeling a desire to get farther away.

These two experiences are mutually exclusive for this reason: it's difficult to get sexually aroused when you're feeling disgusted, and it's
much harder to feel disgusted when you're sexually aroused. This,
again, serves a fabulous evolutionary purpose! Our genitals and excre-
tory organs are very close together, and due to pathogen disgust, we
would normally want to stay very far away from other people's excre-
tory organs. But once we're sexually aroused, disgust fades into the
background. Suddenly, putting our mouth, hands, or genitals so close
to someone else's butthole not only *doesn't* disgust us, but it actually
starts to sound like a great idea! The fact that disgust and arousal are
mutually exclusive allows the human race to continue. But if someone
measures their worth (or ability to get their needs met) by how well,
and how often, they can create the experience of sexual attraction, desire, or arousal in others, it makes sense that they would then regard
making someone feel disgusted as the worst thing they can do. It is,
after all, the exact opposite experience; it's as far away from attraction
and desire as a person can get.

This can all inform why a self-objectifier might worry so much
about being gross, or associate the feeling of "being disgusting" with
shame or failure. It can shed light on why they might scrutinize their
appearance constantly, looking for anything that *might* disgust someone, and then trying to change or hide it, and also why they might re-
play every moment of disgust they ever received, big or small, in their
minds, solidifying those memories into permanent insecurities. And it
can also help explain why "I feel gross or disgusting" is so often the
self-objectifier's most common body image complaint.

Do you resonate with this relationship to disgust? Maybe you'll
never forget how that kid in the third grade said, "Ewww!" when they
saw your birthmark, or that guy in high school who said your arms
were fat and gross, or how you once heard someone make a joke about
how disgusting cellulite is. Maybe your biggest body insecurity is your
thighs, because a partner once expressed disgust at how muscular they
were, or your weight, because you've internalized the idea that it's a

moral violation to be fat. Or maybe you, like many self-objectifiers, feel disgusted by aspects of the human body that have been stigmatized, labeled as repellent, or generally seen as yucky more broadly, like period blood, body odor, genital taste or smell, body hair, pimples, cold sore or herpes outbreaks, or anything related to pooping or farting!

Granted there *may* be a small amount of pathogen disgust involved in some of these, but that theory tends to fall apart when we consider that, men (straight men, at least) are generally allowed to go around stinking, farting, having body hair, and making poop jokes without everyone wanting to crawl out of their skin. It's only when these aspects of the human body occur in a person whose "job" it supposedly is to be attractive and desirable that they are met with so much disgust. This is why so many women feel like they can never, under any circumstances, allow anyone else to see these "disgusting" pieces of them. It's why a woman might *never* fart in front of her partner, even if he comfortably farts all day long in front of her, and why she might be too insecure to have sex if she hasn't shaved her legs or just gotten out of the shower to make sure there's no odor of any kind, while he might think this is ridiculous and feel perfectly comfortable having sex with no hygienic preamble. But even when a self-objectifier keeps these parts of themselves hidden from others, they often still feel disgusted by their own bodies for having them. After all, if the goal is to be a perfect sexual object—to turn people on, and give them pleasure—then having a functioning human body is, in and of itself, an embarrassing failure.

In my early twenties, I had food poisoning while living with a partner from whom I had been carefully hiding the fact that I even had a digestive tract, let alone that I pooped. While doubled over in agony in the bathroom, sweating profusely, and wrecked with cramps, I ran the sink as loud as I could and pretended to him that I was just doing girly spa stuff like face masks and body scrubs. I was sure that if my then boyfriend knew I was actually having cataclysmic diarrhea, he would be so disgusted that he would never see me the same again—which meant he would stop desiring me, stop thinking I had value, and stop loving me. Looking back now, I'm sure he would have just been worried about me, but a lifetime of objectifying myself had led me to develop a completely out-of-proportion self-disgust response; I was convinced that if anyone ever found out I had a fully functioning human body, the charade of my desirability would crumble, and I would end up abandoned and alone.

Given all of this, it probably won't surprise you that many self-objectifiers have a hypersensitive disgust reaction in general, feeling far more frequent and intense disgust than the average person, even when it's *not* about their bodies. Sometimes it's an inborn sensitivity, but more often it's because they've inflated the importance of disgust in their own mind, for all the reasons above, and also because they tend to see the entire world through a lens of objectification. After all, when you believe it's *everyone's* responsibility to look as attractive as possible, then it feels like a moral violation every time someone fails your standards, and you'll often end up feeling disgusted by people. And while this is a totally normal response given the culture that surrounds us, it's also a way in which casual objectification of people is upheld and passed on.

I once had a client write out everything she felt disgusted by when looking at other people. She sent me a four-page single-spaced document including items like "wearing socks with sandals," "wearing the wrong kind of silhouette for their body type," "not putting on concealer when they have bags under their eyes," "wearing sneakers anywhere but the gym," "when women wear dresses without shapewear underneath," "people who don't dye their grays," "skinny eyebrows," and "not getting Botox even though they're in their thirties or forties."

Whew.

This woman believed she needed to maintain extremely high aesthetic standards in order to have any worth, and "literally gagged" when other people—especially women—didn't try to look their best. In her mind, doing everything in your power to always look as attractive as possible was a moral obligation, so people who "cut corners," as she put it, seemed to be committing a grave moral violation, and made her feel absolutely disgusted. (Unsurprising, she was often disgusted by her own body as well.) She didn't *want* to be so judgmental and critical, but she had so deeply internalized her own objectification that she was policing and enforcing the objectification of others.

Considering the many layers at play, disgust plays a starring role in the body image experience of many self-objectifiers. They consider their bodies to have committed a moral violation, and therefore have a feeling of repulsion toward their bodies and a desire to get far away from them, as if their bodies themselves were a source of toxicity. But they *can't* get away from their bodies, of course, which leads to a deeply unpleasant situation—like how you might feel if you encountered a rotting animal carcass crawling with maggots, and then for some reason discovered that you have to spend the rest of your life in constant close contact with that carcass. For this reason, the phrases "I feel gross" and "I feel disgusting" are often actually cover-ups for the self-objectifier's deeper unpleasant feelings, like fear, contempt, shame, anger, anxiety, panic, helplessness, worthlessness, or claustrophobia.

If this sounds like you, it might be helpful to explore which specific feelings might be underneath *your* disgust, and which perceived moral violations are creating your disgust in the first place. Think about which factors might have informed or cultivated your sensitivity to the feeling of disgust, and what they have to do with objectification. Then try to zoom back and see the situation with clear and neutral eyes (i.e., with no stories, interpretations, lies, or significance layered on top of it), and identify the actual toxic force in this scenario. Because there probably *is* something toxic and bad for you here—something yucky that *will* make you sick and you *should* move away from—but *it's not your body*.

If you feel disgust about your weight, for example, the real source of toxicity might be fatphobia. If you feel disgust about the fact that you get gassy and bloated sometimes, or that you were born with body hair, the real sickening poison might be self-objectification. If you feel grossed out by your saggy breasts, acne, or cellulite, the real repulsive factor might be unrealistic and oppressive beauty ideals. And if you feel most disgusting around someone who is critical of you and your body, then it might be their abusive behavior that is the real source of your revulsion. Exploring your relationship to disgust this way can help strip away a lot of the stories, interpretations, and false meaning you've been attaching to your body, bringing you a lot closer to being able to see the objective and neutral truth.

They Feel like They Need Everyone to Think They're Attractive

Wanting to feel attractive and desirable isn't exclusively a self-objectifier trait; it's actually something that *most* people can relate to. The difference between a self-objectifier and someone else, however, is that the latter doesn't attach false or excessive meaning and significance to their attractiveness or desirability, while the former *does*.

A non-self-objectifier might find themselves occasionally wanting to be attractive to someone *they're* attracted to, for example, or wishing desperately to feel desired by a partner they've drifted apart from. They might crave the excitement and confidence boost of dressing up, going out, and flirting with a stranger sometimes, or feel hurt when someone isn't attracted to them. But their response to these scenarios will be proportional and appropriate, because they haven't attached their self-worth to their attractiveness, and therefore are responding only to the scenario at hand, rather than a powerfully negative interpretation of what the scenario *means* about them, their body or appearance, self-worth, or life. The self-objectifier, on the other hand, attaches so much false significance and excessive meaning to their appearance that they end up having wildly disproportionate and inappropriate responses in these kinds of scenarios, often spiraling those feelings into a story about how they're worthless, disgusting, unlovable, or doomed to be alone forever.

This is why the self-objectifier craves the validation of others finding them attractive and desiring them: because that, too, has an inappropriate amount of meaning and significance in their minds and reassures them that they have worth, are valued, are safe, and can get their needs met. But because they're seeking the *validation* rather than the actual *desire*, no amount of people finding them attractive can actually satisfy them. As soon as they know someone finds them attractive, that person becomes little more than a checked box, and they're on the hunt again, looking for their next hit, the next person to give them the attention and validation they crave. This isn't usually conscious, of course, but on some level, the self-objectifier is seeking out another hit of validation in the hopes that maybe *this time* it satisfies them and slakes their thirst.

Many self-objectifiers in this position admit to feeling like a "bottomless pit" for this kind of attention, approval, and validation for how they look—especially from men—and to constantly wanting more. Because they don't understand why this is, and they've learned from cultural messages and media that it's bad to want that much attention and validation, they might feel embarrassed by it, or ashamed of it, believing themselves to be vain, shallow, needy, or pathologically attention seeking. But still, in their most private and vulnerable moments, a huge number of self-objectifiers confess to feeling like they need *everyone in the entire world* to find them attractive.

This might sound silly to someone who hasn't experienced it, but it actually makes perfect sense. The self-objectifier believes their worth is based on people finding them attractive, but that's a particularly difficult metric to measure. Which people? How many people? To a person just trying to figure out whether they have worth or not, there is a frustrating lack of clarity around this, so the brain comes up with a concrete solution and measurement: *everyone*. If everyone on the entire planet found you attractive, *then* you'd know you had worth.

Plus, the self-objectifier often feels a lot of scarcity around their ability to get their needs met by other people in general, because they see relationships as transactional, and attractiveness as currency. They believe a pleasing appearance is what they have to provide in exchange for getting what they want and need in the world, like connection, attention, kindness, respect, opportunities, loyalty, money, security, intimacy, or even love. And because so many self-objectifiers have a long history of chronically unmet needs, they blame their body or appearance. Wanting everyone in the entire world to find them attractive, then, can just be an expression of their desire for their needs to be easily and abundantly met. After all, when we've been bitterly deprived of something, it's completely normal to crave a disproportionately high amount of it.

Think about a person who has been on a super-strict diet for several months: it's totally reasonable and normal for this person to find themselves craving a mile-long smorgasbord of food, and fantasizing about eating *all the doughnuts in the world!* There's nothing wrong with them for craving such abundance, it's just the brain and body's natural response to food scarcity. And the same is true when it comes to emotional needs. If you've been suffering from a shortage of feeling truly seen, being genuinely valued and celebrated, deep intimacy, freedom, dignity, agency, or power—and, if we're being honest, a lifetime of self-objectification leads to *all* of these needs going chronically unmet—then it's normal to fantasize about a ridiculous abundance and to feel like a bottomless pit for it. And when you've learned that the only way a person like you can get those needs met is to be attractive, it makes sense for the fantasy to be everyone in the world finding you attractive!

As anyone who has gone through an anti-diet or intuitive eating journey knows, when it comes to food, you really *do* have to eat all the food and all the doughnuts for a while in order for your body to believe the famine has ended, and for your food cravings to return to a more reasonable place. This has to be done repeatedly over time for the brain to decide that it's safe and that food is abundant again, so it won't happen after one big meal or one box of doughnuts. But with time (and a shit ton of food and doughnuts), the hyperbolic fantasy will fade, and your relationship to food will become clearer and more neutral.[14]

The solution to fantasies of getting your *emotional* needs met with hyperbolic abundance is often exactly the same. If it's possible to find ways of getting those emotional needs met in prolific and abundant ways for a decent stretch of time, you're likely to find that you no longer feel like a bottomless pit anymore, because your brain has decided the famine is over, and feels safe again. When the brain feels safe and satiated, there's no reason for it to send you signals of heightened awareness, obsessive alertness, or alarm about the shortage anymore.

Of course, this doesn't mean you have to get an abundance of validation for how you look, because the shortage was never actually about that kind of validation. The shortage was of the emotional needs you *associated* with that validation, and it's *those* emotional needs you'll need to get abundantly met for this fantasy to recede.

What would it look like to spoil yourself with an abundance of attention, for example, in ways that don't rely on your appearance, and that actually feel satiating to you? Maybe it would look like taking an improv class, starting a blog or YouTube channel, asking your loved ones to listen and hold space for you more often, volunteering to read books to kids at the local library, asking your partner to not be on their phone when you're together, advocating for the kind of attention you most crave, applying for a leadership position, or teaching lessons on your favorite hobby. Maybe it would look like all of the above and more! Would you still need the same amount of validation for how you look if you were regularly being spoiled with attention for these other aspects of yourself? If you've been using your body to get your need for attention met, probably not.

They Tend to Be Women and Femmes, but They Can Be Anyone

You might have noticed that the majority of the examples I gave in this chapter have featured women, and that's because in my experience, the vast majority of self-objectifiers are girls, women, and femmes. While self-objectifiers of all genders exist[15] (and plenty of women don't objectify themselves at all), there just seems to be a lot of crossover between the experience of being a woman in a patriarchy, and the experience of self-objectification. There is also a lot of crossover for people of any gender who are attracted to, sleep with, or partner with cisgender men, because self-objectification is so often linked to the male gaze. (Hence why more gay men seem to connect with this avatar than straight men, while more straight women than gay women do the same!)

The simplest explanation for this pattern is that, thanks to the cis-heteropatriarchy, women and femmes are the people most likely to be sexualized or objectified by others—or to see people *like them* being sexualized or objectified—and then internalize that. We live in a culture that regularly sexualizes and objectifies women, because we live in a culture that was built by and for men who didn't see women as whole autonomous humans, or equals. And even now, despite how far we've come toward gender equality as a culture, women *still* learn to see themselves through the male gaze, and measure their worth through male attention and approval. The combination of women and femmes being *under*represented in positions of power, influence, and leadership, while also being *over*represented in positions of supporter, caretaker, sexual object, and eye candy, sends a very specific message about where they belong, and what gives them value.[16]

Women learn that they are predominantly valued for one thing in our culture: their ability to give other people a positive or pleasurable experience. Sometimes this means the woman taking on a caretaker role, being nurturing and selfless, providing everyone with free emotional labor, making the home feel cozy, raising children, doing domestic labor, or generally tending to everyone in her life. Other times it means being pleasant to look at, being sexy and desirable, titillating or arousing people, or providing men with the sexual pleasure and gratification they need and "deserve." Either way, women and femmes seem to be far more likely than others to adopt a lifelong habit of self-objectification.

On top of all that messaging, many women and femmes have personally experienced one or more of the following:

- Objectification, sexualization, dehumanization, or unwanted sexual attention.

- Having their body or appearance scrutinized, commented on, ranked, critiqued, shamed, or assessed for attractiveness or desirability, *unsolicited.*

- Sexual abuse, sexual assault, or rape.

- Sexual harassment or sexual coercion.

- Doing things sexually that they didn't really want to do, because they were being pressured, felt like saying no would cause problems, or felt like they "owed" it to the other person.

- Sexual experiences with men in which *his* pleasure was central and obligatory, while *her* pleasure was an afterthought, optional, or nonexistent.

- Abusive, manipulative, controlling, or violent (male) partners.

- Sexism, misogyny, gender inequality, discrimination, or even violence just for being a woman.[17]

With all this in mind, it shouldn't come as a surprise that so many women and femmes seem to believe things like:

- Their bodies don't really exist for *them*, they exist for other people to enjoy, and particularly for *men* to enjoy.

- They "owe it to people" to look as attractive as possible.

- They "owe men" sexual pleasure and gratification.

- They have to do whatever people want them to do, in order to have worth.

♦ Their personal needs, feelings, and desires don't matter. In order to have worth, they have to push those down, and always be focusing on other people.

♦ People are entitled to their time, energy, labor, and body . . . so advocating for their needs, setting boundaries, or saying no is unacceptable.

♦ The measure of their worth is men's approval, validation, and desire.

♦ They need to achieve and maintain a very high aesthetic standard in order for a man to choose them, partner with them, treat them well, or stay loyal to them.

None of those beliefs are objectively true, of course, but they tend to *feel* true to the self-objectifier, and to inform the false meaning and significance they layer onto their bodies. And while each belief on its *own* would block a person's ability to see their body objectively or neutrally, many women believe most or even all of them. This is why, when the self-objectifier is a woman or femme, their body image issues seem to be connected to nearly every aspect of their lives, and also why their path to body neutrality tends to involve the deconstruction of big topics like gender and gender roles, worth and value, obligation, purpose, sexuality and pleasure, and relationship dynamics.

When I've worked with *men* who identify with the self-objectifier, however, their body image issues seem to generally take on a narrower scope. Instead of a man connecting his body to his worthiness for love in general, for example, he might just focus on his ability to get what he wants sexually or romantically, or on being attractive to the kind of person he is attracted to. This could possibly be the case because men are more likely to have been valued for who they are as three-dimensional people, and therefore don't feel like they need to "earn" their worthiness with their bodies. It could also be because men are more likely to have gotten their needs met for power, respect, influence, safety, resources, opportunities, money, and autonomy, and again don't need to rely on their appearance to get those things. (This is truer the more privileged identities men have, and less true the more marginalized identities they have, but when matched for those other identities, men have more privilege on average than women.)[18] Either way, this isn't an attempt to downplay a man's body image suffering in any way, because it can still be intensely distressing, but rather to draw your attention to the difference (in how body image issues tend to show up) between folks who have been objectified, exploited, fetishized, dehumanized, and devalued their whole lives, versus folks who haven't.

Women (along with nonbinary, gender nonconforming, and marginalized folks in general) are far less likely to have the majority of their needs already secured, so their hidden body image purpose seems to more often be about getting something *other* than what they want sexually or romantically. With fewer paths available for them to get these needs met, it makes sense that they would view their appearance as a way to earn social power and influence, safety, resources, opportunities, money, respect, and autonomy. (And this fact gets exponentially magnified if the person has multiple marginalized identities, or has been dehumanized, sexualized, or fetishized for multiple aspects of who they are, such as an East Asian transgender woman, a fat Black femme, or a Latina woman with a disability.) It makes sense, then, that people in this situation would become more fixated on their appearance or sex appeal than those with more privilege and power.

It also makes sense why women, femmes, nonbinary, and gender nonconforming folks more often find themselves wanting to be attractive to people they're not even remotely interested in, sexually or romantically. I've worked with several asexual self-objectifiers, for example, who felt immense pressure to look attractive to others, despite not feeling attracted to *anyone*! And a lesbian client, whose body image issues were centered completely on what men thought of her, put it this way: "Men are the gatekeepers of the world. We still have to make them happy." The quality of her personal and professional life was heavily affected by men, so despite not wanting to be intimate with one, she still felt obligated to conform to conventional beauty ideals of "what men like."

Speaking of men, I'd like to pivot for a moment and talk about the objectification of men, because *all* genders are vulnerable to objectification and fetishization, it just tends to look a bit different.[19] And because of the specific cultural messages we learn about where a man's value comes from, some men come to understand themselves as an object or resource to be consumed by others for totally different reasons than women do.

The first way men are often objectified in our culture is *financially*: a dynamic that can be seen playing out everywhere, from women or young gay men going to bars in the hopes of a man buying them drinks, to the old-fashioned expectation that men pay for dates, outright "gold diggers," and the expectation that a man only has value as a partner if he's financially successful. When I lived in New York City, I knew quite a few people who wouldn't even go on a date with a guy if he wasn't rich, or dumped someone when they found out he was broke. And while each person is entitled to make whatever decisions they like, and there *is* a historically good reason for this dynamic (i.e., the distribution of power and wealth has always been, and still *is*, skewed heavily in men's favor), I want us to name it for what it is: *objectification*. A whole person, reduced down to and valued exclusively for the resources they can offer.

The second way men (especially men who partner and sleep with women) are often objectified is for their *height*. You don't have to spend more than a few minutes scrolling through a dating app before seeing how many women write things like "no short men" or "if you're under six feet, swipe left." A lot of tall men list their height in their bios because it's the first thing someone asks them when they match, and a lot of short men get unmatched or ghosted when they reveal their height to an interested party. There's no other way to put it: tall men are fetishized in culture, as are men who are extremely big, lean, and muscular.[20]

While some of this just comes down to what people find sexy, a lot of it comes down to subconscious biases, and a desire for increased social privilege. After all, height matters when it comes to more than just the dating pool. Taller men are far more likely to get more opportunities, make more money, become CEOs, and be offered many other privileges and advantages in life, compared with shorter men. Height privilege and height discrimination are real, and apply more to men than anyone else.[21] A person who sees partnering with men as an opportunity to increase their own social capital and resources, then, would naturally prefer a tall, muscular, and conventionally attractive man, without any awareness that they're objectifying him for both his body and his social capital.

The last way men tend to be objectified in our culture is for *penis size*: many people who are attracted to cisgender men will fetishize and glorify a big penis, while scorning and disparaging a small one.[22] Black men in particular, whose penises are stereotyped to be bigger, are often sought out and fetishized for this reason,[23] while Asian men, whose penises are stereotyped to be smaller, are often denigrated and mocked.[24] Either way, when a man's worth and value as a potential sexual or romantic partner is being measured by the size of his penis, he is being stripped of his full humanity and being valued entirely by the experience he can offer someone else. And what can we call that other than objectification?

Any time someone is intentionally seeking out a particular trait or quality in a potential partner, with that trait or quality being of primary importance, and the person themself being somewhat secondary, that's objectification and fetishization. Anytime a person is deemed attractive because of what they represent or what experience they can offer, that's objectification and fetishization. This includes people who are exclusively into Asian women, transgender women, or fat women (three historically fetishized populations), people who seek out only Black women or Latina women (both populations who have been stereotyped as "hypersexual"), and people who seem to date only identical, rail-thin, twenty-five-year-old blond models (I'm looking at you, Leo DiCaprio).[25]

Of course, people will be turned on by whatever turns them on, and can make whatever choices they want, but it's worth exploring the role that objectification plays in this kind of attraction, desire, and arousal.

They Tend to Experience Body Image Differently When Partnered or Single

+ *The Single Self-Objectifier*

When a self-objectifier is single, but wants to be partnered, their body image issues tend to focus on their lack of a partner. They might think and say things like "I'm so disgusting, who would ever want to be with me?" or "obviously I'm hideous or I would have a partner already" or "nobody is ever going to love me looking like this, and I'm going to die alone." They seem to imagine that if only they had a partner (or got their sexual or intimate needs met), all their body image issues would disappear, because it would prove that they were desirable and worthy after all.

Single self-objectifiers in this situation often feel insecure and disempowered about dating in general. They might go into a date with the mindset of "I hope they like me" instead of "I hope I like them," for example, which gives the other person an inappropriate amount of power and responsibility. Influenced by a lifetime of social conditioning, the self-objectifier tends to imagine their role in the dating game to be fairly passive: show up, and let someone else assess them. Then, if they "pass the other person's test," the other person is responsible for making the next move. Is it any wonder these folks find dating so stressful? They imagine the other person has all the power and responsibility, and that *their* job is to just be desirable enough to motivate the other person to choose them. They often even feel like they don't (or shouldn't) have to do any of the hard, vulnerable, or scary work of "making things happen" with a potential partner, because someone who was attracted to them enough would do all that. But then, if they end up feeling rejected, or not getting what they wanted, they blame it on not being attractive or desirable enough, and become even more convinced that the key to overcoming their body image issues would be to find a partner.

Some self-objectifiers use being single as an intense motivation for change, however, like when someone tries to get a "revenge body" after a breakup, or when someone decides to start dating again, so they get their hair cut and colored, their nails done, and buy all new clothes. These kinds of experiences tend to be full of hope, so they can actually make people feel pretty euphoric and confident for a while, but the effects unfortunately never last. Eventually the person will fall back into their normal routine, get busy with work, shift priorities, or otherwise just stop putting in so much effort, and lose their "improvements." Nobody stays in the motivation phase forever, and these folks tend to suffer a devastating hit to their confidence and body image when it ends.

Lastly, because the single self-objectifier tends to think their lack of intimate connection is the result of not being attractive enough to be chosen, they will sometimes express intense confusion and feelings of jealousy, outrage, or injustice when a less conventionally attractive friend or peer is able to go on dates, have sex, find love, get engaged, or get married. These moments subvert the self-objectifier's entire worldview, which feels deeply unsettling and unfair. *If being chosen is about being hot, and I'm hotter than they are, then I deserve to be chosen first!* So the single self-objectifier often lives in a state of ongoing frustration, injustice, and confusion.

+ *The Partnered Self-Objectifier*

Many single clients imagine that finding a partner would be the "cure" to their body image issues, but it almost never works that way. It's true that finding a partner who adores your body can boost your confidence and reduce your body anxiety, and that finding a partner who loves and values your whole self can improve body image by helping cultivate a stronger sense of self-worth. But having a partner does *not* automatically mean a person will stop self-objectifying, or suddenly feel confident and secure. In fact, in my experience, some of the most intense self-objectification and feelings of insecurity occur *inside* long-term partnerships!

The reason for this, I believe, is that loving someone—letting them into your heart, and entwining your life with theirs—is extraordinarily vulnerable. Many people are terrified of being cheated on or abandoned, and even if they trust their partner completely, there's always the risk of something happening to them, and ending up heartbroken anyway. Opening your heart to another person, and then entwining your life with theirs, makes a person extraordinarily vulnerable to heartbreak, no matter who they choose or how loved they are. And I find that many partnered self-objectifiers simply do not tolerate this fact well.

When a self-objectifier first enters a wonderful new partnership, and is enjoying the oxytocin-packed chemical joyride of falling in love and having lots of sex and feeling intimately connected to someone new, they tend to have the *least* body image issues.[26] I've even known people who claimed during this phase that their body image issues were cured, because they felt so sexy and happy in their bodies! (Spoiler alert: they weren't.) The abundance of attention, validation, compliments, desire, sex, intimacy, touch, romance, and love all tend to quiet the insecure voice in their mind, and the accompanying chemical high makes them feel like it will be like that forever. But when the chemicals balance back out, usually a few months to a few years later, the self-objectifier's old insecurities and patterns are right there again, waiting for them.

That's why I want to talk about the pattern I see among self-objectifiers who have been partnered for a while, *after* that early newlove phase. These folks tend to struggle to ever feel secure enough in their partnership, and to crave constant reassurances that they're safe, loved, desired, and not going to be abandoned. They'll often describe themselves as "needy" or "clingy," because no matter how much reassurance they get from their partner, they always feel they need more. And that's important: the self-objectifier is focused on getting reassurance from their partner to feel safe and secure, but it doesn't last very long because their partner actually *can't* offer them the safety and security they crave; it doesn't exist. No matter what their partner does, they're still likely to feel insecure, unloved, anxious about the relationship, and worried their partner is upset with them, on a regular basis.

Why is this? Sometimes it's a reflection of the self-objectifier's anxious or insecure attachment style,[27] but sometimes it's a reflection of the self-objectifier's inability to tolerate the excruciating vulnerability of loving someone. This vulnerability tends to feel unbearable to the self-objectifier, so their mind concocts a fantasy to protect themselves from it—a fantasy in which, if they can just be attractive enough, they'll never be rejected, heartbroken, abandoned, or alone. Sure, this fantasy places so much extra meaning and significance on their appearance that they might constantly feel insecure about how they look, but at least it gives them a sort of plan to protect themselves, and that makes them feel less vulnerable.

Interestingly, this pattern of self-protection can look completely different from person to person. One self-objectifier might seek attention and validation for how they look *outside* of their partnership, for example, as a kind of constant reassurance to themselves that even if they were rejected or abandoned, they wouldn't actually end up alone, because other people still want them. They might even find themselves breaking their relationship agreements in an effort to prove to themselves that they are still desirable and "have options," but then wonder why the hell they did such a thing when they love their partner!

Other times, a self-objectifier might seek the attention and validation of their partner's desire for them, which generally means they want their partner to compliment their appearance a lot, as well as to frequently, passionately, and eagerly express a desire to have sex with them. Many partnered self-objectifiers feel most secure and confident during (and right after) sex with their partner, because sex validates and reassures them that they are wanted and loved,[28] and they feel the most anxious, insecure, and body negative when they haven't had sex for a while or when their partner seems less interested in sex in general.

Of course, people want (and don't want) sex for any number of reasons, so this perspective puts a ridiculous and unfair amount of pressure on the self-objectifier's partner to always be wanting sex. Too bad for you if you have a gassy belly, or just watched a disgusting video on how to gut a fish, I guess! Your partner's entire sense of relationship security and self-worth is based on your wanting to fuck them all the time, so you better hop to it!

Despite how obviously unhealthy this is, a lot of partnered self-objectifiers rely on their partner's desire for sex and intimacy to feel safe and loved, and therefore they also feel like the relationship is in danger during periods of less sex and intimacy. This is why, when the partnership feels distant or insecure, the self-objectifier is likely to find themselves blaming their body, and obsessing over ways to become more attractive. They're also likely to believe it's their responsibility to "stay attractive" for their partner, and to spend a lot of time, energy, and money maintaining or trying to improve their appearance, even if their partner would be just as happy with, and aroused by, their natural state.[29]

A common insecurity and fear among partnered self-objectifiers is "losing their looks" as they age, get pregnant, or gain weight, and their partner no longer being attracted to them. This makes sense, even if they're not aware of what's underneath this fear. They believe their value comes from their ability to please and arouse their partner, so the fear of becoming less attractive is actually the fear of being abandoned. And while it's totally normal to want our partners to desire us, sexual desire itself is about *so much more* than how we look. Desire and arousal are informed by connection, body language, familiarity, pheromones, a feeling of safety, compatibility, hormones, a person's energy and personality, reciprocal interest, and smell, taste, and touch.[30] People of all ages, shapes, gender, races, abilities, and sizes can both feel desire *toward*, and spark desire *in*, others. But the self-objectifier tends to ignore all of this and get stuck in the belief that the key to a secure relationship is sexual desire, and the key to desire is conforming more closely to beauty ideals.

This all puts a huge amount of pressure and inflated significance on a person's appearance, but it also ignores the underlying issue. There is literally *no amount* of desire or validation that could ever make a self-objectifier feel completely secure in their partnership, because complete security is a fantasy. Choosing to partner with someone is inherently vulnerable, and loving someone comes with the inherent risk of heartbreak. So in order to see their body with clear and neutral vision, the partnered self-objectifier will often need to acknowledge and accept that vulnerability, and learn to tolerate the ever-present possibility for heartbreak, instead of living in a fantasy where it doesn't exist.

THE SELF-OBJECTIFIER'S NEXT STEPS

I'll be offering you specific action steps for how to move toward body neutrality in the last part of this book. For now, just be aware that if you resonate with the self-objectifier, you will eventually need to identify—with clarity and specificity—*exactly* what meaning and significance you've attached to your appearance, and what the subconscious goal of being attractive or desirable is actually about for you. What are you subconsciously trying to get or earn by looking hot? What problems are you subconsciously trying to solve? Here are a few more questions to get your wheels turning before going on to read about the rest of the avatars:

- What are you imagining or hoping would happen if you could achieve or maintain the "perfect body"?

- What are you most afraid of, about not being attractive *enough*?

- What might you *really* be seeking when you want attention, compliments, or validation for how you look?

- Why is looking good so important to you?

- What is the purpose of people thinking you're attractive?

CHAPTER 9

The High Achiever

THE HIGH ACHIEVER IS FOCUSED ON using their body to prove their moral excellence to others, improve their social status, and earn *external* validation—usually in the hopes of achieving an *internal* feeling, such as goodness, worthiness, safety, or relief.

PATTERNS OFTEN SEEN AMONG HIGH ACHIEVERS:

♦ They see worth as relative, rather than absolute, which means they consciously or subconsciously believe a person's worth and value comes from their excellence, impressiveness, dominance, status, or superiority compared with others.

♦ They tend to be highly competitive, perfectionistic, and hard on themselves.

♦ They don't necessarily care about looking attractive, but they care a lot about controlling the shape and size of their body, leading many to develop a disordered relationship with food and exercise.

- Their biggest fear is other people thinking they're "lazy."

- Their "dream body" tends to be exceptionally lean and fit: a body that they think "looks" sculpted through discipline, hard work, willpower, and self-control.

- They associate having more social capital, power, privilege, and influence with feeling happy, fulfilled, and worthy, and strive to increase their social status through any means available to them.

- They often see decisions through the binary lens of moral judgment, believing there is always a "good" or "right" choice, and a "bad" or "wrong" choice.

- At some point, their life may have revolved around strictly regimented fitness and nutrition plans. If so, they're likely to think of that lifestyle as "ideal," even if they can't maintain it.

- They believe people generally get what they deserve (morally speaking), based on the content of their character, and the decisions they make in life.

- They often have a very intense anti-fat bias, falsely believing fat bodies are the result of laziness or some other character flaw, and that they signal poor health, poor moral character, or low intelligence.

- Despite wanting so badly to be good and moral people, they tend to be critical, judgmental, and disapproving when it comes to other people's bodies and choices.

- They see everything as a power struggle, and are preoccupied with making sure they come out on top—or at least that they don't end up at the bottom.

While these are common characteristics of the high achiever, each individual will, of course, have their own experience. The unifying factor for this avatar, as with all of them, is how their body image issues are trying to help them.

THE HIGH ACHIEVER'S HIDDEN BODY IMAGE PURPOSE

The high achiever is always trying to prove or demonstrate their "goodness" and ensure other people think highly of them, by working to get higher up on the social hierarchies and confirming to social ideals. This can be a pattern in many areas of the high achiever's life, but tends to be especially true when it comes to the body. By attempting to conform to conventional beauty and body ideals, the high achiever hopes to earn external validation, increase their social status, and gain social privilege, as well as avoid the challenges of discrimination faced by marginalized folks.

In a culture built on systems of oppression like anti-fat bias, ableism, racism, ageism, and sexism, the high achiever is understandably focused on using their body to seek upward social mobility (or, at the very least, to avoid downward social mobility!) and to secure their social status, social privilege, and feeling of importance or worth. Having learned that a person's position on the social hierarchies is a true indicator of who they are and what they deserve, and that we live in a meritocracy where everyone gets what they deserve, the high achiever often turns to extreme habits of body control, like food restriction and over-exercising, to get there. After all, in a culture that celebrates extreme levels of discipline, willpower, hard work, and self-control (think Olympic athletes, billionaires, celebrities who do their own stunts, and folks who lose huge amounts of weight), the high achiever is understandably convinced that demonstrating those qualities in an indisputable and public way will be the key to getting what they want. And what could be more indisputable and public, they think, than having the kind of body everyone wants but few can achieve? In this way, many high achievers are often desperately trying to sculpt their body into what they imagine to be a walking billboard for their goodness, character, status, or worth so that people think highly of them, and they're rewarded with a good and easy life.

Whew! Talk about adding excessive meaning and significance to the body! It's no wonder so many high achievers can't see their bodies neutrally, and struggle with body anxiety, preoccupation, shame, negativity, and insecurity. They see their bodies as a sort of public statement about who they are, and what they deserve.

This whole plan is based on fatphobic lies, of course. Even if everyone ate and exercised *the exact same way*, natural body diversity would still make everyone's body look different,[1] so a person's body can't actually tell us anything about what they do, who they are, or what they deserve. But the high achiever tends to be loyal to the existing cultural body hierarchies, having never felt like it was their place to challenge something that "everyone else" seems to agree upon, so their hidden body image purpose is to try anyway.

What's important to understand about the high achiever, however, is that they *always* have a deeper motivation for this plan. After all, it might feel good to know that other people think you're impressive, but there's no intrinsic benefit to impressing people. So the high achiever might be consciously seeking social status and external validation, but what they're really seeking is something deeper: something they think increased social status and external validation will lead to, or get them.

This is why it's true, but incomplete, to say the high achiever's body image issues exist to just prove their goodness, improve their social status, or earn them external validation. The deeper thing they're seeking forms a key part of their hidden body image purpose, so it's important to acknowledge that there is always a deeper problem the high achiever is hoping to solve, a deeper need or desire they're trying to meet, or a deeper experience they're chasing *through* goodness, status, and validation. Interestingly, despite how externally focused these goals are, what many high achievers are actually seeking is an internal experience, such as a feeling of happiness, contentment, fulfillment, relief, meaning, purpose, or self-worth.

The deeper thing the high achiever is seeking can vary dramatically from person to person, but they always believe the key to getting there is to prove their goodness and worthiness to others, and to climb the social hierarchies. And they're always trying to use their body to do that.

This is important to understand, because it's why many high achievers have to go through a two-step process when identifying their hidden body image purpose.

All avatars will start out with the same questions on the path to body neutrality: *How are my body image issues trying to help me? How might body anxiety be helping (or trying to help) me get my needs met? How might body hatred be solving (or trying to solve) a problem? What am I hoping a particular kind of body will help me get, avoid, or feel?*

In the third section of this book, you'll learn why finding this answer (i.e., identifying your hidden body image purpose) is a critical step toward letting go of your body image issues, and how to actually do it. But while finding this answer can be difficult for everyone, the other avatars tend to see it as one cohesive exercise, while the high achiever is far more likely to see it as *two nearly unrelated* exercises.

The first time a high achiever tries to identify their hidden body image purpose, they're likely to come up with kind of true-but-not-complete answers to the questions. They might even strike the high achiever as very silly questions, with incredibly obvious answers.

What are my body image issues trying to earn me? Easy. Attention, validation, praise, admiration, respect, access, opportunities, and confidence. What are my body image issues trying to help me avoid? Discrimination, judgment, exclusion, missed opportunities, being treated badly by people, and feeling bad about myself—duh.

But after identifying this true-but-not-complete hidden body image purpose, the high achiever has to then go back in and ask themselves about the underlying purpose, goal, desire, or need for each individual answer, as well as what false assumptions or biases it might be based on. For example: What are you hoping (or expecting) would be *different* in your life if you got all the external validation, praise, or admiration that you crave? And is it actually true that having a certain kind of body would automatically make you feel fully confident as a person? If not, where did this story come from, and what are you *really* seeking?

This kind of deep and radically honest self-inquiry tends to be challenging for the high achiever, both because they've been taught to ignore their intuition (and therefore their subconscious), and because they tend to be rule followers who have been taught not to question the authority of the masses. *Everyone* wants to be thinner, they say, because being thinner is just *better*! It's *obvious* why they want to have a certain kind of body, because that body is celebrated and important—and who would want a body that everyone makes fun of or thinks is bad and gross?

In this way, the high achiever might be able to easily identify that underneath their desire for a lean and toned body is a desire for, say, admiration, but then not know that underneath their desire for admiration is a desire for purpose, self-acceptance, or permission to rest. In a world that treats some people better than others, the pursuit of upward social mobility is just a given to the high achiever, even if they don't know what exactly they're chasing, or why it's so important. All they know is that people are judged by how they look, and it feels crucial that they be judged positively.

Hopefully you can see why the high achiever's hidden body image purpose is often deeply hidden and hard to identify. There is always a superficial version, a true-but-not-complete version of what they're trying to gain or avoid by looking a certain way, that fits somewhere in the realm of external validation and praise, increased social status and privilege, upward social mobility, or being seen as "good." But then there is also always a deeper and more complete version, explaining *why* exactly they're chasing those things, and what they're hoping those things will get them.

It's important that we pause here for a moment and acknowledge that lots of people change the way they look to gain the benefits afforded to people who look that way . . . and that in a world that systematically advantages certain people and disadvantages others based on how they look,[2] this makes total sense. Manipulating your appearance *is* a valid way of pursuing upward social mobility in some ways, and if you can increase your access to opportunities (and decrease your risks of discrimination) just by altering the way you look, why not do it? A Black woman might get her hair relaxed before a job interview, for example—not because she necessarily prefers it that way, but to appeal to the manager's racist biases about work-appropriate hair, and increase her odds of getting the job. A man might push himself to get super muscular, just to have an easier time dating, and a woman might get a boob job to make herself more appealing to men.

We can probably all agree that things like these shouldn't have to happen, but given the society we live in, it makes sense that they do. People have always, and will always, attempt to climb up the social ladder to escape the disadvantages of marginalization and access the benefits of privilege, and how we look plays a role in that.

So what's the harm, a high achiever might ask, in just trying to play the game to win? Aren't we just acknowledging the unjust truth of the world we live in, and making decisions accordingly?

Not really. That *can* be a valid way of moving through the world, but it's not what the high achiever is doing, for two reasons.

The first reason is that the high achiever is often operating under the false belief that our bodies and appearances are entirely within our control, and that an "ideal" and impressive body can be achieved by anyone, if only they display enough hard work, discipline, willpower, and self-control. Because of this, many high achievers refuse to accept the boundaries of what a person *can* and *can't* do to alter their body or appearance safely, wisely, and sustainably. Instead, they either believe themselves to be, or desperately want themselves to be, the exception to these boundaries. As a result, they often end up trading everything—physical health, mental health, social life, relationship happiness, pleasure, joy, embodiment, rest, and the ability to be present—in pursuit of something impossible. Is this seeing the truth of the world we live in and acting accordingly? I don't think so.

The other reason the high achiever is doing something other than just "playing the game to win" is that they're never just making calculated and strategic decisions based on seeing our unjust world clearly. I say that with certainty, because the amount of emotional distress the high achiever experiences around their body image is wildly inappropriate and out of proportion for that goal.

The high achiever's vision is always clouded by layers of deeply ingrained prejudices, false interpretations, and untrue biases about what different bodies *mean*, because they genuinely believe a person's body can reveal what kind of person they are, and what kind of life they deserve. On some level, they believe the system is fair, and that if everyone would just work harder and follow the rules, they would all be rewarded equally. So they're not *working* the system, they're *upholding* it.

A HIGH ACHIEVER CASE STUDY: CATE

Cate, a grad student whose parents were Chinese immigrants,* told me that her parents were very hard on her growing up, and had very high standards and expectations. "Anything less than perfect was a failure," she told me, so she learned to push herself at everything. She practiced cello until her fingers were raw, worked so hard during track practice

---

*You might be wondering why I include certain identifying details like race when introducing *some* clients, but not others. I do this because, outside of career title, I try to stick to the details that each person felt were particularly relevant to their own body-image and self-image.

that she sometimes vomited or passed out, studied late into the night, and had practically no social life.

In the ninth grade, Cate discovered she could go long stretches without eating, and that doing so made her feel proud, impressive, and *successful*. She heard all the other girls talking about how they didn't have the willpower to skip lunch, or that they just loved carbs too much to give them up, even though they wanted to lose weight, but Cate found that both of these things were surprisingly easy for her. The other girls were incredulous, which felt amazing, and they regularly told Cate how impressive and "inspirational" she was as she continued to skip meals and get smaller.

Cate's behavior developed into a full-blown eating disorder within a year; the less she ate, the more successful and impressive she felt. Eventually, she came to associate the feeling of a full belly with failure, shame, and weakness, and the feeling of a hollow belly with being strong, special, and "good."

Cate and I started working together when she was twenty-four, ten years after her eating disorder developed. In that time, she had undergone two hospitalizations for being severely underweight, spent several months doing in-patient recovery treatment, and had gotten a ton of therapy and nutrition support to get her eating disorder under control.

When we met, Cate described herself as still "anorexic at heart," but her body was at a healthy weight, and she hadn't restricted food in years. She told me she was glad to be healthy, and proud of how hard she fought to get there. She said she genuinely wanted to *live*, and to someday get married and have babies, and she understood she needed to eat and be healthy for those things to be possible. And yet still, when Cate looked in the mirror and saw her healthy body, all she felt was hatred.

Cate told me, with absolute contempt in her voice, that she just looks so . . . *average*. So *normal*. Not special at all. Not impressive. The body of "a person who gave up." And this all made her feel so unhappy that sometimes she just sat in front of the mirror, crying.

When I asked Cate what she missed most about being unhealthily thin, she talked about the attention and praise she received from other girls and women. They were constantly complimenting her willpower and strength, exclaiming over how good she was for passing on dessert, and expressing their envy and admiration. It felt great, she said. Never having had close friends growing up, Cate came to think of admiration and jealousy as even better than friendship, and it gave her a sense of power, worth, and social place. Her hyperthin body placed her above other women, and everyone seemed to recognize it. She could walk into a room full of women and instantly be given the status of their superior, their alpha, their leader. It made her feel confident, empowered, and valued, because her body was a walking representation of her will-power, self-control, and discipline. It made her feel like she had *earned* the praise and recognition, and *deserved* the power it got her.

As Cate had gained weight during recovery, all the praise, attention, recognition, and power slipped away. Now that her body was just "normal and average," she was both mourning the loss of all that praise, attention, recognition, and power, *and* mourning the loss of the feeling that she deserved those things. Cate didn't think she was good enough at anything else to earn that kind of attention, power, or confidence another way, and so she believed she'd have to spend the rest of her life feeling unworthy and undeserving, unable to access the things she most desired.

Cate's hatred toward her body started to make sense in this context: she had subconsciously assigned her body the job of "earning" her praise and admiration, status, envy, power, the feeling of being special and worthy, and connection with other women. Who could feel neutrally about a body they believed was preventing them from getting so many things they wanted and needed?

When I suggested we consider other ways Cate might be able to get some of her needs met, she balked. The kind of status, power, and attention she craved could only be made possible if you were the *best* at something, she said—if you were *special*—and she couldn't think of anything else that made her superior or special. This led us to consider what the underlying point of that status, power, and attention was. Sure, it felt good to be put on a pedestal, but what needs had that pedestal actually helped her meet, and what problems had that pedestal actually helped her solve?

By considering it this way, Cate was eventually able to identify that being treated as special for her body had made her feel seen and valued, and like she was good enough, which were experiences she hadn't gotten much of growing up. It had also made her feel *connected*, because everywhere she went, people (especially women) seemed to like her and want to talk to her—another experience she had been lacking. Plus, the act of not eating itself made Cate feel powerful, proud, and strong, which made her feel confident and good about herself, and restricting food had given her life a sense of meaning and purpose in a way that nothing else had. Knowing all that, we were able to see that Cate's hidden body image purpose had been to get all of those needs met (to feel seen, valued, good enough, connected, confident, and like her life had meaning and purpose) by making her body so thin that everyone saw her and treated her as important, impressive, superior, and special.

Cate had learned from her parents that it's important to be the best at things, that only "perfect" was good enough, and that being normal, average, or "like everyone else" meant she had failed. This made it impossible for her to connect with others as equals, so she sought out a dynamic of connecting with them as their superior, and it convinced her that only people who are impressive, special, or perfect get to feel good about themselves. Once we recognized all of this, it became clear that in order to stop hating her body so much, Cate would both need to find alternative ways of getting these actual needs met, *and* to dismantle her belief system around the importance of perfection, dominance, and superiority.

Over the next year and a half, that's exactly what Cate did. Through reeducation, exposure to new perspectives, and constant self-inquiry, she was able to shift her ideas about what makes a person worthy and confident, and let go of her competitiveness and perfectionism. She explored her *own* values instead of mindlessly upholding the values she had been taught, and in so doing, she learned to break solidarity with her parents and think for herself. She cultivated a new sense of self-worth, based on her own system of values, and discovered the warmer and gentler joy of feeling good about herself *without* first feeling better than someone else. She learned to connect with people from a place of equal footing, and cultivated several strong female friendships. In those friendships, she experienced a deeper and more genuine feeling of being seen, valued, and "enough" than she ever had before.

In the beginning of our work together, Cate reported never having a day go by where she wasn't affected by how much she hated her body. As she started the process described above, however, she started having the occasional day here and there where she wasn't affected by it, and didn't get upset. These days became more frequent as her mindset shifted and her needs got met, until they became the majority.

COMMON CHARACTERISTICS AND EXPERIENCES OF THE HIGH ACHIEVER

Now that you have an idea of how a high achiever's body image journey might look, let's explore some of the most common patterns, characteristics, and experiences seen among high achievers.

They Seek Upward Social Mobility

Our society teaches us that we live in a fair and equal meritocracy, and that people get what they deserve. This often leads to a belief that people at the top of the social hierarchies *deserve* to be at the top, and that people who are at the bottom deserve to be at the bottom too. From that perspective, the pursuit of upward social mobility is not just possible, it's *mandatory*, because it's how we communicate to everyone what kind of person we are and what kind of life we deserve.

Being the dutiful rule follower that they are, the high achiever often adopted the lessons, values, and beliefs that they were taught growing up, without asking too many questions. That means that their worldview is heavily influenced by our capitalist, colonialist, white supremacist, and ableist patriarchy, and their implicit biases—which is to say their unconscious stereotypes and preferences for or against certain types of people—tend to reflect those systems.[3] They imagine a person's value can be measured by their productivity, industriousness, dominance, power, and—of course—wealth. Masculine-coded work is more valuable than feminine-coded work. Individuality is superior to collectivism. Power is more important than kindness, and logic trumps emotion. Any sign of weakness is seen as an invitation to be exploited or attacked. Everyone must prove their worth and earn their respect through hard work, discipline, self-control, rugged individualism, and the careful eradication of all signs of personal weakness.

Inside of this belief system, each individual's actions and character determine their fate, so all you have to do to ascend the ladder and be rewarded is follow the rules, always do the right thing, and demonstrate impeccable moral judgment and character. And that's exactly what the high achiever is trying to *use their body* to do.

Because the high achiever considers a person's social status to be "proof" of their character and worthiness, they're nearly always trying to increase their social status by having "the kind of body" people revere and respect. This most often means a body that is visibly athletic, lean, toned, thin, or muscular, but sometimes it means having a body capable of performing impressive achievements and accomplishments, like playing professional sports, running marathons or triathlons, doing CrossFit, or powerlifting. Anything that makes other people think highly of them, increases their status, or earns them external validation.

It also has to be said that the high achiever may seek upward social mobility using whatever means they have access to, not just their body. They might seek out notable career success, for example, rack up big achievements and accomplishments, pursue impressive accolades, or acquire status symbols like a fancy car or "trophy spouse." But given the society we live in, where a person's body and appearance have a huge impact on their social status and levels of privilege, the body often becomes the high achiever's main strategy and tool for upward social mobility.

If only they work hard enough, the high achiever thinks, they'll get exceptionally lean, thin, or muscular. Then everyone will be able to see how good, industrious, hardworking, and disciplined they are, and they'll soar to the top of society and reap their rewards.

They Adhere to a Strict Moral Binary

The high achiever believes everyone gets what they deserve, so the key to getting what they want is to first prove themselves worthy of getting it . . . and the key to proving themselves *worthy* is to climb the social hierarchies, through a demonstration of superior moral character. For this reason, the high achiever tends to be a very black-or-white thinker, with very little tolerance for nuance or gray area, who adheres to a strict moral binary. This means they imagine that every single choice in life has a right answer and a wrong answer—a good decision and a bad decision—and that a person's moral standing is the result of how well they choose.

This view that all actions are intrinsically right or wrong is sometimes called moral absolutism, and is often a tenet of organized religions, like Christianity.[4] As a result, high achievers often find themselves preoccupied with the morality of every choice they make, and every choice *other* people make, in an ongoing effort to figure out who is good and who is bad.

Moral absolutism can cause the high achiever to find it wildly stressful, and even paralyzing, to make decisions. There's a sense that a person's character is a sort of pass-or-fail situation: you're either good or you're bad, and there's nothing in between. Even a decision that seems small and unimportant can feel high stakes, if you believe you must constantly be choosing the right thing, or else you yourself are bad.

In order to ensure they're always making the right choices, avoiding mistakes, and maintaining a position of moral excellence and righteousness, the high achiever will often rely on rules, routines, and structure. After all, the fewer choices they have to make per day, the fewer opportunities they have to mess up. And because there's no shortage of messages about the "right way" to do things, they often don't even have to come up with their own. Whether learned through family culture, organized religion, school or higher education, corporate culture, social etiquette, or somewhere else, following a set plan allows the high achiever to rest easy, knowing so many of life's decisions will be made for them. It also allows them to sidestep the fact that they don't quite trust themselves to properly decipher what's right and what's wrong. They may believe in moral absolutism, but they're not always 100 percent clear on the exact rules and don't want to get anything wrong.

By adhering to rigid rules and strict structures, the high achiever minimizes the number of choices they have to make (therefore minimizing their risk of making mistakes), while also getting to maintain a feeling of superiority, pride, and righteousness, which they tend to mistake for confidence and self-worth. They might feel smug and self-satisfied, for example, if they successfully followed the "no sex before marriage" rule, and enjoy the feeling of looking down on people who didn't. Or, like Cate, they might imagine feeling better than others to be the absolute height of self-esteem.

Of course, there's a downside to moral absolutism too. Many of my high-achieving clients report feeling most confident and calm when they've been sticking to all their rules, and being "good," but feeling a massive amount of anxiety, distress, guilt, and shame when they've been breaking their own rules, or being "bad." And even if their emotional reaction to breaking a rule seems totally unnecessary and out of proportion to *other* people's—like my client who had a complete breakdown on vacation because she broke her "exercise every single day" rule—it makes sense to the high achiever, because each choice carries so much moral significance in their mind.

It might not surprise you that the diet and fitness/wellness industries *intentionally prey* upon people with this all-or-nothing mindset. They seek out people who are trying to do everything right and be good but don't trust themselves, because those people are easier to sell to. They also seek out people who are looking for structure and rules to feel safe, or who have mistaken a feeling of moral superiority for a feeling of genuine self-worth, because *these* are the people who will become the most dedicated, buy the most products and programs, and most strongly enforce the moral binary in their communities. The diet and fitness/wellness industries intentionally moralize food, exercise, and bodies, and encourage people to think of themselves as "good" or "bad" depending on which choices they make, because people concerned with moral salvation spend more money. And the high achiever, who is already primed for this kind of marketing, is especially likely to fully commit themselves to a plan designed to keep them from making mistakes, and do whatever it takes to get a body that demonstrates their moral excellence.

The problem with this plan, however, is that the "information" out there about which rules a person should follow to get this kind of body are at best confusing, complicated, and contradictory, and at worst impossible, dangerous, and absurd. As a result, the high achiever is provided with endless opportunities to mess up and feel guilty. *I have to exercise, but it only counts if I do it for an hour, five days a week, and push myself hard—otherwise I may as well do nothing. I can't drink soda or juice, but kombucha is okay because it has probiotics. I'm supposed to eat lots of healthy fats like nuts and seeds and fish, but fat is also high in calories, and I don't want to gain weight, so I can't eat too many.*

For this reason, a lot of high achievers seem uptight or high strung when it comes to food, exercise, and other body stuff. Their partners and friends can't understand why they get so upset if they break one of their rules, because the rule doesn't make sense, or seem particularly important, to anyone else. So the combination of the high achiever's preoccupation with moral goodness, and their rigidly binary sense of right and wrong, tends to make them feel isolated and alone—a fact that can be perceived by them as either proof they *are* special and superior to everyone else, or as proof that they're broken and worthless. Again, there's no room for nuance.

Let's go back for a moment and explore why the high achiever often either believes, or *wants* to believe, that the universe is organized around a system of moral justice and equity, and that the morality of a person's character and actions always leads to a fair and fitting outcome. The belief that the world is fundamentally fair, and that people therefore always get what they morally deserve, is actually a cognitive bias called the just world fallacy,[5] and it's very appealing to someone who is looking to erase all nuance, outsource all decision-making, and avoid making mistakes.

The big problem with the just world fallacy is, of course, that it's demonstrably, categorically, and catastrophically false. We don't live in a fair and equal world, we don't live in a meritocracy, and people don't get what they morally deserve. People in positions of social dominance and power are not automatically more moral or deserving than those in positions of marginalization and suffering, and to say that they are is to actively uphold a system of violence and oppression.

But while this cognitive bias can be easily disproved (just go ahead and try to tell me that a child with cancer "got what they deserved"), the high achiever still tends to be very attached to the idea that if they prove their moral goodness through their actions, they will be rewarded with everything they want and need, because people get what they deserve. So they spend their lives not going after whatever it is they actually want and need directly, but instead trying to prove they are worthy of it, by following a million tiny rules they have attached moral significance to, many of which end up focused on the body.

Admittedly, the idea that the world is fair and just is a much nicer alternative to reality, and it offers comfort and peace to the person who believes in it. It even allows them to ignore or tolerate the presence of so much oppression, violence, and brutality in the world, because they believe those people must have done something to deserve it. It allows them to feel safe, knowing that bad things happen only to bad people, so if they're good their whole lives, nothing bad will happen to them. It's a lie, but it's a comforting one, and it protects the high achiever from facing both the chaotic randomness of suffering, and the many systems of injustice and inequality our society is built on.

The high achiever's habit of black-and-white thinking serves another valuable purpose too. Evolutionarily speaking, it's incredibly useful to be able to instantly boil a situation down to just two options. In an emergency, we don't have time to consider nuance; we have to come to a snap decision as quickly as possible about the safest option.

If a bear were about to attack me, for example, I wouldn't sit there weighing the nuance of the situation. I would take about a half microsecond to boil the situation down into a binary. Bear attack: bad. Me getting the hell out of there: good. No subtlety, no gray area, just two options. This is what binary thinking is meant for: moments of danger or urgency, when you don't have time for nuance, and just need clarity *fast*. It's the reptilian part of our brains trying to help us survive,[6] which might explain why it seems to show up so often for the high achiever, who tends to be very anxious in general.

Thanks to growing up with critical or manipulative caretakers, organized religion, or some other source of morality-based fearmongering, the high achiever often learned to live in constant fear of the moral consequences of their own actions, and that showing signs of weakness is an invitation for someone stronger to attack. With immense pressure to be morally "good" or else suffer some kind of catastrophic consequence, and the constant fear of being dominated, the high achiever ends up terrified of failing, making mistakes, or being imperfect in any way, and riddled with guilt and anxiety. Is it any wonder their brain thinks they're constantly in danger, and tries to boil everything down to a simple binary of "good" and "bad" to help them get to safety? There may be no room for nuance in the high achiever's life because every moment is a potential threat.[7]

That said, the habit of rigid all-or-nothing thinking, a belief in a meritocracy, and an adherence to moral absolutism all block the high achiever's ability to see their bodies, themselves, and the world clearly. The high achiever in this position will need to dismantle and release these blocks to make body neutrality a possibility, learning to tolerate nuance, finding another way of feeling good about themselves (without feeling superior), and facing the injustice of the reality they live in. Unfortunately, however, this process can be scary, uncomfortable, and even painful, and a lot of people just aren't ready for it.

More likely than the other avatars to have a fair amount of social privilege to begin with, the high achiever has often attached their entire sense of identity and self-worth to their ability to be better than others: more moral, more hardworking, more virtuous, more impressive, or just *more worthy of good things*. This is true even when the high achiever has terrible self-esteem or feels like a failure all the time, by the way, because they are still measuring themselves against a strict moral binary in which the possibility of their being perfect exists, and the only way for them to be good enough is to be better than everyone. There is, after all, a certain amount of ego and self-importance involved in the belief that you're a failure for not being perfect (implying that you, and you alone, had the potential to be perfect in the first place), or that your flaws and mistakes make *you* the worst person, or biggest failure, on the planet.

To clear away these blocks to neutrality, a high achiever may have to do some truly life-altering and earth-shattering work: facing the existence of oppression and inequality, acknowledging their own privilege (and reckoning with the harm they've caused), learning to think for themselves, rebuilding a sense of identity and self-worth, and finding a whole new way of relating to their bodies, themselves, and other people.

They're Judgmental

The combination of moral absolutism, the just world fallacy, and a preoccupation with being seen as "good" puts the high achiever in quite the conundrum. On the one hand, it's extremely important to them to embody the qualities of what they consider a "good person"—kindness, compassion, generosity, selflessness, and tolerance—while on the other hand, they find themselves riddled with thoughts and feelings of judgment, criticism, competitiveness, selfishness, and intolerance.

Thanks to their dedication to climbing the social hierarchies, the high achiever sees other people as competition, and will often compare themselves with others to see who "ranks higher." And because they're so focused on their *own* bodies, they tend to focus on *other people's* bodies, too, trying to figure out whose body is thinner, leaner, more impressive, or closer to the "ideal." They do this from a place of insecurity, of course, and an anxious desire to know where they stand in society, but it immediately creates a moral dilemma.

After all, if they compare themselves with someone else and decide the other person is superior, for example, they might feel jealous, spiteful, or even hateful toward the other person, or find themselves having many critical or unkind thoughts to tear them down. If they compare themselves and decide that they themselves are the superior party, then not only were they critical and judgmental, but now they also feel pleasure and pride (even glee!) in being able to look down on the other person with pity, contempt, or disgust. Obviously, none of these thoughts and feelings square with most codes of morality, which generally center on qualities like acceptance, humility, compassion, and goodwill. So the high achiever, who cares so deeply about being a good person, ends up feeling guilty and ashamed, and worrying that their thoughts and feelings actually make them a *bad* person!

This pattern creates a weird and confusing inner conflict for the high achiever, whose sneaking suspicion that they might be a secretly bad and wicked person lurks right below the surface of their identity as an uncommonly good and virtuous person. I had a client once admit with visceral embarrassment that she regularly looked up her wife's ex, just to confirm that "she's still fat and ugly," and feel better about herself by comparison. Another said that she was secretly envious when her sister lost a bunch of weight during chemotherapy for cancer, because now her sister was "the thinnest person in the family"—a title that she had always proudly held. And while these kinds of stories are uncomfortable to acknowledge, because everyone wants to imagine themselves to be "better than that" deep down, they're also very common. The high achiever might try to shove these critical, uncharitable, and intolerant parts of themselves down and ignore them, but they're still there, and they still cause shame and worry in low moments. *What if I'm actually just a bad person?*

Let's be clear about the fact that these thoughts and feelings aren't really an issue of morality, though, no matter what the high achiever believes. They're a very normal response to the worldview and belief system the high achiever lives in, in which worthiness is *relative*, not absolute. Because only people at the very top of the social hierarchies are worthy of good things in the high achiever's mind, it matters less that you're a good person, and more that you're a better person than everyone else. In this way, everything becomes a rivalry, other people become your competition, and community-mindedness goes right out the window. It's exceptionally difficult to stay in a place of kindness, connection, compassion, and generosity when you think your only chance at getting what you want is to beat everyone else to get there.[8]

Plus, the high achiever tends to believe that if they *don't* beat everyone else, they'll be seen as weak, passive, or easy to take advantage of, and end up exploited or destroyed. This is partly because they believe people lower on the hierarchies must have demonstrated poor moral character, and are therefore inherently less deserving of respect, opportunities, power, kindness, and other good things. It's also in part because they see the world as so cutthroat and competitive—eight billion people on the planet all trying to secure their place at the top—that they think of other people as dangerous: cold-blooded competitors who will do whatever it takes to get to the top. In this way, everyone else becomes a threat in the high achiever's mind, and all trust, or optimism about people's innate goodness, disappears. In fact, they almost expect that people will be vicious and self-centered; that a lack of empathy, compassion, and concern for others is the norm. (This perspective may even intensify the high achiever's desire to be a good and kind person—to *be* what they wish to *see* in the world!)

For this reason, social dominance becomes a key part of the high achiever's strategy for self-preservation, both because they believe it's the key to securing scarce resources, and because they think it's the only way to keep from being attacked or exploited. It's an eat-or-be-eaten world that the high achiever lives in; everything is dominate-or-be-dominated. So much so that they may even believe people who display signs of weakness are "asking" to be attacked or exploited, because they've made themselves a target.

Is it any wonder the high achiever spends so much time comparing themselves, picking people apart, or judgmentally "ranking" everyone? Is it any wonder they're constantly trying to position themselves as superior? These habits might not square with conventional ideas about morality, but they make sense. The high achiever is just trying to ensure their needs will be met, and protect themselves.

The irony of the high achiever's worldview is, of course, that it comes from a subconscious recognition of the systems of inequality and oppression that they work so hard to justify and ignore. They're afraid of having done to them what they're doing to others, if they slip up or relax, even for one moment. This worldview isn't just in the high achiever's mind either. It's something we see encouraged in the mainstream media, especially from the political Right, around rugged individualism: that people are innately untrustworthy and will take any opportunity to dominate or exploit you, so you must stay vigilant and fiercely defend yourself. But this alarmist perspective often leads people to go on the offensive and "protect themselves" by dominating or exploiting others *first*. If that leads to moral conflict, they can always justify it to themselves with the belief that the party who dominated must have obviously been stronger, better, and "more worthy" of being at the top.

This is important to understand, because the high achiever's worldview is self-perpetuating: the more a person dominates others, the more afraid they become of being dominated, and the more a person has been dominated, the more they see domination as the only path to freedom and safety. In the United States, the political Right believes establishing our dominance as a country is the *only* way to keep ourselves safe, and that if we try to "play nice" with the rest of the world, they'll see us as weak and attack us. This perspective is understandable, because politicians in the United States often see the *rest* of the world this way, and have regularly dominated and steamrolled other countries. Projecting their own eat-or-be-eaten worldview onto the rest of the world is what makes politicians in the United States feel afraid of being attacked or dominated, and that fear makes them commit even more fiercely to establishing a position of dominance over everyone else. In this way, the cycle of fear is reinforced and perpetuated.[9]

This is very similar to what a lot of high achievers are doing. *Everyone else is out for themselves, they're all secretly competing with me, and they're trying to defeat me, so I have to defeat them first!* But because other people don't necessarily see the world this way, the high achiever will often spend their entire life defensively trying to one-up everyone in an effort to win at a game that other people don't know they're playing.

They Become Obsessed with Body and Weight Control Behaviors

In an effort to publicly demonstrate their moral excellence and establish their social dominance, the high achiever often wants their body to look like the product of discipline, hard work, willpower, and self-control. This is an unrealistic goal, because body shape and size are determined by many factors unrelated to a person's conscious habits (including health conditions, age, medication, income, location, metabolic changes due to food scarcity or dieting, and natural genetic body diversity[10]), but that doesn't stop the high achiever from trying to reach it anyway. Then, because they think their body can "tell on them" in this way, their body insecurities start to feel like a huge deal, broadcasting their weakness or badness to everyone who looks at them.

It's important to point out here that the belief that a person's body shape and size accurately reflect their habits or character is not only *false* but also wildly fatphobic. (After all, if you believe thin bodies automatically represent people with a strong work ethic and lots of self-control, what do you believe fat bodies automatically represent?) This might not seem like a big deal, but actually the anti-fat bias tends to play a massive role in the body image issues of the high achiever, who is often either terrified of gaining weight or obsessed with losing it.

Given how omnipresent the anti-fat bias is in our society, it's no surprise that the high achiever learned to think of folks with thin bodies as good, hardworking people, and folks with fat bodies as bad, lazy, and gluttonous. While research shows us that this is nothing but unsubstantiated bigotry, these kinds of messages endure.[11] And given how the anti-fat bias leads to the discrimination of, marginalization of, and violence toward folks with fat bodies, it's understandable why someone would want to avoid or escape that. But this is just the rugged individualism mindset at play again. The high achiever looks around and sees how fat people are being harmed by the anti-fat bias, and instead of getting motivated to fight against the bias and create a safer and more equitable society for us *all*, they're only motivated to make sure that harm doesn't happen to *them*. They'll try to climb to the top of a hierarchy that they know causes harm to the people at the bottom, because it's every person for themselves. Plus those fat people must deserve to be there, right? Everyone gets what they deserve, and the size and shape of a body is determined exclusively by the person's habits and character, so they should just work harder if they don't want to be discriminated against!

This is the stance a lot of high achievers take, and while it's incredibly harmful and violent toward folks in fat bodies, they feel justified in it. In the end, however, this stance is also harmful and violent toward the high achiever themselves, because it causes them to become obsessed with controlling their weight, to adopt extremely rigid habits of body control, and, far too often, to develop a completely disordered relationship to food, exercise, and their bodies.

Naturally drawn to rules, routines, and structure, the high achiever will often develop a very long list of rules and behaviors they "have to follow" in order to either lose weight, or keep their weight "under control"—a phrase indicating the aggressive preventive measures they're taking against the weight they imagine their (bad, lazy) body is *trying* to gain. These rules and habits give them structure, order, and a feeling of knowing the "right thing" to do every day, which can temporarily reduce some of their anxiety. But remember how the self-objectifier would engage in body-checking behaviors to reduce their body anxiety, only to end up with more body anxiety later? The high achiever ends up in the same position; the more rigidly and strictly they follow their rules, the more stress, anxiety, and fear build up around breaking them. This is how a high achiever's weight and body control behaviors can come to hold a huge amount of power over a high achiever's life, and spiral into obsessions, compulsions, disorders, addictions, and delusions.

My client Justin had turned to lifting weights as a way of improving his health and filling his time when he decided to quit his job as a bartender to be a stay-at-home dad. But within a year, what started as a healthy routine had completely taken over Justin's life. At first, he just worked out for about forty-five minutes, three or four times a week, drank a protein shake afterward to help with recovery, and cut down on junk food. He felt great, and started seeing results in the mirror—his biceps and shoulders were filling out, and his belly was shrinking—so he got motivated to kick it up a notch. He added in more workouts per week, worked out for longer each time, bought some supplements, and started intermittent fasting.

By the time we started working together, Justin was very lean and fit, but his *entire day* revolved around his fitness and diet routines. He would wake up, do a half hour of fasted cardio before the kids got up, drop the older two kids off at school, and return home to drink a protein shake and work out while his littlest kid napped or watched TV. The workout took about two hours if he could manage it, and then he would make lunch: grilled cheese or chicken strips for his daughter, and a salad full of superfoods and lean protein for him. If he skipped any part of this morning routine, he would feel irritable, guilty, and anxious all day, and make up for it in the evening when his wife got home, even if that meant skipping family time, social time, or sleep. At the same time, Justin was following a strict protocol for when, what, and how much he could eat, scrutinizing his body in the mirror every morning to see what he still "needed to change," and spending a lot of time reading articles, watching videos, and thinking about fitness and nutrition.

Justin's body had undergone a seemingly impressive transformation, but his mental health, marriage, and social life had taken a nose-dive, because instead of fitness and nutrition augmenting his life, they had become the center of it. He had also been adhering to his strict food and body rules for so long that the thought of breaking any of them really freaked him out. He loved having structure and purpose, he loved that other people were so impressed, and he loved feeling like an "alpha" for the first time in his life. Justin was convinced that if he loosened his grip, even a little bit, all of that would disappear, and he would go back to being the aimless, doughy schlub he was before.

Unfortunately, a lot of high achievers experience something very similar to Justin; as their weight and body control behaviors start to stand in for a wide variety of unmet emotional needs, they become completely dependent on these behaviors. What starts as a healthy and balanced habit of exercising and eating nutritiously can easily cross over into a compulsion,[12] if it's the only way a person is getting their needs met, and the high achiever seems to be particularly vulnerable to this happening.

What needs are we talking about here? All kinds! Body control rules and behaviors can give the high achiever something to organize themselves around, providing them with a sense of purpose, meaning, structure, order, and direction. They can also help the high achiever meet their need for stability and predictability, security, empowerment, self-efficacy, or self-determination. Sometimes they just help the high achiever feel productive, like they're in the middle of an important project, which can provide fulfillment, satisfaction, hope, pride, confidence, or a feeling of growth and self-improvement. If controlling their weight or body is the only thing the high achiever believes themselves to be good at, these habits can provide a (somewhat fragile) sense of self-worth and value, or stand in for an authentic sense of self-identity. Sometimes body control behaviors provide the high achiever with a feeling of having "earned" (and therefore being deserving of) the good things in their life, to assuage the guilt they feel for having them.

Whatever needs a high achiever's body control rules and behaviors are meeting, the high achiever will often come to rely on them and believe they *need* them. Sometimes the high achiever will even develop a sort of superstitious approach to their rules and behaviors, believing that the rules and behaviors are responsible for keeping them safe, and that breaking one would lead to something terrible happening. This mindset often causes the high achiever to double down on how rigidly they follow their own body control rules, and develop a severe anxiety or even phobia of breaking them.

This cycle happens because our minds are wired to find patterns to make sense of the world, but sometimes we misinterpret the data and see patterns that aren't there. This phenomenon is called apophenia, defined in Webster's dictionary as "the tendency to perceive a connection or meaningful pattern between unrelated or random things,"[13] and it can lead to perfectly intelligent people believing in conspiracy theories, superstitions, and curses. A great example of this is the cognitive bias of the "hot hand phenomenon" in sports, in which an athlete is believed to be more likely to make a successful shot if their previous shot was successful, despite there being no statistical evidence of this.[14]

Apophenia can lead a person to believe their actions are the cause of some bigger (unrelated) outcome, like a guy who has to wear the same jersey during his team's football games, or else he's bringing his team "bad luck," and it'll be his fault if they lose. It can also lead a person to believe their morning run is the only thing standing between them and complete disaster, that if they eat a single bite of cake, they'll blow up like a balloon, or that skipping their workout will make something terrible happen.

The high achiever—who *may* already have certain predispositions for anxiety, obsession, compulsion, eating disorders, or other mental illness—seems to be particularly vulnerable to these body and weight control behaviors taking over their life. But whether or not the situation ever becomes clinically or medically significant, the high achiever tends to be disproportionately drawn to strict, rigid, intense, punishing, and even dangerous body control rules and behaviors, and often struggles with fluidity, balance, or moderation when it comes to food and exercise.

While many reasons for this have already been discussed, I want to point out that the experience of being a human can also just be wildly overwhelming and exhausting—especially in today's modern, fast-paced, and overstimulating world. Sometimes the high achiever's obsessive relationship with weight and body control behaviors exists to merely simplify things, to shut out all the scary stuff and shrink their world down into something smaller, easier, and more manageable. Either way, though, a high achiever in this position will eventually need to explore their relationship to these rules and behaviors and slowly strip them of the power, meaning, and significance they've been given, if they want to reclaim their ability to see food, movement, their body, and themselves through a clear and neutral lens.

They're Seeking an Internal Experience through an External Process

The high achiever is focused on using their body to signal moral excellence and worthiness to others, but not necessarily in an effort to actually get anything from them. Respect or admiration maybe, and validation, sure, but unlike the self-objectifier, whose plan is to be so attractive that other people are motivated to meet their needs, the high achiever isn't usually trying to motivate anyone to *do* anything.

When I ask high achievers how they imagine life would be if they had the "perfect body," they often describe the experience of knowing other people think highly of them. They say things like "people would look up to me," "everyone would be impressed," "the other moms would be jealous," or "I wouldn't have to worry about people judging me." It's almost as if all the external validation, praise, respect, power, moral superiority, and even improved social status that a high achiever seeks are only important because they're evidence that other people think highly of them. And this is important to understand, because the deeper outcome the high achiever is chasing with their body often isn't so much in the details of this fantasy, but the feeling.

Our culture has promised us that if we work hard, follow the rules, and choose the morally righteous path, we will be rewarded. Rewarded with what, though? With status, power, accolades, external validation, and opportunities sure. But status, power, accolades, external validation, and opportunities hold such a high appeal only because of the internal experiences we've learned to associate with them. We've learned to associate those experiences with a feeling of contentment, satisfaction, significance, or purpose. We've come to think of them as the key to happiness, inner peace, or relief from anxiety. We've been taught they'll make us feel lighter, freer, more joyful, more present, or more fulfilled. And, of course, we associate them with feeling confident, worthy, and deserving of good things.

The high achiever, being fully invested in these associations, often believes that if they can prove to everyone that they are worthy and good (and earn enough external validation for being worthy and good), they will eventually feel worthy and good. That's how it's supposed to work, right? The external is supposed to become the internal, and people are supposed to get what they deserve. So the high achiever might spend their life actively trying to make other people think highly of them, but it's all in the hopes of achieving something deeper and more personal, like happiness, purpose, a feeling of worthiness, or inner peace.

This is why I say the high achiever is often seeking an internal experience through an external process. External validation, social status, and moral superiority aren't really the end goal of the high achiever's hidden plan, they're just the strategy being used to get to the end goal. In the high achiever's mind, the prerequisite for getting what they want in life is to prove themselves irrefutably worthy of it, and climbing the social hierarchies is supposed to accomplish that. But even if the hierarchies had that kind of power (they don't), the high achiever's true end goal tends to be a feeling or internal experience, which can't be "earned" like this. So no matter how hard they work, no matter how "good" they are, no matter how impressive their body gets, the high achiever never reaches their end goal. Despite putting in extraordinary—sometimes even destructive—amounts of effort, the high achiever never receives their reward.

Since this whole thing tends to play out below the surface of the high achiever's conscious mind, they're often completely unaware that anything is going on, and just assume they haven't received their reward yet because they haven't worked hard enough, or have been "bad" in some way.

"Of course I don't feel worthy," they think. "I've been so bad and lazy, lately!" Feeling ashamed of themselves, they try to buckle down, work even harder, and be even more disciplined. This cycle leads to more shame, more self-loathing, and more power and significance being placed on every single choice they make when it comes to food, exercise, or their bodies. With these blocks to body neutrality present, is it any wonder the high achiever can't see themselves or their bodies clearly?

A high achiever who is caught in this cycle and wants to move toward body neutrality will need to identify the deeper experience they're actually chasing, and find a way to go after it more directly so their body no longer carries any role or responsibility in "earning" it. After all, with clear and neutral vision, we can see that none of the internal experiences a high achiever might be seeking actually require them to have a certain kind of body, and also that there is no body capable of automatically generating them.

Plus, even though the high achiever can technically be seeking *any* kind of internal experience via external status and praise, they seem to most often seek experiences that are entirely self-generated. I'm referring here to the emotional tanks that only the high achiever themself is capable of filling, because they come from *inside*, like self-acceptance, happiness, purpose, meaning, inner peace, and a sense of their own identity, worth, and value. The high achiever has, in fact, often been seeking from others the exact thing they desperately need from themselves: approval, acceptance, validation, trust, respect, and love. The truth is that nobody else can make a high achiever feel worthy or "good enough," and nobody else needs to. Self-worth is an inside job, and once you discover that, you can stop trying to earn it, prove it, or win it from anyone else.

THE HIGH ACHIEVER'S NEXT STEPS

Like all the avatars, the high achiever's next steps toward body neutrality center on understanding exactly how their body image issues are trying to help them. But since they tend to connect only with the more superficial, true-but-not-complete version of their hidden body image purpose, they'll often say things like "I want people to think I have my shit together," "I want to feel special, or impressive," or "if I looked a certain way, I wouldn't be as anxious."

This is why, if you resonate with the high achiever, I encourage you to think of your answer in two parts: What are you chasing, and *what's the underlying purpose of chasing it?* What are you trying to get with your body, and *what do you imagine you'll feel if you get it?*

You'll be guided through the exact process of identifying your hidden body image purpose in the last part of the book, but for now just start thinking about what you might be trying to "earn" with your body, and why. Here are a few questions to get the juices flowing!

- ♦ What problems are you hoping to solve by having a body that looks "sculpted by discipline, self-control, and hard work"?

- ♦ Why is being seen as "good" or "right" so important to you?

- ♦ What are you hoping increased social status, privilege, or power will lead to?

- ♦ What is the purpose of everyone being impressed with you, or seeing you as superior?

- ♦ In what way do rigid rules and structures serve you? What needs do they help meet?

CHAPTER 10

The Outsider

THE OUTSIDER IS FOCUSED ON USING their body to either get their need for secure social connections met, or to protect them from the threat of social disconnections (i.e., rejection, judgment, criticism, humiliation, or abandonment).

PATTERNS OFTEN SEEN AMONG OUTSIDERS:

- ◆ They generally aren't focused on wanting to look exceptionally good or better than anyone. They're focused on fitting in, blending in, or avoiding negative attention, so they're often going for a body that's just good *enough*.

- ◆ They're people pleasers, caretakers, empaths, and nurturers. They do a lot for other people, try to make everyone happy, put their own needs last, and live in fear of disappointing, upsetting, or burdening other people.

- ◆ They blame themselves (and their bodies) for other people's bad behavior. For example, if someone criticizes an outsider's weight, they're more likely to get angry at themselves and their body than at the person who made the comment.

♦ They often grew up in a culture where subtextual guesswork was encouraged or required (instead of direct or transparent conversation), and they struggle to be assertive, direct, or honest about their thoughts, feelings, needs, and desires.

♦ They constantly worry about being judged, and spend a lot of time and energy trying to prevent that from happening. (They also worry that people are secretly mad at them, disappointed in them, or don't like them.)

♦ They feel weird, different, wrong, isolated, or alone, even if they seem well-connected and well-liked. They struggle to connect with people the way they want to, and they don't feel like they quite belong anywhere.

♦ They may be conflict avoidant, or have an anxious attachment style, due to a history of insecure attachments, relationships where conflict felt threatening, or relationships where it wasn't safe for them to be their authentic selves.

♦ They identify as highly sensitive, intuitive, or emotionally intelligent—and believe they can accurately tell what other people are thinking or feeling, based on the other person's subtle body language, facial expressions, actions, tone, and word choice.

♦ They find it difficult to stand up for themselves, say no, set boundaries, or ask for help.

♦ They struggle with being and expressing their authentic selves, and sometimes don't even know *who* they would be if they weren't so focused on making other people happy, or being what other people wanted! (This leads to a feeling that nobody *fully* sees or knows them, which makes having deep, nourishing connections difficult, and increases their feeling of isolation.)

THE OUTSIDER'S HIDDEN BODY IMAGE PURPOSE

The outsider's body image issues exist to try to earn them the connection and belonging they crave, or to protect them from the rejection and humiliation they fear, by having a body that is socially acceptable. Unlike the self-objectifier and the high achiever, the outsider isn't usually trying to catch anyone's eye, compete with anyone, or stand out at all. Quite the opposite, in fact; the outsider wants to look *just good enough* to fit in and avoid negative attention. Being singled out for any reason can be uncomfortable for the outsider, so looking exceptionally good can feel just as scary as looking exceptionally bad, and they may strive to look sort of unremarkable and inconspicuous instead.

The outsider's hidden body image purpose has two separate and distinct branches: to earn something they want, or to avoid something they don't.

1. The first branch is where the outsider is trying to use their body to earn social *connection*. Their hidden body image purpose is essentially to have the kind of body that earns them whatever specific form of connection they most desire: acceptance, inclusion, community, nourishing relationships, or a feeling of belonging.

2. The second branch is where the outsider is trying to use their body to avoid social *disconnection*. Their hidden body image purpose, then, is to have the kind of body that prevents or protects them from whatever specific form of disconnection they most fear: judgment, criticism, exclusion, conflict, rejection, humiliation, or abandonment.

These two directions aren't mutually exclusive by any means, and many outsiders will recognize themselves in both, but one direction usually has a bit more power than the other. That's why one of the first things I do with outsider clients is to ask which branch resonates with them most—their answer can help inform and guide the rest of their path to body neutrality!

Outsiders who are mostly focused on earning the connection and belonging they crave will more often report wanting to look a specific way in order to be accepted by a specific person, type of person, peer group, class, culture, industry, or community. A client who worked in finance, for example, told me his body goal was to "look like a finance guy," because the other men at his hedge fund were all tall, lean, and athletic. Similarly, a midlevel social media influencer reported hating her body because her peers in that space were all so much thinner, and she felt like she didn't belong.

Outsiders in this boat are trying to secure their belonging in a particular space, and will therefore focus their attention on the particular kind of body they believe will do that. If they want to fit in with the other PTA parents, they might obsess over the ways their body or appearance differs from the established "PTA parent aesthetic." Whether they're searching for connections at the office, at the gym, in a new city, or through a hiking group or local bar scene—the connection-seeking outsider's body insecurities tend to focus on the ways they perceive themselves to be aesthetically different from "everyone else" in that space.

Sometimes, though, an outsider's insecurities were formed during their childhood and adolescent years, when their sense of difference and outsiderness was the most heightened, and those insecurities just stuck. If everyone else in middle school had straight hair and you had curly hair, for example, your curly hair might have become an insecurity— even if, as an adult, you know plenty of fabulous people with fabulous curly hair. Or if everyone else was petite in the third grade and you towered over them, you might still feel self-conscious about being gigantic, even if you stopped growing in the tenth grade and everyone else shot past you. Even if it's not logical anymore, because you ended up with a below-average height as an adult, you might still find yourself hunching and trying to shrink down to fit in. These kinds of formative insecurities have a way of sticking around long past their relevance, and of whispering that you don't belong here now because you didn't belong there then.

Whether their body image issues are relevant to the present moment or carried over from the past, connection-seeking outsiders tend to struggle most with the parts of their body or appearance that they perceive (or perceived) as making them stand out from everyone else in their chosen comparison group. These differences feel dangerous, and the outsider perceives them as threats to their ability to fit in, be accepted, or belong in the spaces that matter to them. As a result, the connection-seeking outsider tends to feel the most negativity and insecurity around these differences, and to blame them for any lack of connection and belonging in their life.

Outsiders for whom the second branch resonates, however, are focused on avoiding negative social consequences, and don't usually have a specific target or comparison group. More often, they want to fit in everywhere more generally, and say things like "I just want to look normal" or "I just don't want anyone judging me." Sometimes these folks consider attention of any kind to be so dangerous that they're actually hoping to avoid it altogether, wanting their appearance to render them almost invisible. After all, if nobody notices you at all, you're a lot less likely to face rejection, criticism, or humiliation, right?

Outsiders in this boat tend to feel most insecure about aspects of their body they worry could make them stand out, attract attention, invite judgment or criticism, or get them in trouble. They hate the parts of their body they imagine have the power to get them judged, excluded, rejected, laughed at, or kicked out—and this tends to mean any part that breaks the rules of what they consider socially acceptable, "normal," or privileged.

Some disconnection-avoiding outsiders have body image issues because they live in, or *have* lived in, a marginalized body, and they're understandably afraid of the discrimination, disrespect, exclusion, and even violence they know marginalized folks have to face. Others live in fairly privileged bodies, but worry about losing that status and facing the disconnection of marginalization, anyway. After all, marginalized people really *are* judged, excluded, criticized, rejected, and humiliated in our culture, on top of facing other disadvantages and burdens financially, mentally, emotionally, and physically.

Under such circumstances, the outsider's hidden body image purpose might be to protect them from the disadvantages of marginalization and oppression. This can certainly be true for any of the body hierarchies (as it can be true in relation to any system of oppression), but I tend to see it show up the *most* around weight, and the anti-fat bias. The hidden body image purpose for a huge number of outsiders is to protect themselves from people's cruel and violent fatphobia, by losing weight.

Speaking of which, sometimes an outsider's body image issues are the result of specific life experiences or traumas, like someone who hates their belly fat because their partner used to criticize them for it, or someone who associates their large breasts with unwanted attention and harassment. Other times, an outsider's body image issues are the result of *vicarious* embarrassment or shame, meaning, the result of seeing other people be judged, criticized, or humiliated for something about their body, imagining how that person must feel, and then wanting to avoid that experience at all costs. Lastly, an outsider's body image issues can represent a general (or even arbitrary) projection of shame and negativity onto the body, like someone who hates their body because they hate themselves, or someone who fixates on a birthmark, because in their mind, the birthmark represents their immutable *difference* from others.

It's also important to remember that the outsider's hidden body image purpose isn't always focused on their appearance. As is true for *all* the body image avatars, some outsiders struggle with body issues that have nothing whatsoever to do with the way they look. That said, the outsider seems to find this to be true a bit more often, perhaps because there are so many ways a person can perceive their body as a threat to their ability to connect and belong, and so many systems of oppression and prejudice deeming some bodies "good and normal," and others "bad and weird." My client Devon was unable to get his wife pregnant, for example. He struggled with a lot of body shame and resentment, because he felt like his sterility made him a failure as a man, both in his wife's eyes, and in the eyes of other men, with whom he desperately wanted to feel like he belonged. Another outsider's body insecurity was centered on her Crohn's disease, and many neurodivergent outsiders spend their entire lives feeling like outcasts, losers, or the "wrong kind of people," simply because their brains work a little differently.

Whether an outsider is searching for more connection and belonging, or less disconnection and criticism, their hidden body image purpose always centers on the idea that having the "right kind of body" is the key to getting there. The "right kind of body" can either be a body that makes people include you, like you, and accept you, or it can be a body that prevents people from judging you, laughing at you, excluding you, or abandoning you. Either way, the outsider ends up assigning a hugely inappropriate amount of power and significance to their body: the power to control other people's behavior, the power to protect them from harm, and the power to meet their connection needs. And even though the body doesn't actually *have* the power to do any of these things, the added layers of interpretation and meaning make it impossible for an outsider to see their body with clear or neutral vision.

THE OUTSIDER CASE STUDY: LENNY

Lenny, a nonbinary Reiki practitioner, is the kind of person who will always say yes to a favor, always answer their phone in the middle of the night, and always offer a discount to people who can't afford their services. They're a helper and a fixer, with a huge heart and a big smile. Kind and generous to a fault, Lenny prides themself on always being there to uplift others, but struggles to ask for help or support when *they* need it.

Lenny started coaching with me because they hated their self-identified "super-fat" body, and felt a ton of shame about "letting it get so big." This was true even though their weight had very little to do with their habits or choices—Lenny had always lived in what they called a "small-fat body," until they went through a long stretch of serious medical issues, and ended up on lifesaving medications that caused a significant amount of weight gain. Lenny knew the weight gain was the direct result of their medications, but they still saw it as shameful, and blamed themself for being "lazy and out of control" anyway. The weight gain had led to a significant shift in how people treated Lenny day to day, and without realizing it, they ended up blaming *their body* for everyone else's fatphobic and prejudiced behavior.

Body neutrality is impossible when you believe your body has the power to make people be cruel to you, or that your body is responsible for your marginalization and oppression. Unfortunately, that's exactly what Lenny believed, so despite desperately hoping to find some amount of peace in their fat body, Lenny couldn't imagine *not* hating it. They hated their thighs, hated their belly rolls, hated their fat arms, hated their back fat, and hated, hated, hated their double chins. Lenny longed for a body that "made people be nice to them again," and even felt *guilty* about how the size of their body "brought out the worst in people." They told me they thought most people were "good and kind, deep down," but that something about their body had the power to instantly turn kind, warm, and respectful people cold, critical, patronizing, and hateful. Lenny hated being stared at, judged, criticized, lectured, discriminated against, and harassed for their body size . . . but they felt like it would be *unfair and unkind* to blame the people who did all of these things, because they were just "responding appropriately" to a super-fat body.

"It's my fault," Lenny said. "I'm the one putting them in that position by being so big, and I feel bad about it."

This is very common for outsiders in marginalized bodies like Lenny's. They often have a lifetime of experience being rejected, devalued, excluded, and harmed by society, and they come to believe *society* is right and *they* are wrong. After all, if everyone seems to believe something, doesn't that make it true? Lenny believed *they* were responsible for the exclusionary, unfair, and nasty treatment they received on a daily basis, and even though this was happening subconsciously, it made them hate their body.

As you might have guessed, Lenny's hidden body image purpose was slightly more focused on *avoiding* the pain of disconnection than on *seeking* connection, because it was trying to protect Lenny from the contempt, disrespect, discrimination, harassment, and judgment of others. This subconscious plan was impossible, of course, both because Lenny couldn't actually lose the weight and because their body was never responsible for other people's behavior in the first place.

Now, if it had been possible for Lenny to get their needs for respect, belonging, safety, kindness, and acceptance met in the world without changing their body size, doing so would have been a big part of their path to body neutrality, because it would have helped strip their body of inappropriate power and blame. Unfortunately, however, thanks to our society being so violently anti-fat, doing this wasn't exactly possible, so Lenny had to strip their body of power and significance another way: by learning to stop holding it accountable for other people's cruelty, ignorance, bigotry, and violence.

The truth is that nobody's body has the power to "make" another person hurt, disrespect, or oppress them. The blame for such treatment belongs exclusively to the people perpetuating that harm, and to the system of oppression they're upholding, so Lenny spent the next year or so learning more about anti-fat bias and weight stigma, and getting involved with a community of fat-liberation and anti-oppression activists. The more Lenny learned, the angrier they got about the way fat people are treated in our culture, and with that anger came a shift in whom Lenny held accountable for that treatment. Instead of blaming their body, they started blaming the people causing harm; instead of quietly taking responsibility for everyone else's feelings and actions, Lenny started speaking up and holding other people accountable for their disrespect, bigotry, ignorance, prejudice, and violence.

Through this process, Lenny's body image suffering faded—not because they were being treated any better, but because they no longer assigned their body any role in preventing fatphobic people from enacting fatphobic harm. Eventually, Lenny even came to think of their super-fat body as a sort of vetting system, helping them determine *immediately* whether a person is oppressive and toxic so they can get the hell away from them. Navigating the world in a large body is still difficult and painful, and Lenny is still dealing with a lot of anger. But the difference is that they no longer blame *themself* for the pain they're in, and they no longer feel angry at their body.

COMMON CHARACTERISTICS
AND EXPERIENCES OF THE OUTSIDER

Now that you have an idea of how an outsider's body neutrality journey can play out, let's take a look at some of the patterns, characteristics, and experiences most often seen among outsiders.

They Tend to Be People Pleasers

Many outsiders are people pleasers, which is to say they are extremely motivated to make other people happy, and to avoid upsetting other people, at all costs. They tend to be highly sensitive to any disruptions in a relationship, and the thought of someone being mad at or disappointed in them is often so distressing to the outsider that they'd rather pretend to be whatever the person wants them to be than to risk it.[1]

For the record, I'm actually a bit dubious of the term "people pleaser," because I think it's taken on a very negative connotation in pop psychology and is far too often used to pathologize, blame, or denigrate people. I'm using it here because I know so many people will identify with it, but I want to be clear that I am *never* using this term as a criticism or insult, and I invite you to see it as I do: through a totally neutral lens.

The truth is that folks who are people pleasers learned to be that way for good reason; it's one of the brain's many clever strategies for self-preservation. Trying to make other people happy isn't a random character flaw or weakness, and the folks who do it aren't lacking in courage, strength, or intelligence. Some people struggle to speak up for themselves, advocate for their needs, take up space, or set boundaries because at some point they learned that doing so might cost them the connection we humans all need to thrive.[2] So a people pleaser is simply someone for whom tending to the health and security of their relationships is a bigger priority than tending to themselves. People-pleasing is just a coping strategy, developed to help us secure the connections we need to survive.

The term "people-pleasing" also tends to go hand in hand with other labels, like being *conflict avoidant* or *codependent*, or having an *anxious* (or otherwise insecure) *attachment style*[3]—but again, I too often hear these terms used to stigmatize rather than liberate. I'm mentioning them here for reference, because these terms are popular and there is so much crossover between them, but please remember that all of these coping strategies are morally neutral.

If you identify with any of these strategies or patterns, it's likely that at some point in your life, your need for secure attachment and connection wasn't adequately met. And because our need for secure attachment and connection comes *before* our need for self-actualization and self-expression, you did what you needed to do: change yourself, to do or be whatever you needed to do or be, to make (or keep) your relationships secure.

If a child's caretaker was always busy, for example, or unable to show up fully for whatever reason, then the child might have felt like their needs and emotions were a burden on their caretaker, and they needed to keep them hidden to keep their caretaker happy. If their caretaker demanded the child's attention, affection, or emotional labor, the child might have learned that a relationship is safe only when they're doing what the other person wants them to do, and that being loved and valued is conditional, not innate. And if a child grew up in an erratic or abusive environment, perhaps because their caretaker was dealing with domestic violence, alcoholism, addiction, mental illness, or poverty, the child might have become an expert at reading people's moods, walking on eggshells to make everyone happy and to stay safe.[4] When a person feels like showing up as their whole, unfiltered, three-dimensional selves could cause them to be rejected or abandoned, learning to present themselves in a less authentic way that feels safer is a very clever coping strategy.

We humans are social animals who cannot thrive in isolation, so when a person's attachments and relationships don't feel secure, that person will naturally prioritize the needs of the relationship over their own personal needs.[5] This impulse can even be healthy and adaptive, when used appropriately. For example, I normally voice any grievances to my partner as they occur to me in real time, but if my partner is going through something particularly stressful or painful, I'll bench my thoughts for later and just focus on my partner's feelings and needs. Why? Because the health of the relationship is much more important in that moment than my need for, say, the kitchen to be cleaned.

Prioritizing the needs of my partner over my own needs in a moment like that isn't people-pleasing, it's just part of being in a relationship. We *all* do this, in fact; we're constantly navigating between, and weighing out the urgency of our own needs versus the needs of the people we're in relationships with. It's actually a very useful skill to have, along with knowing how to compromise, read a room, pick up on subtle clues that someone is upset with you, offer care, or anticipate someone's needs. So there's nothing inherently wrong with prioritizing someone else's feelings or needs; the issue for many outsiders is just that their need for secure connection overrides *everything else.*

The outsider has often learned from experience that their own feelings and needs are dangerous and unacceptable and must be kept hidden, or else people will reject, attack, or abandon them. They've learned they can never require someone else to do any labor on their behalf, because that would represent a weird (and unsafe) role reversal in the relationship. The people-pleasing outsider's job is to do the labor on everyone *else's* behalf: the labor of noticing, deciphering, anticipating, supervising, tending to, and taking care of everyone else's feelings and needs. Sadly, this kind of outsider learned that the key to earning someone's love and loyalty is to do and be whatever the person wants them to do and be, and never ask for anything in return.

As heartbreaking as this is to say, experiences like this teach the outsider that their *value* is based on what they can provide to other people, that they are worthy of love only when they "earn" it, and that they don't deserve to have their own feelings or needs. This pushes them even further toward people-pleasing behaviors, like always acting cheerful (no matter how they feel), never saying no to anything, apologizing even when it wasn't their fault, having absolutely no boundaries, performing free emotional labor with no reciprocity, or always bringing baked goods into the office.

Essentially, the people-pleasing outsider is just doing whatever they can to make others happy, avoid being a burden, and keep people from rejecting or abandoning them. (This can include what they *don't* do, too, like never speaking up for themselves, never advocating for their needs, never taking up space, never asking for help, never sharing their true feelings, and never expressing their whole authentic selves.) And while this pattern can show up in any part of life, the outsider is often trying to use their body, consciously or subconsciously, to manage other people's thoughts and feelings, secure their connections, and avoid rejection and abandonment.

With all this going on, the outsider often never even gets to develop a sense of themselves outside of people-pleasing. How could a person come to discover who they are, what they need, or what gives them worth, when they're constantly thinking about other people? There's no space for self-actualization or self-expression, because their constant need to prioritize and secure their relationships overrides their individual and personal needs. In this way, people-pleasing habits can become the outsider's identity, and their ability to make other people happy can become their source of self-worth, making it even more difficult to ever put themselves first.

Given how intensely the outsider holds themselves responsible for other people's feelings and experiences, it probably won't surprise you that the outsider's body image issues tend to focus on the ways in which their body or appearance might be a disappointment to others or give others a negative experience. I had a client once tell me that she felt incredibly guilty that other people had to look at her, because they "deserved" to look at someone thinner and more attractive. She imagined that anyone looking at her would have a negative feeling (like disappointment or disgust), and then get mad at her for ruining their day.

People-pleasing obviously goes a lot deeper than body insecurity, but it *can* play a major role in the outsider's body image suffering, because it encourages a wildly inappropriate amount of meaning and significance to be placed upon their body (and behavior). An outsider who wants to see their body (and themselves) with clear and neutral vision will have a lot of work to do, examining and dismantling their people-pleasing patterns, and cultivating an authentic sense of their own identity and worth.

They Often Identify as Empathic, Emotionally Intelligent, Intuitive, or Highly Sensitive

Nia, a pediatric nurse in her early thirties, told me during our first coaching session that her body image issues were the result of being "extremely intuitive" about what other people think and feel, because she could always tell when someone was judging her. When I asked her how she could know for certain that people were actually judging her if they never said anything, she responded with: "I'm really good at reading people, so to me, it's just obvious. I'll pick up on something subtle, like a facial expression or eye move, and I just know."

Many outsiders, like Nia, seem to self-identify as intuitive, empathic, emotionally intelligent, or highly sensitive, and pride themselves on their ability to figure out what other people are thinking and feeling. And in some ways, they may be right! After all, a lifetime of people-pleasing can help a person get pretty good at reading others. Unfortunately, however, they also seem to consistently overestimate the accuracy of what they can "figure out" through this kind of subtle detective work, and end up creating more problems for themselves.

Because the outsider is so sensitive to the threat of disconnection or abandonment, they often try to figure out what other people are thinking and feeling, using their heightened awareness of the subtle messages being communicated through the other person's body language, vocal tone, facial expressions, word choice, or even punctuation in a text. The ability to do this with any amount of accuracy is a skill, and while it may involve some amount of inborn sensitivity, that's rarely the full story. More often than not, it develops out of necessity, to help a person better predict (and manage) someone else's mood or feelings and avoid getting hurt.

There's no denying that developing extreme sensitivity to other people's feelings is a very useful coping strategy, especially for someone dealing with the unpredictable, erratic, or abusive behaviors of others. Particularly if they grew up with people who communicated through passive-aggression or emotional outbursts, the outsider often needed a way of knowing, moment to moment, whether they were in someone's good graces (and therefore safe) or upsetting them (and therefore in danger). Constantly searching for hints or clues about how people are feeling allowed them to better predict what would happen next, so many outsiders may actually be unusually tuned in to and aware of other people's moods and feelings. But being *tuned in* doesn't make the outsider's interpretations of what they see *correct*. Sometimes, in fact, the exact opposite is true.

Because this hypersensitivity was developed to keep the outsider safe, their interpretations of other people tend to err on the side of negativity. This leads the outsider to regularly misinterpret real signals, and sometimes even to imagine they're seeing signals that aren't there. And accuracy is likely to be even worse when a person feels insecure or distressed, because anxiety makes our brains especially sensitive to negative facial expressions and body language signals. Trying to play detective while feeling anxious will literally make us think we're picking up on neutrality where there was actually positivity, and on negativity where there was actually neutrality.[6] So despite the outsider's confidence in their own people-reading accuracy, they're disproportionately likely to think someone doesn't like them when they do, or that someone is mad at them when they're not. Plus, lonely people have been shown to be more critical of the people around them, which leads to a greater feeling of separation and outsiderness, making them then feel even more disconnected, isolated, and lonely.[7]

As you can probably imagine, this leads to a very painful self-perpetuating cycle. The outsider, who has a history of disconnection and is therefore trying to figure out how people feel in order to better secure their connection, interprets what they see as negative and ends up believing everyone is judging, disliking, or mad at them—even if that's not true. This makes the outsider feel even more disconnected, which increases their anxiety, insecurity, loneliness, and desperation to be liked. They decide to work even harder to do or be whatever it is the other person wants, which also means working harder to interpret the other person's mood, thoughts, and feelings. But of course, at this point, the outsider's anxiety makes their interpretations even more negative (sometimes even making them feel like the other person hates them!), and their loneliness makes them start picking the other person apart anyway, ensuring that *no* connection has the possibility to bloom there.

After this, the outsider will often face an even more isolating experience if they try to share their observations and interpretations. If they share them with the person they've been analyzing, for example, they're likely to be met with the person's confusion, denial, defensiveness, or irritation, making the outsider feel incredibly disoriented, panicky, misunderstood, or alone in the world. But even if they share with someone outside the situation, they may still come up against dismissal, invalidation, disinterest, or criticism, making the outsider feel stupid, "crazy," or broken. At the very least, it's disorienting and upsetting to be *so* sure of what you're seeing and then have the other person deny it. This is, after all, what gaslighting feels like.[8]

My client Jayla used to regularly ask her boyfriend what was wrong, because she was *so sure* he was giving out little clues that he was secretly upset, and she just wanted to make it better. He'd be oddly quiet at dinner, for example, or have a grumpy look on his face while watching TV, or wash the dishes in what she considered a hostile manner. Jayla's attention would be completely overtaken by trying to figure out what was wrong, and paying closer attention to her boyfriend's nonverbal signs, until she had gathered enough evidence to be sure: he was angry with her for something she had done earlier.

But Jayla's boyfriend was always bewildered by her assertion that he was upset, and maintained that he was never giving out any secret signals, he was just living his life. He promised her over and over that if he *were* mad at her, he would just tell her. Eventually however, after this dynamic had played on repeat for years, Jayla's boyfriend started actually getting angry when she asked if he was mad, because the question seemed to be a sign that she didn't trust him. Her detective work, which had been intended to help Jayla safeguard and protect her relationship, ended up being completely counterproductive and causing tension between them.

This is a very common experience for the outsider. They'll tell someone the results of their secret detective work, and the other person's response will make them feel confused, ridiculous, broken, stupid, needy, or even more alone. As a result, many outsiders report struggling to trust themselves and their own reality, because it's so often called into question. They might even spend a lot of time and energy replaying such situations, and trying to get to the bottom of it: *Was I making things up, or were they lying?*

This cycle of disconnection and loneliness begetting more disconnection and loneliness is at the heart of why so many outsiders report feeling fundamentally broken, bad, wrong, or unlovable, and why their body ends up taking on so much significance and importance. When you're ashamed of who you are, having the kind of body that makes people like and accept you can almost feel like a bribe, a way of "making up for" the parts of yourself you see as bad and broken.

It also has to be said that the ability to read people is sometimes the result of coming from a family or community culture in which doing the subtextual detective work that Nia described was encouraged and required, rather than one in which verbal directness and transparency were the norm. According to a 2010 article in *The Atlantic* by Alex Eichler—which in part quotes a 2007 response by writer Andrea Donderi to an Ask MetaFilter post—these two cultures have come to be called guess culture and ask culture[9] respectively, and a person's communication style can be greatly influenced by which culture they grew up with.

While there are pros and cons to each communication style, there is an undeniable pattern of outsiders having grown up in guess culture.

But before we dive into why that is, let's first take a moment to understand ask culture.

In ask culture, it's socially acceptable (and even encouraged!) to ask for the things you want, even if the answer might be no. As a result, in this kind of family or cultural dynamic, it's perfectly fine to say no when someone asks you for something you can't or don't want to do. There are no extra rules to follow or labor to be done in ask culture, because everyone is encouraged to be transparent and speak honestly and directly, both when making requests and when accepting or denying requests.

In ask culture, you might ask your friend if you can stay at her place when you visit her city, and she can tell you that it's actually not a good weekend for her, so a hotel would probably be better. You wouldn't be offended, and she wouldn't feel guilty, because both of you are following the rules of ask culture. Plus, if she says yes, you can accept her invitation without any further thought, because you trust that she wouldn't have said yes unless she genuinely meant it.

Does the dynamic of ask culture feel familiar to you? If you're an outsider, it might not. I've even had some outsiders gasp in horror when I describe it, because the thought of everyone just *voicing* their needs and desires all the time, and regularly being rejected, feels so awkward, painful, and dangerous to them. Folks who didn't grow up in ask culture sometimes critique this kind of communication style as aggressive, rude, mean, or even shameful, because it flies in the face of "polite social etiquette."

Now let's take a look at "guess culture." In guess culture, *niceness and politeness* are paramount, and social etiquette exists to uphold a feeling of community warmth and bondedness, which means it's very important to avoid making other people uncomfortable. As a result, you can't ask for something unless you're already almost *positive* the answer will be yes.

Asking for something, without already knowing the person will want to say yes, is a social faux pas in guess culture for serval reasons.

The first is that you risk getting rejected, which is seen as shameful or embarrassing, and would also just suck for you because people in guess culture get very little experience with rejection, and therefore end up with hardly any tolerance or resilience for handling it. Plus, even if the person was polite and apologetic in their rejection, you might also be left wondering if they're secretly mad at you, or if something else is going on, making this rejection a subtextual message you're meant to decipher. The second reason it's a faux pas is that it risks putting the other person in the uncomfortable position of either saying yes when they don't want to say yes (and therefore inconveniencing them), or of saying no, which could be awkward for them, because saying no is considered selfish, rude, and even mean.

In guess culture, asking for something without first knowing what the other person wants to do is like putting the other person in a social trap. There's a lot of social pressure for them to say yes even if they want to say no, which can make a simple question feel more like coercion. By putting in some extra detective work beforehand (through subtly probing questions, dropping hints, or asking around for information), everyone can maintain the veneer of selflessness and pleasantry—but this dynamic also has a way of eroding trust.

If you ask your friend to stay at her place, for example, she might say yes because it's the polite thing to do, even if it's a terrible weekend for her to host someone. And if you and your friend are both coming from guess culture, you might accept her yes, but then worry that she only said it to be polite, and that actually your visit would be a huge burden on her. So you check in multiple times to be sure it's *really* okay before you visit, giving her lots of options to back out without guilt, offering to stay in a hotel instead, and seeking reassurance that she really wants you to come. She then has to reassure you, over and over, that yes she wants you to come—even if she doesn't—because she doesn't want you to feel guilty or unwelcome.

Despite the fact that guess culture is based on the desire for pleasant relationships and generous community support, it can also breed guilt, anxiety, insecurity, inauthenticity, and the feeling of being a burden. *Did they want to say yes, or were they just being polite? What if they wanted to say no, and now they're mad at me for asking? I know they would never speak up for what they need, so I have to identify the problem and then solve it on their behalf.* Guess culture can reinforce the belief that you are responsible for secretly managing the feelings, needs, and experiences of other people, and they are responsible for secretly trying to manage yours.

Guess culture encourages, and even requires, a significant amount of subtextual detective work to fish for information indirectly, to guess what someone else feels or needs, and to avoid social impropriety. It encourages you to imagine that other people should be able to read your mind, anticipate your needs, or know what you're feeling without your communicating it, which sets you up to be constantly disappointed (or to feel unloved) when they don't or can't. It encourages you to spend a lot of time thinking about other people's thoughts, opinions, feelings, and experiences, and tending to their needs and desires instead of to your own. And it encourages distrust between people, because social etiquette is often at odds with a person's truth, leading to a lot of second-guessing and anxiety. When few people in your world directly advocate for their own needs or overtly voice their opinions, your developing a debilitating fear of being a burden, or people secretly judging you, makes *sense*.

All of this is to say that being intuitive, emotionally intelligent, sensitive, and empathic can be wonderful gifts, but overreliance on these qualities causes more problems than they solve. The outsider, for example, might desperately crave reassurance that people still like them and aren't mad at them, but they can't ask for it because they don't want to be rude or needy, and they wouldn't believe the other person if they said yes *anyway*, because social etiquette obligates them to lie. Then when someone else asks the outsider if *they're* upset, the outsider, too, is obligated to lie, which means they can never air what's bothering them or ask for what they need, so their relationships remain less deep, connective, intimate, or nourishing than they wish for.

And that's the ironic tragedy here: often, the outsider is working so hard to connect that they actually keep connection from being possible. Someone who relies on their ability to read subtext, for example, probably won't have developed many other communication and connection skills, and their relationships will suffer for it. They'll end up too preoccupied with their detective work and anxiety to ever be fully present, authentic, or vulnerable with someone, and they'll be too convinced the other person is lying or hiding something to fully trust and receive what they're being offered. Placing too high an emphasis on intuition, empathy, and emotional intelligence actually tends to create roadblocks to connection that rob *everyone* of the ability to build the deep, honest, authentic, and nourishing relationships they crave—and unfortunately, this will only continue to reinforce the outsider's feeling of outsiderness.

Despite these consequences, however, the outsider will often insist that these skills and behaviors are based in kindness, care, generosity, and bigheartedness . . . a belief that reinforces their identity and self-worth as a caretaker or people pleaser, and makes it feel even scarier to give up. But even if the outsider can't imagine a world in which they just said what they felt, asked for what they needed, set boundaries without guilt, or trusted other people to advocate for and manage *their own* needs and feelings, that is exactly the kind of world that encourages, supports, and helps cultivate body neutrality.

They're Terrified of Humiliation

Zaima, an introverted and conventionally attractive artist in her thirties, had spent her entire adult life trying not to "get in trouble," upset anyone, or let anyone down. She was married to a man she loved, considered herself very lucky to not have a nine-to-five job, and took pleasure in creating art for her Etsy shop. But Zaima came to me for coaching because she suffered from ongoing body anxiety, insecurity, and dysmorphia that would spiral into panic and ruin her entire day on a regular basis.

When I asked Zaima why she wanted so badly to look different, she said it was so that nobody would ever judge her. I reflected that people could *still* be judging her, for any number of things, no matter how her body looked, and also that other people's judgment isn't actually dangerous. It might not feel good to find out (or imagine) that someone was judging us, but that judgment doesn't actually mean anything about us, or require any action. So why was Zaima so afraid of other people's hidden thoughts? What power did she imagine they had that it felt so important to keep it from happening?

Eventually Zaima realized she associated people judging her with them talking about her behind her back, which she thought could lead to everyone sort of ganging up on her, and she was terrified of them either publicly blindsiding her in some way, or just deciding to reject and exclude her from the group or community without her knowing. This was an important insight: Zaima wasn't so much afraid of the judgment, but rather of being caught unaware, and publicly humiliated. Every time she imagined everyone coming together as a group to trash-talk her, decide to exclude her, or confront her, it made her want to crawl under her bed and never come out. When I asked what the worst part of this scenario would be, Zaima said it would be the humiliation that she hadn't seen it coming.

Can you see how secretly brilliant it was for Zaima to develop body anxiety? To prevent the unbearable humiliation of not having seen something like that coming, Zaima imagined it every single day. She was constantly criticizing and putting down her body, so that she would never be caught unaware when other people did. By trash-talking her body in her own mind, she'd have "seen it coming" if someone else did it. Constantly picking her body apart made Zaima feel dignified and savvy in a way, secure in the knowledge that she would never play the fool when it came to her appearance. She even said it seemed *dangerous* to ever like how you look, because if you dare to think you look good, especially as a woman, you're setting yourself up to be attacked and humiliated.

It's interesting to me that the words "humility" and "humiliation," which have such opposite connotations, share the etymological root "humilis." Humiliation—a universally negative experience—is about suddenly (and painfully) having other people think less of you, which of course *does* become far more possible if you have an arrogant or inflated sense of your importance or status. The higher you climb, the farther you fall, as the saying goes. Humility, however—a widely respected and even revered quality—is about maintaining a modest (or even low) opinion of oneself. And because humility is the exact opposite of arrogance or inflated importance, it *would* be significantly more difficult to humiliate someone who already has humility, right?

This is the source of a lot of the outsider's body image issues: a subconscious desire to hold themselves in such low regard that nobody else can humiliate them. If you constantly cut yourself down, nobody will ever feel the need to "cut you down to size," and if you never think highly of yourself, nobody can claim you've "gotten too big for your britches," or you "think too much of yourself." This is important for the outsider, who defines their value by their ability to make other people happy and tend to other people's needs. In other words, their worth is based on their selflessness, so any sign of selfishness, ego, or arrogance feels threatening to both their identity and their self-worth. Plus, as Zaima once said, "Already hating yourself means nobody else has the power to knock you down."

Fear of humiliation, especially in response to perceived arrogance, plays a role in many outsiders' body image issues. Sometimes their hidden body image purpose isn't even so much about trying to *change* their bodies as it is about trying to stay aware of all potential threats. A seventeen-year-old I worked with once told me she thought her body-critical voice existed so that if someone ever went up to her and said, "You're disgusting, fat, and ugly!" she would have the dignity of responding with "Yeah . . . I know."

When I asked her why she wouldn't say something like "wow, you are a real jerk," she said it had never even occurred to her. She was more focused on keeping the person who tried to hurt her from having the satisfaction of humiliating her. In this way, hating her body was like reclaiming some power over her pain. *If someone is going to hurt me, it's going to be* me, *damn it!*

This is often the case for outsiders. They abuse themselves to prevent or prepare for abuse from others. And if you've learned that standing up for yourself, advocating for your needs, or setting boundaries is dangerous (or might threaten your relationships), this, too, is a very clever coping strategy. Striving to discover and keep track of all of your "flaws" gives you the opportunity to try to change them or hide them, and therefore prevent criticism, rejection, or humiliation at the hands of abusers and jerks. But if that doesn't work, you can at least learn to make those abusers and jerks more tolerable and predictable by doing their job for them first and robbing them of the element of surprise. This can help restore a feeling of agency and power, make you feel less vulnerable overall, and even possibly make you a less attractive target to abusers, because they won't "get the satisfaction" of watching you be humiliated.

A lot of outsiders are also just exceptionally sensitive to embarrassment and humiliation in general, considering these to be the all-time worst feelings on earth, and doing whatever they can to avoid them. Many even feel intense embarrassment on behalf of other people, cringing with discomfort whenever someone else makes themselves vulnerable to judgment or humiliation, like singing karaoke, publicly trying something new, or dancing when nobody else is dancing. Even if the person doing the thing doesn't seem to be bothered or embarrassed in the slightest, the outsider might still feel wildly embarrassed on the person's behalf. Being so sensitive to these experiences, outsiders in this boat would often rather live in *constant fear of embarrassment* than to occasionally end up embarrassed.

Sometimes this hypersensitivity to embarrassment is the result of having gone through traumatically embarrassing or humiliating experiences that stuck with the person, but in my experience, it's just as often not. The first one makes intuitive sense, because if you've ever been publicly blindsided or humiliated, it's perfectly reasonable that you would develop a hypersensitive alarm system to avoid feeling or facing that again. Often, though, the outsider is just terrified of these emotions and experiences because they represent their biggest fears: social disconnection, exclusion, and isolation.[10] And by spending their lives avoiding it (through people-pleasing, tuning in to other people's feelings, avoiding risks, and keeping their self-regard low), the outsider has never actually gotten the chance to develop any tolerance or resilience for those experiences—which makes them sound all the more terrifying.

This is the position many outsiders find themselves in when it comes to body image. They're terrified of being humiliated or blindsided, and their hidden body image purpose is to prevent or prepare for that (or reclaim some measure of power and dignity), by rejecting, criticizing, disapproving of, and hating every inch of their bodies first.

They Blame Themselves (and Their Bodies) for Everything Bad That Happens to Them

At some point or another, *everyone* will feel disliked, judged, criticized, rejected, erased, excluded, and abandoned. The more marginalized identities a person has, the more often these experiences are likely to occur,[11] but *nobody* gets to completely skip them altogether. That's probably why the outsider seems to have less privilege, on average, than the self-objectifier or high achiever—but it also highlights the unique way that the outsider tends to respond to these moments.

The outsider is used to taking responsibility for other people's feel-ings and behaviors, so when these experiences happen, they don't tend to blame the person who caused them harm. Instead, they blame them-selves or their bodies, taking all the negative feelings they had about the experience and turning them inward. If they were bullied for how they look, for example, they turn their anger and disgust toward their body for "attracting bullying," instead of toward the bully. Instead of getting angry at the system of oppression that marginalizes them, they get angry at themselves for somehow "deserving it." They think of all the ways they could have worked harder to prevent it, and sometimes even feel bad for "making the other person" do the harmful thing.

In this way, the outsider imagines that every bad thing that ever hap-pened to them was their fault. Probably because holding other people accountable for their behaviors would involve self-advocacy, taking up space, demanding labor, and facing the potential for conflict or aban-donment, the outsider tends to feel much more comfortable holding themselves accountable instead. They still feel all the anger, disgust, shame, outrage, or grief about the situation, but because they can't dir-ect any of it outward toward the person who caused them harm, they direct it inward instead, toward themselves and their bodies.

Like Lenny, from the beginning of this chapter, many outsiders come to blame their bodies for every single painful moment of criti-cism, harassment, discrimination, humiliation, and violence that has ever been aimed at them. And especially for those in marginalized bodies, through enough experiences of feeling like their body was at-tracting danger or getting them hurt, the outsider subconsciously re-casts their body from the role of a neutral companion or friend to the role of an evil or villainous enemy. The outsider themselves might only be aware that they feel anger, disgust, shame, outrage, or grief toward or about their bodies, however, and not even realize they've been interpreting these moments of harm as their body's fault, or hold-ing it accountable for other people's actions. Luckily, though, once an outsider can identify exactly what they've been blaming their body for, the whole story starts to lose power.

Cameron, a smart and successful lawyer in her late fifties, lost her mother to breast cancer when she was nine years old. She consciously knew that her mother's cancer had nothing to do with her, but during our work together, it became clear that she had a subconscious association between body size and abandonment. Right around the time she gained weight (her body's healthy way of preparing for adolescence), her mother died; these two experiences had become linked.

Cameron never blamed herself for her mother's death on any kind of conscious level, but she felt that her weight was something she needed to meticulously control to avoid ending up abandoned and alone. This deep subconscious link between weight and abandonment meant that whenever Cameron thought about giving up dieting, a massive surge of grief and panic seemed to rise up out of nowhere, and stop her. (Note: this is a great example of how the body neutrality journey can reveal a need for professional mental health care!)

Through our work together, and Cameron's work with a trauma-informed therapist, she was finally able to recognize the link between these two experiences, unpack her tangled beliefs, and release some long-held shame. She was finally able to see that her body had never actually done anything wrong. Her obsession with her weight and hatred of her body had essentially been the self-preservation strategy of a nine-year-old who missed her mother and didn't want to be abandoned again. After finding forgiveness for her body, Cameron also realized she owed it a huge apology, because it had been not only her mother who "abandoned" Cameron when she died, but also *Cameron* who had abandoned herself and her body.

As damaging as this is to our body image, blaming ourselves and our bodies for bad things that happen to us comes with a lot of perceived benefits too. It lets us completely absolve the other party of any blame, anger, or criticism, for example, which is very helpful if we're trying to reconcile the harm someone caused us with our love for them, or maintain a conflict-free relationship. Our bodies can stand in as a scapegoat for our suffering when we need one, and blaming them for making bad things happen can even give us a false sense of power and control over the situation. After all, if we're the problem, then we can also be the solution. If Cameron's mother died because Cameron gained weight, then at least she would know how to prevent that from ever happening again. So misguided or not, blaming their body for bad things that happen to them can offer the outsider a feeling of empowerment, hope, and even safety.

Do you see the absolute genius, and the extraordinary heartbreak, of this plan? We do whatever we need to do to survive, and blaming ourselves (or our bodies) for relationship ruptures, hurt, and harm done to us can be a very clever survival strategy.[12] Unfortunately, it leads a lot of outsiders to live in a fantasy world in which they (or their bodies) have the power to actually prevent bad things from happening in the first place.

With such a belief system in place, it makes sense that the outsider would feel so much negativity, anxiety, obsession, or dysphoria about their body. They associate their body with danger and harm, hold their body accountable for other people's feelings and behavior, subconsciously assign their body the task of preventing bad things from happening to them, and then blame it when bad things happen anyway. And as you can probably guess by now, all this inappropriate and false significance, meaning, and power placed on the body make it completely impossible for the outsider to see themselves with anything even close to body neutrality.

They're Often Seeking *Permission* to Be (and Express) Their Authentic Selves

When the outsider imagines how life would be if they had the "right kind of body," they tend to imagine life would be easy and wonderful—they'd avoid hurtful social experiences and have many intimate, authentic, and secure connections and relationships. Part of that fantasy is that, once their body is "right," they would finally feel safe enough in their relationships to let their true selves take up space. They imagine they would finally stop feeling so afraid of rejection or abandonment, and be able to focus on themselves for once: What do *they* like? What do *they* need? What do *they* think and feel?

Having spent a lifetime tending to others, the outsider often has no idea who they are deep down, but they're dying for an opportunity to find out. Self-actualization may have been on the back burner for decades while they try to nail down the feeling of relational security, but the plan was never to abandon themselves forever. We all crave a secure and intimate connection with ourselves, and it's extremely uncomfortable and unsettling to feel like we don't know ourselves at all.[13] So underneath all their efforts to secure connection with *others*, the outsider is often seeking permission to finally connect with *themselves*. Underneath the pursuit to blend in, they're often just waiting for someone to tell them they've finally "earned" the ability to be unique.

It's almost as if, in the outsider's mind, there were a video game–esque parameter for life, in which you have to beat the first level before progressing to the second. You can't move on to the "standing out" level until you first beat the "fitting in" level. You won't be granted access to the "self-actualization" level until you've properly won at the "people-pleasing" level. So the outsider paradoxically tries to get their need for individuality met by first seeking conformity; they seek permission to focus on themselves by first focusing on everyone else.

This may sound a little silly, but it actually makes perfect sense when we consider how attachment theory works. As babies, we develop attachment to others before we do anything else. Our sense of identity and self is developed within the container of those early attachment relationships. Put another way, we learn who we are through the eyes of our attachment figures before even considering who we are through our own eyes. Children require secure attachment to feel safe going off and exploring the world on their own, because they need to know someone will be there to comfort and care for them if they get hurt, which is why toddlers will do a sort of back-and-forth dance between independence and neediness. In this way, secure attachment *is* a literal prerequisite to the development of individuality.

As adults, we sometimes still prioritize the security of our attachments and relationships over our individuality, especially if we didn't get the secure attachments we needed when we were younger.[14] If an outsider feels their relationships are constantly insecure or under threat, they will naturally spend all their time and energy trying to nail those down first, in the hopes that once those feel secure and safe, they can then go off and develop, explore, and express their identity, individuality, and independence. The subconscious hope is that by doing whatever it takes to make other people happy, they'll secure the social acceptance and belonging they crave, and then finally be free to figure out who the hell they themselves are, and what would make *them* happy.

There is another unmet need lurking underneath even this one, though, and that's the need for authentic self-expression. We humans are wired with a deep need to feel seen, heard, and known, and that can't happen if we're never expressing our authentic self to others. (Granted, it's rather difficult to express our authentic selves when we don't even *know* our authentic selves, so a good amount of self-exploration tends to come first here.)

As adults, authentic self-expression is actually a prerequisite to meaningful bonding; we require some amount of it to feel connected to other people in the first place.[15] This makes sense—imagine trying to get to know someone who was fake, superficial, guarded, repressing their own feelings and needs, or just always trying to say and do what they think you want to hear or see. How easy would it be for you to form a deep and meaningful bond with this person? And what are the odds that, no matter how kind and patient and interested you are, this person would ever end up feeling seen by, accepted by, and connected to you?

If we're too busy trying to figure out what other people think, manage their feelings, avoid conflict, and be whatever they want us to be, then we never get to express anything remotely authentic in our relationships, and then we never feel like we're being truly seen, heard, or known. Even if the other person adores us under these circumstances, we probably won't fully receive it or internalize it, because it isn't really *us* that they're adoring. There's a missing element of vulnerability and honesty that blocks true intimacy in this situation, and makes the outsider feel even more isolated, insecure, and alone.

So on top of seeking permission to focus on and get to know themselves, the outsider is also seeking permission to express that self to others, and have it held, accepted, and loved. It's like they're hoping that by having the right body, and being what people want, they will finally be allowed to let people see who they truly are. Underneath their desire to fit in, the outsider wants to feel seen, known, and understood, and for their connections to feel genuine and meaningful.

This ends up being a bit of a trap for the outsider, who imagines they first have to master the "be what everyone wants" level, to progress to the "authentic self-expression" level. Expressing our truth to someone, and having it be witnessed, accepted, and loved, is what makes our relationships feel deep, intimate, and secure,[16] but the outsider is waiting for their relationships to feel deep, intimate, and secure enough *before* they're willing to express their truth. As a result, they end up stuck and unhappy with their current level, but unable to level up.

This is another reason the outsider feels as if there was "something wrong with them." They spend their entire lives looking around and seeing how easy it seems to be for other people to form deep, intimate, and secure relationships, while struggling to do the same. They observe other people embracing their unique weirdness without apology, embodying and expressing their full authentic selves, and letting their freak flags fly. They may even become fixated on such people, involuntarily drawn to them, while also facing big emotions like jealousy, confusion, admiration, or awe in their presence.

There's nothing wrong with the outsider, of course, and it makes perfect sense that they would end up in this situation; they've just gotten the order of events backward. The outsider has been seeking permission to be and express their authentic selves by first building secure relationships and belonging, when actually, being and expressing their authentic selves is the *key* to building secure relationships and belonging.

The outsider has assigned their body the job of earning them enough secure connections that they finally have permission to explore and express themselves, but that day never comes; without first knowing and sharing their true selves, their connections will never quite feel secure enough. This leads the outsider to then blame their body for standing in the way of everything they dream of, and everything they most desire. With so much false significance, meaning, and power assigned to the body, the outsider ends up with rich and fertile ground for body anxiety, preoccupation, negativity, dysmorphia, and hatred to grow.

Objectively speaking, the outsider's body plays no role whatsoever in getting their need for meaningful connection met, or in avoiding painful disconnection. There's not a single body on earth that can make up for a person's lack of authentic self-awareness and self-expression in a relationship. There's not a single body on earth that can make a person invulnerable to judgment, rejection, humiliation, or abandonment either. And there's not a body on earth that can make the vulnerable and scary work of self-discovery and self-expression feel safer or easier. Bodies are, frankly, just not that powerful.

Luckily, a body doesn't have the power to *block* any of this either. If the outsider is looking for permission to be themselves, they can give themselves that permission in any shape or size body. Self-permission is an inside job, just like self-approval, self-worth, and self-love. Only the outsider themselves can grant it.

If the outsider wants to connect with others on that deepest and most intimate level, they'll have to stop trying to be what other people want, and instead grant themselves permission to first figure out, and then show people, who they truly are. And if they want to feel truly accepted, appreciated, and like they belong, they will have to grant themselves permission to be polarizing, and be rejected, in service of finding their people. After all, *nobody* is universally liked and accepted, so once an outsider starts showing up in the world with more authenticity and vulnerability, and refusing to hold themselves accountable for everyone else's feelings, some people probably will reject them. But others will get really freakin' excited about them, and *those* relationships will be the ones to eventually make the outsider feel truly and deeply seen, accepted, and loved, as well as providing the mutual trust, depth, belonging, intimacy, and security they've been chasing for so long. And when that happens, the body is stripped of its excess significance and power, and can finally go back to just being a body.

THE OUTSIDER'S NEXT STEPS

Just like the other avatars, the outsider's path to body neutrality requires them to figure out how their body image issues have been trying to help them. If the outsider resonates with you, start by considering whether your body image issues seem to center more on trying to earn something, or trying to avoid something, and what that specific "something" might be. What role have you "assigned" to your body when it comes to connection, acceptance, or belonging? How about when it comes to rejection, criticism, humiliation, or abandonment?

The last part of the book will teach you how to identify your specific hidden body image purpose, so don't worry if you still have no idea. For now, just try answering the following questions.

- What problem are you hoping to solve by having the "right" kind of body?

- What are you most afraid of, about having the "wrong" kind of body?

- What is the purpose of making people happy or making them like you?

- What might you have been subconsciously blaming your body for?

- What might you really be seeking or hoping for when you're trying to fit in, be what people want, or manage people's emotions?

CHAPTER 11

The Runner

THE RUNNER IS FOCUSED ON USING their body—along with body image behaviors and body image suffering itself—just to survive. They tend to use body control and other behaviors to cope with pain, stay numb or distracted, feel in control, armor themselves against vulnerability, or avoid their inner self.

PATTERNS OFTEN SEEN AMONG RUNNERS:

+ They're nearly always trying to avoid, ignore, or repress something that lives deep inside them, whether it's their emotions, needs, desires, pain, sexuality, vulnerability, or intuition. That is to say the thing they're most terrified of, and running from, is almost always *themselves*.

+ They're highly anxious, and try to control everything (especially their bodies), because control makes them feel safer.[1]

+ They've learned their emotions and desires are bad, shameful, or dangerous and must therefore be kept hidden, pushed down, avoided, numbed, or strictly controlled to stay safe.

- They struggle with vulnerability, often finding it very difficult to trust other people or let them get too close.

- They tend to find deep intimacy overwhelming and uncomfortable, sometimes even pushing people away or sabotaging relationships to avoid it.

- They often struggle with what they call "self-destructiveness" or "self-sabotage," referring to behaviors that go directly against their goals but that they can't seem to stop or control.

- They have a variety of numbing and coping behaviors to help them stay distracted, avoid their feelings, push down their truth, or dull their pain. Some of these relate to the body (e.g., dieting, exercising, bingeing) and some don't (e.g., alcohol, porn, endless scrolling on social media).

- They feel disconnected from their bodies, and sometimes even totally numb, which makes the advice to "listen to your body" very confusing and difficult for them.

- They may be disconnected from their emotions, too, unable to identify or talk about what they're feeling in any given moment.

- They tend to have a history of trauma, which is to say, at some point in their lives, the stress or distress they experienced overwhelmed their mind and body's ability to adequately cope with it. (Sometimes this even causes them to dissociate from their bodies, which can play a role in their disconnection from it later on.)

- Because vulnerability and trust are difficult for the runner, they often develop a kind of hyper-independence, trying to never rely on people, and just doing everything themselves instead.

- They rarely have a strong relationship to their intuition or inner wisdom, leading to a lot of stress and confusion when making decisions.

- They seem to always be sure, on some level, that facing or feeling whatever it is they've been running from would kill them. They are, subconsciously, running for their lives.

THE RUNNER'S HIDDEN BODY IMAGE PURPOSE

The runner seems to always be living in fear (even if they're not consciously aware of what they're afraid of), and always trying to avoid pain (even if they're not consciously aware of what hurts). Their body image issues exist to help them solve one or both of these problems—to either help them feel safer and less vulnerable, or to help them avoid (or cope with) whatever is hurting them. The exact details of the runner's hidden body image purpose can vary widely, but there is always fear or pain (and often the fear *of* pain!) at the heart of it.

The runner is trying to avoid or escape something. Very occasionally it's an external source of danger or pain that they're running from, like a person who wants to look different to avoid their partner's abuse, but that kind of purpose and motivation is generally better represented by the outsider. Instead, the runner is nearly always running from a source of pain or perceived danger that lives *inside themselves*. Maybe they consider their deepest desires too vulnerable and scary, for example, or maybe they don't think they would survive it if they let themselves fully feel and face the depth of their grief, anger, or need. Maybe they don't feel capable of fully facing the little voice inside them telling them something needs to change.

Either way, the runner is usually running from some deep-down part of themselves that feels too big, too scary, too out of control, too painful, or too dangerous to be allowed. They don't have the skill, resources, or capacity to deal with that part of themselves directly (or at least, they don't *think* they do), so they just try to avoid it, repress it, numb it, escape it, control it, or defend against it. And as it turns out, body image issues provide the runner with about a million opportunities to do exactly that. There are so many ways to distract yourself when it comes to the body, and so many options for numbing, controlling, and armoring. Body image issues offer the runner endless opportunities to feel safer.

It's important to note here that it's generally the feeling of being safer that the runner is chasing, not the actual safety itself. Actual safety tends to be largely impossible (given that the thing they've deemed dangerous lives inside them), so it's more the *feeling* of being protected, or at least less vulnerable, that they seek. And while that might sound silly, it's actually something we all do!

When I had to get a very painful procedure done in my twenties, I was so anxious about it that I wore heavy black lipstick and eyeliner to the appointment. My makeup obviously had zero effect on the actual procedure, but it gave me the *feeling* of wearing battle armor. When I looked in the mirror that day, I saw someone tough, strong, and capable of handling anything. I was still scared, and the procedure still hurt, but I honestly think the makeup helped me get through it.

Many runners are doing a similar thing, using diet, exercise, skin care, hair, makeup, clothing, or body language to give themselves the feeling of being safer, stronger, or less vulnerable. They may also try to exert control over their bodies, in the hopes of both developing a certain (supposedly safer) aesthetic, and of controlling, repressing, or numbing the scary thing inside them.

If a runner is scared of their sexuality, for example, they might be able to successfully suppress their libido with a very restrictive diet and too much exercise. If they're terrified of their own emotions, they might be able to avoid them by obsessively tracking calories all day instead. If they're feeling too vulnerable before an event, they might be able to avoid it by instead having a meltdown about how fat they look in all their clothes. If they're trying to ignore the little voice whispering, "This isn't right," they might be able to stuff it down each night with food.

The runner's body image thoughts, feelings, behaviors, and even the pain of body image suffering *itself* can all form a part of their avoidance and survival strategy. They're rarely consciously aware of this hidden body image purpose, though, and unlikely to know they're running from *anything*, let alone how their body image issues are trying to help them do it. Most runners just know that they hate their bodies, they feel "out of control" in their bodies, and they just prefer to look a certain way. These statements are true, but they don't represent the whole story. But this is the whole point: the runner never actually lets themselves see the whole story, because seeing the whole story would mean seeing all of *themselves*, and they're far too afraid of themselves to do that.

Body image suffering can sometimes function as the runner's cover story, justifying the many ways they numb, hide, distract, ignore, protect, or avoid themselves. For this reason, the runner can come to actually rely on their body image issues to survive and feel safe, even if they also make them miserable. (This is why the runner tends to "self-sabotage" too! No matter how badly a runner consciously wants something, their subconscious mind is always, "I'm not letting that happen, it would kill you!") The very *existence* of body hatred is what the runner is attached to in this case, because it gives the runner permission to keep engaging in the thoughts, feelings, behaviors, and coping strategies they believe they need to survive. For this reason, the runner is often very attached to the added meaning, significance, and power they've assigned to their body, and resistant to letting it go, even when they know doing so is the only way to make body neutrality possible.

THE RUNNER CASE STUDY: AALIYAH

Aaliyah came from a family where nobody talked about feelings, ever. She told me that her parents were good people, but they were busy, and practical, and never understood why she seemed to need so much or feel so much. She had a pretty "uneventful" childhood,[2] in her words, and didn't have her first taste of heartbreak until she was twenty-four, when her fiancé, whom she had been with since she was sixteen, died in a car accident. The other driver had been drunk, and her fiancé had been completely sober, coming home from work.

The scope and senselessness of this tragedy, and the sheer horror of realizing everything could be taken away from her in a flash, completely destroyed Aaliyah's life. She told me that the next few years were a blur of crushing grief and severe depression, and that when she started to come out of it and rebuild her life, she noticed she seemed to have a lot more walls up and found it difficult to connect to herself or others. When she eventually started dating again, she struggled to trust anyone, be vulnerable, and let anyone get close to her. Despite someone seeming "perfect on paper," at some point Aaliyah always started nitpicking, or losing interest. She moved to a new city, and fell out of touch with the high school friends she had shared with her fiancé. Her new friends were people from work, who seemed most comfortable talking about reality TV, gossiping about people they knew, sharing the details of their new diet or exercise plan, and body bashing.

When I met Aaliyah, she was thirty-six and had spent what she described as "a truly disturbing amount of time and energy" thinking about her body and appearance. She never quite stuck with a health or fitness routine, but would sometimes eat healthy and do yoga every day for a few weeks before falling off the wagon and going months eating takeout and lying on the couch. She hated how she looked but could never seem to keep up the momentum or motivation needed to change it. As a result, Aaliyah spent a lot of time criticizing her body in the mirror, feeling frustrated and out of control, and being too insecure about her appearance to go on dates or out with friends.

While exploring how her body image issues were trying to help her, Aaliyah first thought she wanted to look better to fit in with her appearance-focused friends and coworkers. But she didn't seem to connect much with those people, and had never given me the impression that she cared much what they thought. Why try to earn their approval, then? "Maybe to keep me busy," Aaliyah finally said. But busy from what?

As we dug deeper, several deep and painful insights emerged.

The first was that Aaliyah had never received the proper care and support she needed after the loss of her fiancé. Her family didn't talk about feelings, so not only were her parents unable to offer her adequate support as she grieved, but she also hadn't been taught the skills needed to properly process the experience. After the first few months, everyone seemed to expect her to be back to normal, so she tried to just shove everything down and ignore it. Aaliyah felt like there was something wrong with her for not being able to get over it faster and for still being messed up by something that had happened so long ago, but all that grieving was still stuck inside her, unnamed and unhealed, because she hadn't had the language, tools, resources, or skills to deal with it back then. Nobody had been there to normalize and validate her experience, or recommend she get the support she needed from a therapist, grief group, or medication. Her ability to cope had been thoroughly overwhelmed by the pain of her loss, and she had been left to deal with it completely alone.

By developing a fixation on food, weight, exercise, and her body's "flaws," Aaliyah had been able to keep her mind busy, which helped her avoid thinking about the unbearably dark stuff that lived in the corners of her mind. Thinking about food and her body provided a distraction from her grief, her anger, her shame, and her feelings of helplessness and despair. Unsurprisingly, her body-critical thoughts always seemed to be the loudest and most urgent when she got home from work, between 6:00 and 9:00 p.m., because those were the hours with no other distractions available. Aaliyah's body fixation was most present during her quiet moments alone, because that's when she needed the most protection from the grief and pain that lurked below the surface of her mind.

The second thing that emerged for Aaliyah as we worked together was that she had closed her heart off after the accident and never again let herself be vulnerable with someone. Her fiancé had been her best friend, the person Aaliyah told everything to, and the only person who she felt understood her. Her fiancé's death caused Aaliyah to build up walls to protect herself from ever feeling pain like that again, and to decide (subconsciously, of course) that letting someone into her heart like that again just wasn't worth the risk.

This led Aaliyah to push people away, and to bail if they started to get too close. She dated casually but was quick to break it off if it got too serious, and she allowed herself only superficial friends who engaged in superficial conversations. "Better to talk about reality TV and the latest diet craze than to go deep, get vulnerable, and risk getting too attached," she joked. But with this new insight, Aaliyah was able to finally acknowledge that she was *deeply* lonely, and that even though the thought of letting someone in was scary, she was *starved* for intimacy and connection.

Aaliyah's body image issues had been helping her in so many ways. By feeling too insecure about how she looked to go on dates or out with friends, she could successfully avoid building close relationships with anyone or risking falling in love again. When she *did* go out with people, she was too distracted by thoughts about her body to be present or connect. And the endless project of berating her body, planning to change her body, and then feeling guilty when she couldn't stick to her plan kept Aaliyah's mind constantly occupied so she never had to feel or face the deep well of pain she was running from.

Aaliyah's hidden body image purpose was at least twofold: it was trying to protect her from vulnerability (and therefore from the potential risk of future heartbreak), and it was helping numb and distract her from the unprocessed heartbreak that still lived deep inside her. Her body image issues were making her miserable, insecure, and lonely . . . but because she didn't believe she could survive facing heartbreak (new or old), she clung to them for survival.

To release these huge blocks to body neutrality, Aaliyah had to build the skills, resources, and capacity to face, feel, and process her vulnerability, pain, and heartbreak directly, without protection or distraction. But because there was so much standing in the way of her ability to do that, Aaliyah had to spend the better part of *three years* working on it: reconnecting with her body; processing her old grief; learning to identify, feel, and share her emotions; practicing vulnerability; connecting with her intuition; creating a mindfulness practice; improving self-trust; and cultivating a sense of resilience in the face of heartbreak.

During the first year of our work together, Aaliyah's body image issues didn't change one bit, and she sometimes doubted the process entirely. But the further into the journey we got, and the more of those new skills she acquired, Aaliyah found herself slowly thinking about her body less often, and feeling less upset when she did. Within three years, she reported spending most of her time in a state of body neutrality, and that body-negative thoughts and feelings would emerge only when she felt especially vulnerable about something. But by that point, Aaliyah knew exactly what was going on when that happened, and had all the tools and skills she needed to face her vulnerability directly, so even those thoughts and feelings no longer had the power to cause suffering.

COMMON CHARACTERISTICS AND EXPERIENCES OF THE RUNNER

Now that you have a sense of how the runner's body image journey can play out, let's explore some of the patterns, characteristics, and experiences that many runners have in common.

Control Makes Them Feel Safe

We humans are naturally drawn to control, because control makes us feel safer. When we "feel in control," we're confident in our ability to have an impact on the outcome of things, which makes us feel more optimistic and hopeful, boosts our self-image, gives us a sense of purpose, and makes the future seem more predictable and certain. Believing we have this kind of control over our lives feels good; studies have even shown that people who feel like their actions have an impact on future outcomes at work tend to be much happier, and mentally healthier, than those who don't.[3] Feeling in control is also very reassuring, because it means we're not under the control of someone else—it means we're *free* (rather than subjugated), which is a requirement for us to thrive.

While a desire for this kind of control is perfectly healthy and natural, I'm not sure the word "control" is accurate or specific enough. What we're lumping together into the category of "control" would probably be better broken down into a person's individual needs for self-determination, self-efficacy, agency, autonomy, purpose, freedom, and independence. Those are all inborn emotional needs that we require to thrive: the belief that our actions have an impact, that we're free to make our own decisions, that we have a reason for existing, and that our lives (and bodies) are our own.[4] But that's not always where our desire for control stops, is it?

The runner, for example, often feels like they need to control *everything*—not just because they're searching for a sense of their own efficacy, meaning, or liberty, but because control is one of their main tools for feeling safe in a world where they constantly feel unsafe. They'll often say things like "I'm a control freak" or "I have a hard time letting go" or "I'd rather just do everything myself" and then try to control things that are far outside their scope of responsibility (or possibility) to control, like other people's behavior, the exact details of how everything gets done, their health, or the passing of time.

But why is this? Why do some people cross over from the human need for self-determination, self-efficacy, agency, autonomy, purpose, freedom, and independence into a place where they feel the need to control everything? And why is the runner so terrified of feeling *out* of control?

In order to understand those questions, we must remember that, while none of us were born with an innate need to control everything, we *were* all born with an innate need to feel safe, and that in order to feel safe, we need to believe our basic needs will be met. Unfortunately, many people grew up in situations that taught them the exact opposite: their basic physical and emotional needs won't be met, and therefore they're not safe.[5] Under such circumstances, when the thing we need isn't available, we naturally start looking for substitutes. Feeling in control can sometimes function as a useful substitute for feeling safe in this way: a sort of replacement or alternative that we can call upon when the real thing is unavailable.

From that perspective, the runner's need to control everything starts to make sense. But it doesn't stop there. Control can also function as a substitute for other emotional needs, like power, which is especially gratifying for anyone who has felt helpless, powerless, or subjugated, and productivity, which can stand in for a feeling of meaningful forward progress, or a full life. Plus, if someone has been chronically unable to get their needs for self-determination, self-efficacy, agency, autonomy, purpose, freedom, or independence sufficiently met, they might overcorrect (as we often do after such scarcity) by pursuing an excess or overabundance of power and control.

As you can see, control can be a useful substitute for a variety of emotional needs and stand in for a lot. The runner may be drawn to control, then, both because it offers them an alternative way to get some of their underlying needs met, and because they always feel like danger is right around the corner. Controlling everything can offer runners a (false) feeling of safety, or just help them cope with the stress of feeling chronically unsafe.

With all of this in mind, it shouldn't come as a surprise that the runner hates to feel *out* of control. They hate feeling vulnerable and often find it intolerable to surrender control to someone else (or even just to the universe!), because it feels too scary and dangerous, and requires a level of trust they can't muster. They would prefer to do everything themselves rather than allow someone else to have all the power, and they find it nearly impossible to just let go and surrender, whether they're working on a group project, having sex, doing housework, or even just riding in a car with someone.

Feeling "out of control" is the runner's most common and most distressing complaint with respect to their lives in general, but even more so when it comes to their bodies. On a particularly bad body image day, the runner might beat themselves up for letting their body get so out of control, or express a burning need to get it *under* control. They tend to think of their bodies as insubordinate and unruly children, as if the body's "bad behavior" were the result of being allowed too much agency, freedom, or power and must therefore be met with stricter rules and a firmer hand. This of course implies that the body has a will of its own, along with nefarious intentions, which isn't true, but it represents how the runner sees their body: like an unmanageable adversary in need of taming or conquering.

This view of the body, combined with an overall need for control, leads the runner to develop a rather authoritarian, if not outright tyrannical, relationship with their body. There are an infinite number of body control behaviors the runner can call upon, from dieting and exercising, to taking supplements and adopting a nine-step daily skin care routine, to feel like they're getting their body "under control." Many of these behaviors provide the runner with an immediate feeling of safety, comfort, agency, power, purpose, productivity, or relief, which makes them incredibly useful coping and self-soothing tools.

These types of behaviors are intrinsically rewarding and self-perpetuating—sometimes even taking on a compulsive or addictive quality—because they provide the runner with that instant hit of good feelings. So the runner often ends up both obsessed with the concept of getting their body "under control" *and* heavily reliant on the various body control behaviors they use to numb, cope, and feel better.

Just because the runner is obsessed with getting their body "under control," however, doesn't mean they actually succeed. Certainly some do, but for many runners, the harder they try to crack down and control the body, the more out of control they feel. This often happens because they're trying to force their body into unhealthy or unsustainable behaviors, like a crash diet that leads to bingeing, or an intense daily workout habit that ends up getting them injured. It also sometimes happens because the runner subconsciously relies just as much on their "out-of-control behaviors" as they do on their "in-control behaviors," for the hits of the comfort, coping, or relief they crave. That is to say, some part of the runner might believe they actually *need* behaviors like bingeing, zoning out with their phone or TV, using substances, nail biting, skin picking, hair pulling, or always being busy, to survive.

Unaware of their hidden purpose, the runner perceives these "out-of-control" behaviors as acts of self-sabotage, confirmation of their weakness, or proof that they actually *are* shamefully out of control. For many runners, however, arriving at the outcome they think they want—a "totally under-control body"—would be far too dangerous for their brain to ever allow it, because that would mean they no longer had a justification for, or access to, the various behaviors they rely on to cope and feel safe. That's why the runner will often vacillate wildly between periods of strict control and periods of being totally out of control, when it comes to their bodies.

The truth is that our brains and bodies don't handle oppression very well, even if (and perhaps especially if!) we are trying to be our *own* oppressors. The harder we try to control our bodies, the more our bodies push back: food restriction leads to bingeing, overexercising leads to illness or injury, and pushing ourselves too hard leads to burnout. Plus, regularly forcing ourselves to do things we don't want to do, like over-exercising or eating salads exclusively, tends to make us hate that thing, which makes us need even *more* self-control and discipline to get ourselves to keep doing it.[6]

This cycle reinforces the runner's belief that discipline and willpower are the only things keeping their body from spiraling cata-strophically out of control, and that obviously they just need *more* willpower, *more* discipline, and *more* self-control to get their body where they want it. Eventually, though, those resources just run out. When they do, the runner slips up, falls off the wagon, or quits—which of course makes them feel like failures, berate themselves for their weakness, or spiral into shame and self-loathing. And all this shame and blame just makes the runner want to crack down on their body even harder.

In short, the worse and more out of control a runner feels, the harder they try to control themselves, and the harder they try to control them-selves, the worse and more out of control they feel. But they'll still try to control everything anyway (especially their body), because they sub-consciously rely on those control behaviors to meet so many of their needs, to cope, and to survive.

They Are Masters of Numbing and Escaping

Whatever it is the runner is running from, they are highly motivated to shut it up, push it down, and get the hell away from it. Whether it's emotions, sexuality, hunger, vulnerability, or pain that the runner doesn't feel capable of facing or feeling, they develop a vast arsenal of tools, behaviors, strategies, and habits for numbing, escaping, or avoid-ing it.

Seeking out ways to avoid being present in our bodies or lives isn't exclusively a runner thing, of course. Most of us find ourselves escap-ing the present moment on a regular basis, through things like phone scrolling, alcohol, video games, porn, or constant busyness.[7] It's a movie trope for someone to eat an entire container of ice cream after they get dumped, because being stuffed full of fat and sugar helps tem-porarily numb the pain of heartbreak, and many of us now bring our phones with us into the bathroom to avoid even two or three minutes of sitting alone with our thoughts. But while the habit of numbing and escaping our inner selves isn't unique to the runner, it does tend to *be particularly dialed up* for them.

One big reason for this seems to be that the runner is so afraid of vulnerability, and struggles so much to trust people, that they try to go at life alone, without relying on other people for anything (understandably so, as many runners seem to have a history of neglect, and therefore learned that nobody else was going to come through for them when they were in need). But we humans are communal animals, and our nervous systems are wired to find comfort, security, and support in our relationships. When we feel stressed, sad, overwhelmed, lonely, or scared, connecting with another person (either physically or emotionally) can quickly help us feel calmer, safer, and better.[8]

But the runner often doesn't feel safe seeking out that kind of comfort or support, because they would feel far too vulnerable to, say, ask to be held while they cry. As a result, they miss out on our most potent tools for regulating the nervous system and feeling better, and have to rely instead on tools that allow the runner to be totally self-sufficient. Unfortunately, that means they often can't access any *actual* feelings of comfort or safety, and are stuck instead with options that just help them numb, escape, suppress, distract from, or avoid their uncomfortable feelings.

Some of these options have nothing whatsoever to do with the body or body image, but many do. A person might choose to escape through gambling, drugs, online shopping, or mindlessly scrolling social media, for example, or they might escape by restricting food, overeating, obsessively tracking what they eat, training for a half marathon, or picking themselves apart in the mirror. Whatever tools they use, the runner is often just trying to cope with life alone.

Another big reason the runner seems to rely so heavily on numbing and escaping behaviors is that they have come to believe, on some level, that they wouldn't be able to survive facing or feeling the thing they're running from. We all want to numb our pain sometimes, because pain is unpleasant, but the runner tends to believe their pain is so *powerfully dangerous* that repressing it is a matter of life or death. Sometimes this belief is the result of trauma, in which the runner quite literally did not (or does not) have the skill, support, or capacity to face or feel something safely, and other times it's simply a lifelong lack of encouragement, education, practice, and resilience for facing and feeling things in general.[9]

If a child learns that their emotions upset or irritate people, for example, they might try to keep their emotions hidden, even from themselves. Over time, as they keep hiding, numbing, or pushing their emotions away, the thought of directly facing those emotions starts to sound more and more scary and impossible. Unfortunately, this is a very common experience for the runner; after a lifetime of avoidance, they have no skills and no capacity for facing themselves. After all, if you had completely avoided exercise your entire life, you might reasonably conclude that getting up one day and running a marathon could quite literally kill you, right? That's what it often feels like for the runner: after a lifetime of avoiding their pain (or needs, desires, emotions, or truth), they believe trying to face and feel it all now would literally kill them.

So what does the runner do? They *survive*. They adopt numbing or avoiding behaviors that make it tolerable for them to be themselves, without relying on anyone else, and without facing or feeling the parts of themselves they're too afraid to face. And before you go judging any of the runner's behaviors as "unhealthy" or "bad," let me remind you that numbing and escaping behaviors are all just a part of the brain's brilliant plan for survival. They help us get by when we need them, and they deserve our gratitude, not our derision. At the very least, we must consider them neutral, and refrain from draping any interpretations, meaning, or significance over them. That said, at a certain point, relying on these kinds of behaviors leads to more problems than it solves.[10]

One fairly obvious (but huge) problem with chronically numbing or avoiding our pain is that then we never give ourselves the opportunity to learn how to deal with it. The less practice a person has doing something, the harder and scarier it seems. Learning to tolerate (and bounce back from) pain is an important life skill, and if we never practice it, we never get to build up our skill, capacity, confidence, or resilience for next time.

This is the cycle the runner often finds themselves in: they're scared of pain, so they avoid it, and then the thought of pain gets even scarier. The same is true for the other aspects of themselves they might be running from. If they're so scared of their sexuality that they avoid it altogether, for example, their fear is likely to just worsen over time. If they consistently ignore or repress their emotions (or needs, or inner wisdom), those emotions will seem even scarier.[11] That fear reinforces the runner's desire to avoid it, of course, so the cycle continues.

The second big problem with using numbing and escaping behaviors as a crutch is that *survival* becomes our brain's primary goal, and our brain will go into autopilot mode to keep us safe, even if that means completely overriding our conscious minds. Thought you were going to stop bingeing at night? "No way," your subconscious mind says. "Bingeing is helping us survive." Thought you might go to the gym today? "Sorry," it says. "Staying sedentary keeps our emotions under wraps." Thought you'd quit smoking weed or drinking alcohol for a month? "I don't think so," it says. "We can't risk facing sobriety."

This cycle tends to make the runner feel completely dependent on their numbing, escaping, coping, and avoiding behaviors. Even if the runner wants to stop the behaviors, they can't. After all, no amount of willpower or effort can override a behavior you subconsciously *depend on to survive*. For all of these reasons, the runner is the most likely of all the body image avatars to report compulsive behaviors and addiction, "self-sabotaging" in ways they don't understand, and feeling completely out of control.

Obviously, none of this is conducive to the runner's mental or physical health, self-worth, or body image. The more afraid they are of what lives inside them, the more they seek to control and escape their body, and the more they seek to control and escape their body, the more afraid they become of what lives inside them. They also tend to feel weak, broken, and bad about themselves for not being able to change their behaviors, and those additional negative feelings can either get channeled into body control behaviors, or projected onto their body in the form of hatred and disgust. Plus, because of how often the runner bumps up against their psychic "override" mechanism, it can feel like the body has a mind and will of its own, and that it's actively trying to sabotage the runner's goals. This makes them distrustful of their body and reinforces the belief that the only way to get what they want is to be even more strict and tyrannical in their body control efforts.

A runner in search of body neutrality will need to learn how to survive *without* numbing or escaping. They'll need to identify, explore, and address the many ways they run, while simultaneously cultivating the tools, capacity, and confidence in their ability to feel and face everything inside them in order to dismantle their reliance on such behaviors and to strip the body of significance and power.

They Are Often Disconnected from Their Bodies (and Emotions)

The runner's habit of numbing, avoiding, and escaping themselves tends to disconnect them from their bodies. They're usually just trying to disconnect from *specific* parts of themselves, but the body comes as kind of a package deal. As Brené Brown writes in *The Gifts of Imperfection*, "When we numb the painful emotions, we also numb the positive emotions."[12]

This means we can't numb our pain without also numbing our pleasure, we can't turn down the volume on grief without also turning it down on joy, and we can't tune out our inner no without also tuning out our inner yes. So the runner who tries to numb their pain can end up numbing their entire body, and the runner who tries to separate from their feelings can end up separating from their entire inner self.

For this reason, the runner is likely to report feeling deadened, dull, numb, detached, or desensitized physically or emotionally. They have no idea what people mean when they say things like "listen to your body," either because they're so out of practice that they no longer know *how* to listen, or because at some point their body stopped talking.

The body is designed to be in constant communication with us, sending us continuous signals through the language of sensation. When we need food, for example, the body sends us hunger signals through the *sensation* of a growling, achy, or empty-feeling belly, or other sensations like weakness, nausea, and lightheadedness. When we need to drink water, it sends us the sensations of thirst; when we need to move our bodies, it sends the sensation of restlessness; and when we need to rest, it sends us the sensation of fatigue. It's a genius design, really—each person was born with their own instruction manual! The issue is that this was never supposed to be a one-way conversation.

It takes energy for our body to talk to us, and it doesn't want to waste energy for no reason. If we acknowledge and respond appropriately to our body's message, it knows that was a message worth sending and will continue to send that kind of message in the future. If we don't, though, the body has essentially just wasted energy trying to talk to someone who isn't listening. If that keeps happening, those messages tend to get quieter and quieter, and eventually they can even disappear completely.

This is what happens to a lot of runners: they numb, suppress, or ignore their body's messages for long enough that the messages fade away. Someone who has spent decades trying to ignore or override their hunger and fullness signals, for example, might eventually lose access to those signals altogether. After all, why should the body try to tell you to eat when there's clearly a food shortage? What a waste of energy that would be. And someone who always holds their pee until the last second might eventually not even *know* they have to pee until, suddenly, out of nowhere, they feel like they're going to burst. If all the earlier, more subtle "gotta pee" signals are just getting ignored anyway, then sending them is a waste of the body's energy.

But the runner isn't just disconnecting from little messages, like needing to pee. They're trying to avoid painful, scary, *big* things, like grief, anger, jealousy, heartbreak, desire, intuition, and vulnerability. And the bigger the thing is they're running from, the bigger the disconnect is likely to be.

The human experience can be exquisitely painful, scary, and uncomfortable (both physically and emotionally), and the runner lacks the adequate information, tools, skills, resources, support, or capacity to safely and confidently handle such experiences. But by choosing to constantly repress, ignore, numb, or avoid them, the line of communication between the runner and their body gets weaker. Plus, our bodies are where we feel and experience everything, both good and bad, and where we form our sense of *how it feels to be us.*[13] The runner, who seems to have experienced either a particularly high number of unpleasant life experiences, or a particularly low number of pleasant life experiences, is likely to report the very experience of being themselves, and of having a human body, to be an unpleasant and uncomfortable one. So in their mind, inadvertently disconnecting from their body might be more of an added bonus than a drawback.

It's no wonder the runner wants to escape their body so badly. After a lifetime of numbing, controlling, pushing away, avoiding, and repressing various parts of their experience, many runners end up feeling like "walking heads," with no connection to their bodies at all. The experience of disconnection is different for each individual, of course, but many runners report struggling to "hear" messages like hunger, fullness, fatigue, thirst, or needing to pee, as well as difficulty identifying or differentiating between emotions. Sometimes their sense of taste or touch feels dull and distant, or they're physically clumsy and uncoordinated, because they're disconnected from proprioceptive feedback.

Sometimes certain body parts are numb while others aren't, like a client who said she could feel everything from the waist up, and everything from the knees down, but nothing in between. Some experience genital numbness, or are so disconnected from their sexuality that they struggle to get aroused, feel sexual pleasure, or reach orgasm. And many runners have an unusually high pain tolerance, because somewhere along the way they learned to ignore, repress, or disconnect from physical pain.

There are other reasons the runner might end up disconnected from their body too. For example, if they were shamed or criticized for their emotions or were never taught how to tolerate or process them, then their emotions might have felt too dangerous to be allowed. As a response, they might have tried to shove their emotions down, ignore them, control them, or build a kind of psychic dam to keep them at a distance. And because our emotions are felt in our bodies pushing down or numbing our emotions distances us from our bodies as well.[14] The same applies if the runner learned that their *intuition* conflicted with the reality they lived in, hurt people, or got them into trouble. My client Asher, for example, started to shut down and disconnect from his body when his parents were going through a divorce. He was a sensitive kid, and he *knew* something was going on; he could feel it in his body. But everyone kept saying things were fine and he was being silly, and when Asher tried to point out the stuff he was noticing, his mom got upset. Having learned that his inner wisdom must be either wrong or dangerous, Asher slowly learned to block it out over time, and eventually became an adult with absolutely no connection to his intuition, and very little to his body.

It's also important to point out that while disconnection from the body's messages is *frequently* built slowly and over time, as described above, it sometimes happens in an instant, and all at once. During trauma, for example, when a person's experience overwhelms their ability to cope with it, a person may experience an instantaneous and involuntary dissociation from their body. In these moments, the brain is pulling a sort of last-ditch-effort protective rip cord to help them escape mentally or emotionally from a dangerous or painful situation that they can't escape physically. Often called an out-of-body experience, these moments are sometimes described as a feeling of instant separation between the body and the conscious self, as if a person's mind and spirit were floating away from their body, or that the person's consciousness were looking down on the scene from a distance.

Dissociation is a protective bit of genetic coding, a merciful mechanism to prevent unnecessary suffering.[15] Imagine someone has been caught in the jaws of a hungry lion, for example. They tried to run, but the lion won. There's no way to escape now; if there were still a chance they could escape, the brain would still be pumping out adrenaline and sending fight-or-flight messages, but that time has passed. The lion is going to eat them, and there's nothing they can do. So their brain's built-in mercy mechanism kicks in, and gently removes *them*—their *conscious self*—from the situation. They might freeze and go physically numb as their consciousness disconnects from their body so that they don't have to *be there* to feel the pain of what's going to happen. In our modern environments, we tend to experience dissociation under very different circumstances, of course, but the process is the same.

What's interesting is that when an animal goes through this kind of experience but then somehow survives, it has an instinctual understanding of how to close the stress response cycle that led to its freeze-and-dissociate experience, so it can immediately "come back" to its body. It'll shake its body violently to discharge the build-up of adrenaline, and then sleep or rest for a long time, to signal to its brain that the danger has passed. The human brain, on the other hand, *inhibits* this instinct, so we don't automatically close the stress-response cycle and reintegrate our consciousness with our bodies after trauma. And because trauma is so poorly understood in our culture, a person can easily go years or even decades in a state of lingering dissociation, disconnection, or numbness.[16]

However the runner's disconnection occurred, without the wisdom of their body, heart, and gut to guide them, they tend to end up the same: disoriented, adrift, unhappy, and *terrified*. It's very difficult, after all, to take good care of a body without knowing what it needs, or to make good decisions for your life without knowing your own heart. How do you ever know what to do? How do you choose a career, find friends, improve your health, or even decide what you should eat or wear today? Without access to their body's wisdom, the runner has no choice but to rely on *logic* for all of these decisions and more, and while logic can be helpful in many situations, it's notoriously terrible at helping us build a life where we can be happy and thrive. Plus it's incredibly stressful to be confused all the time about how you feel, and it's wildly unpleasant to never be able to get what you want and need.

Living this way is also a bit like trying to drive a car while blindfolded: it leads to worse and worse consequences the more you do it. Because the runner is disconnected from their body, they're more likely to ignore or misinterpret important signals, and therefore likely to end up with more injuries, illness, unmet needs, mental health issues, pain, and suffering. Naturally, though, because they have no idea why any of this is happening, it all tends to make the runner feel even worse about themselves, and to hate their body even more for malfunctioning or being so "out of control." That means that not only do they end up with *even more* reason to numb, control, or disconnect from their body, but also the runner's belief in their body being bad, broken, or in need of punishment is continually reinforced.

They Emotionally and Physically Armor Themselves

Let's say, for a moment, that throughout your entire life, people randomly shot at you with a BB gun. For whatever reason in this scenario, you can't stop them from doing it, and you never know when it's going to happen. It's reasonable to assume that you might start wearing some kind of armor, shield, or physical barrier day to day to protect yourself from BBs, right?

Now what if, throughout your entire life, people randomly hurt your feelings, took advantage of you, or broke your heart? What kind of armor, shield, or barrier might you develop to protect yourself *then*? Unfortunately, this is the reality most of us live in, and we *do* find ways of armoring ourselves mentally, emotionally, and physically. The runner in particular, who is so afraid of pain, tends to armor themselves on two fronts: they build external walls to protect themselves from other people hurting them (seen both in behavior and in habitual muscular tension), and they build internal walls to protect themselves from their own feelings, needs, desires, and inner wisdom.

Armoring can sometimes come in the form of mental patterns, like obsessing, criticizing, blaming, ruminating, imagining the worst-case scenario, being cynical or negative, being a perfectionist, or feeling like a failure. Other times it comes in the form of emotional patterns, like getting angry about everything, repressing the urge to cry, or pushing down all emotions except happiness. Armoring can also come in the form of relationship behaviors, like lashing out, creating conflict, people-pleasing, withdrawing, avoiding conflict, refusing to be vulnerable, or being hyper-independent. And many of our coping, controlling, and numbing behaviors, like tracking calories, bingeing, body checking, shopping, obsessing over skin care, being a workaholic, comparing ourselves with others, and overexercising, are actually forms of armor as well, either because they make us feel safer and better or because they allow us to avoid relying on other people for comfort, soothing, and support.

The runner tends to call upon all of these various types of armor, as well as armoring themselves *physically*. Sometimes physical armor is just the natural extension, or involuntary side effect, of a person's mental or emotional armor, like in the case of someone whose neck and shoulder muscles are constantly tight and achy because the person spends long hours at their work computer every day to avoid going home and being alone with their thoughts. Other times the armor is a subconscious response to an experience or threat, like if someone gains a significant amount of weight after a sexual assault to feel less sexually visible. Sometimes armor comes in the form of chronic muscle tension, tightness, numbness, or postural imbalances,[17] and other times we can see it in the changes to a person's body shape or size. Even those body shape or size changes can sometimes exist in their own right as armor (like in the case of a guy who decides to get big and muscular to feel more powerful), and sometimes they can just be the result of the habits or behaviors the person is using to armor themselves (like in the case of a teenager with an eating disorder).

You can think of this kind of *involuntary* physical armor as the person's subconscious inner world being represented physically, and we all have some form of it. A person who is self-conscious about being tall, for example, might develop a hunched or stooped posture due to years of trying to shrink themselves, and a person with a history of sexual abuse might have exceptionally tight and inflexible hips from years of subconscious hypervigilance. Other times, however, a person's physical armor is cultivated more consciously and intentionally, through the way a person chooses to hold themselves, move, stand, breathe, speak, eat, or exercise, and the type of body shape or size they choose to cultivate. Think of a muscular gym bro, for example, who walks around with his chest puffed up, pelvis rigid, and arms sort of standing out away from his sides. This kind of body and posture might be a conscious choice on his part to feel more masculine and powerful; it might be the armor he's chosen to avoid feeling small, weak, or vulnerable.

With endless options for how a runner armors themselves, no two individuals are likely to have the exact same kind of armor. One might develop powerful body language to look intimidating, like the gym bro, while another hunches and collapses to appear meek and nonthreatening. One might starve themselves to be a smaller target of attack, while another binge eats to quell their anxiety about getting attacked. Armor doesn't have to be obvious, though, and it doesn't have to make sense to anyone else. It doesn't even have to be particularly effective! It just has to make the runner *feel* safer, consciously or subconsciously, for at least a moment.

When I was twenty-one, I fell in love with strength training and powerlifting. Having always been fairly small and out of shape, and with a history of sexual trauma, I *loved* making my body both look and feel strong and powerful. The more muscular and lean I got, the more intimidating I was to guys, which meant I was harassed less often, *and* for the first time in my life felt like I actually stood a chance of fighting off, or running away from, an attacker. In this way, my body became my armor.

This probably wouldn't have become a problem, if that had been the extent of my armor. It wasn't, though, because I, a runner myself, had already spent decades feeling unsafe and afraid all the time. So on top of my fitness routine, I also had a chronic habit of holding, clenching, and tensing various parts of my body, and my nervous system was stuck in the "on" position, so I was always on the lookout for danger and could never fully rest or relax. That was all mostly involuntary, but to top it all off, I also spent every minute of every day sucking my stomach in as hard as I could, to look like I had a flat belly. This made my breathing rapid and shallow, and after years of this, I found myself completely unable to breathe deeply or diaphragmatically, which led to some serious issues, including anxiety, a neck injury, and long-lasting gastrointestinal and reproductive system issues.

This is the problem with relying on our bodies to armor us: it's not what the body was designed for, at least not long term, so it tends to be unsustainable and lead to some unpleasant consequences.

Like I used to, many runners feel anxious, breathe rapidly and shallowly, struggle to rest and relax, and carry an unhealthy amount of chronic muscle tension, clenching, tightness, or stiffness in their bodies. This is because, for one reason or another, they live with the constant sense that danger is lurking, and their bodies are responding accordingly.[18] After all, it wouldn't be appropriate to trust your environment, let your body totally soften, or go into a deep sleep if you thought you might get attacked at any moment, right?

That is, unfortunately, how the runner lives: like they're in danger of an attack at any moment. But when the kind of attack they're defending against comes from *inside them*, feeling safe is unlikely. On some level, they're constantly aware that something bad and scary lives down there—even if they don't know exactly what it is—and it's constantly threatening to break free and kill them. So they employ their survival strategies; they numb, control, avoid, repress, disconnect, and armor themselves, all in the hopes that the thing they're running from never finds them.

It's important to recognize that even though the runner's armor makes them *feel* protected, it's often functionally useless. Tensing up our shoulders doesn't actually protect us from anything, being very fat (or very thin) doesn't actually make us invisible, and people-pleasing doesn't actually prevent heartbreak. Letting go of armor is difficult, but I think it's a bit easier when we can acknowledge that it wasn't really doing anything, anyway.

That said, there *are* times when a person's armor legitimately offers them some kind of protection. The way we look can affect our odds of discrimination, attack, or other danger, and sometimes our armor plays a role in keeping those things from happening. That gym bro's big muscular physique might legitimately reduce his odds of being attacked, for example, and a person of color who armors themselves with a more "white-looking" presentation very well might face fewer instances of discrimination, and a transgender person who armors themselves by "passing" as cisgender may be able to reduce their risk of transphobic violence. There is no right or wrong answer when it comes to this kind of armor; choosing to hold on to it can be a valid choice, even if it's causing pain or making body neutrality more difficult. The only person who can decide whether or not it's worth keeping is the one experiencing it.

Certain kinds of armor are also genuinely effective at helping the runner cope. We feel our emotions more intensely when we're breathing slowly and deeply into a soft belly, for example, than when we're breathing fast and shallow, with the belly held tight. So if the runner's goal is to avoid their feelings, shallow breathing and muscle tension can help them do it.[19] But even though the runner developed armor to feel safer and less vulnerable, there is a certain point at which the armor *itself* becomes a source of vulnerability and danger. Chronic muscle tension makes us vulnerable to injuries, imbalances, and joint pain, and living in a state of hyperarousal makes us vulnerable to adrenal fatigue, burnout, and any number of physical and mental health issues.[20] Plus, the longer a runner wears their armor, the harder it is for them to imagine facing life without it.

Eventually, an overreliance on armor will hurt us. It will also reduce the quality of our lives, get in the way of our ability to thrive, and make body neutrality impossible. You can't see your body as neutral, after all, if you also see it as a constant source of *danger.* And you can't see your body as neutral if you believe it's the only thing protecting you from danger either. So the path to body neutrality often requires the runner to do the impossible: To face death, over and over, until they are no longer afraid of it. To remove their armor, and brave the world without it. To stop running, look inside, and finally face (and feel) *everything.*

They See Their Bodies as the Enemy

Avery, a college student with fibromyalgia, was furious with her body. Her illness had come out of nowhere, and destroyed everything she was working toward. She had always tried to take good care of her body, and this is how it repaid her: with cruelty and pain. Her interpretation, that her body was untrustworthy and malicious, made Avery literally see something grotesque, vile, and repugnant when she looked in the mirror. Her feelings of shock, hurt, and rage about her body's unforgivable betrayal led Avery to develop intense body hatred and dysmorphia.

The runner tends to see their body as their enemy for a variety of reasons. As already discussed, they sometimes attempt to control their body, which already encourages an adversarial relationship, and then when their body resists being controlled, their perception is solidified: *This body is trying to ruin my life.* Sometimes they're so afraid of what lives inside them that their *body itself* comes to feel like their attacker or oppressor, while they feel like the victim being terrorized. And sometimes their inability to hear their body's messages leads to injury, illness, unmet needs, pain, or other suffering, making them feel like their body is "out to get them." Whatever the reason, though, many runners come to see their bodies as enemies endlessly waging war against them.

The runner might also come to see their body as the enemy because, like Avery, they perceive their body to have betrayed them in some way. Something happens, like an injury or illness, for example, and the person interprets it as an open declaration of war on them by their body. From then on, they view their body as a hostile traitor, saboteur, or villain, and any chance of a peaceful or neutral relationship is gone.

This response makes sense, in a way, given the interpretation. If someone I knew kept hurting me, getting me in trouble, inviting danger into my world, threatening me, or attacking me, I sure as hell wouldn't trust or like that person either. I'd be pissed, defensive, and resentful. I would definitely see that person as my enemy, and there's no way in hell I'd feel neutrally toward them.

The problem, however, is that the runner has made a *subjective and false* interpretation of their body's behavior, and that false interpretation is now clouding their vision entirely. Going back to Avery, for example, her interpretation of events was that "everything was fine one minute, and then BAM, everything hurt all the time, and [she] couldn't get out of bed." She remembered her illness hitting her out of nowhere, but when we talked about the period of time leading up to her illness, it was clear that she had been under a ton of stress, pushing herself too hard at work, overexercising, and not sleeping. Based on the various little injuries, illnesses, and issues that had been popping up during the year or so before the onset of her fibromyalgia, it actually sounded to me like Avery's body had been screaming out to her, literally begging her to slow down. Her body had tried to be a good, protective teammate, but Avery didn't listen, and eventually she pushed herself too far.

Given all that, is it objectively true that Avery's body betrayed her? Is it true that her body was some kind of malevolent evildoer who attacked out of nowhere, because it wanted to see her suffer? No, of course not. Her illness developed in response to the overwhelming stress she was under, both physically and emotionally, in a desperate attempt to get Avery to finally, forcibly slow the hell down. What else was it supposed to do? She hadn't been listening.

Looking at it this way, Avery was able to see that her body had been on her side the whole time, trying to communicate and keep her healthy. And believe it or not, this is nearly *always* the case. Our bodies and brains are constantly fighting to protect us, even when it feels like they're attacking or betraying us. They're on our side; we just can't always see it in the moment.

The stories we tell ourselves, and the ways we interpret these kinds of experiences, can have a huge impact on our health, happiness, and body image. If a runner sees their body as the enemy, they're more inclined to try to numb it, control it, disrespect it, punish it, and push it away. Plus, because their enemy is their body, and they can never get away from it, they might end up feeling trapped and panicky, powerless and weak, or full of rage, resentment, hatred, or disgust toward it.

On the other hand, when we can see the truth—that our bodies are always just trying to help or protect us—all that negativity disappears, and our feelings of safety and power are restored. Obviously, this means that a runner who wants to access body neutrality will need to challenge and dismantle the various layers of false interpretation, meaning, and significance that made them feel betrayed and pitted them against their body in the first place. And because there's such a wide variety of experiences that can cause a runner to feel betrayed by their body, I want to give you a few examples from my coaching practice, of both the perceived betrayal *and* the neutral and objective truth we eventually replaced it with.

THE PERCEIVED BETRAYAL:

A woman felt betrayed when her budding prepubescent body got her unwanted sexual attention and harassment and caused her to feel ashamed, guilty, dirty, and afraid.

THE NEUTRAL AND OBJECTIVE TRUTH:

Her young body was just doing what it was designed to do. The boys and men who sexualized and harassed her when she was a child were doing something disgusting and evil. *They* were her real enemy, along with the patriarchy and the objectification of women: two systems of oppression that upheld the disgusting and evil behavior she encountered.

THE PERCEIVED BETRAYAL:

A person felt betrayed because they waited until marriage to have sex, and then when they did, they didn't get any pleasure or enjoyment from it. It made them feel broken, guilty, and worried that God was mad at them.

THE NEUTRAL AND OBJECTIVE TRUTH:

The sex wasn't pleasurable because they had no idea what they liked or wanted, but they *did* have sky-high expectations, a ton of guilt and anxiety, and a lot of pressure to have a magical experience. That's a lot to deal with at once, and their body was just navigating the moment. If there was an "enemy" in this situation, it would be the sex-negative messages of purity culture, and the unrealistic expectations set up for them by their church, *not* their body.

THE PERCEIVED BETRAYAL:

A woman believed her body "tempted" her rapist to rape her, and then betrayed her by freezing instead of fighting or running.

THE NEUTRAL AND OBJECTIVE TRUTH:

Her body did nothing wrong whatsoever. A body is *never* responsible for tempting anyone to rape; the *only* responsible party for rape is the rapist. Her rapist was her real enemy (and the patriarchy that upholds rape culture), not her body. Also, the freeze response kicked in to protect her, because that's what the freeze response does after assessing the situation in an instant and recognizing that any attempt to fight against or flee from someone so much bigger and stronger than her probably would have failed, or led to even more suffering.

THE PERCEIVED BETRAYAL:

A person saw their body as their enemy because it made their parents criticize and verbally abuse them.

THE NEUTRAL AND OBJECTIVE TRUTH:

A body doesn't have the power to "make" anyone choose to be critical or abusive. Their parents are the only parties responsible for the abusive behavior. And their parents may not be "their enemy," exactly, but the parents were the ones who did the betraying, *not* the person's body.

THE PERCEIVED BETRAYAL:

A woman saw her body as the enemy because it made her partner cheat on her.

THE NEUTRAL AND OBJECTIVE TRUTH:

Again, a body doesn't have the power to "make" anyone break their relationship agreements, lie, or hurt people. Her partner was the one who betrayed her, not her body.

THE PERCEIVED BETRAYAL:

A man felt betrayed by his body for getting injured and ruining his chances of being a professional athlete.

THE NEUTRAL AND OBJECTIVE TRUTH:

His body tried to do everything he asked of it during years of intense training, while also trying to keep him safe. There is a random genetic component to professional sports, because people have to have especially resilient and durable bodies to make it that far, and they also have to get a bit lucky. His feelings of grief at his loss, and the identity tailspin his injury led to, are completely valid—but his body didn't do *anything* wrong.

THE PERCEIVED BETRAYAL:

A person felt like their body was constantly trying to ruin their plan to lose weight or to keep weight off.

THE NEUTRAL AND OBJECTIVE TRUTH:

Our bodies tell us to eat a whole bunch of food after being in a state of food scarcity and restriction (i.e., dieting) to protect us from starvation or malnourishment. After all, the body doesn't know the difference between a famine and a diet, and its focus is to keep you healthy and alive, not help you fit into society's unrealistic beauty and body ideals. So, again, this person's body was just trying to keep them safe, not ruin their life.

THE PERCEIVED BETRAYAL:

A woman felt betrayed by her body because first she couldn't *get* pregnant, and then she couldn't *stay* pregnant.

THE NEUTRAL AND OBJECTIVE TRUTH:

Her grief and pain were valid, but her body wasn't doing this *to* her. She could keep trying, but some bodies just can't get pregnant, and that neither means anything about her, nor is something she can control. That said, we live in a culture that stigmatizes the topics of infertility and miscarriage, so if she was betrayed in this situation, it was by a society that made her feel broken, ashamed, or alone on her fertility journey.

Hopefully these examples demonstrate how easy it can be for a runner to blame their body, feel betrayed, and come to think their body is the enemy, as well as how inaccurate their interpretations are. The sad truth is that many runners spend the majority of their lives engaged in warfare with a body that has *only ever* been trying to protect them. And body neutrality is completely impossible under such circumstances.

THE RUNNER'S NEXT STEPS

The runner's path to body neutrality will require them to first acknowledge they've been running from something and that their body image thoughts, feelings, and behaviors have been helping them run. Then they have to figure out what it is they've been running from, and eventually find a way of facing it head-on: no numbing, no avoiding, no controlling, and no armor.

In the next section of the book, you'll be given specific steps to help you identify your particular hidden body image purpose and face your inner demons, but if you resonate with the runner, here are a few questions to consider in the meantime:

- In what ways do you use your body (or body behaviors) to control, numb, escape, distract from, or disconnect from your body, your feelings, or yourself?

- What might you be running from, avoiding, repressing, or staying distracted from? What are you afraid of facing or feeling?

- What do your body image issues (or body-related behaviors) protect you from feeling, thinking, doing, knowing, or being?

- Why did you need your body image suffering, or body-related behaviors, when they first developed? (Do you still need them now? Why or why not?)

- In what way do you perceive your body to have betrayed you or to be your enemy? Why?

Part III

THE PATH TO BODY NEUTRALITY

CHAPTER 12

The Body Neutrality Blueprint

NOW THAT YOU'VE BEEN INTRODUCED to the main concepts of body neutrality and to the four body image avatars, you're probably wondering what the hell you should do next. How do you apply this information to yourself? What are the actual steps needed to see your own body through a neutral lens?

The answers to those questions are as complex and unique as every individual human being is, but in the following chapters, I'll outline the practical steps for you to find *your* answers. Whether or not you fit perfectly into one or more of the avatars doesn't matter, as we'll just be using the avatars as a jumping-off point anyway. From here on I'll be sharing the exact methodology I created to help clients move from body image suffering to body neutrality, including specific steps, tools, and concepts to keep you on track. When I started developing this method, I mostly just wanted a clear and effective way to explain the body neutrality journey to my clients so they could conceptualize what was about to happen and why. But over time it evolved into a pretty concrete system or process, which I now call the body neutrality blueprint.

You can think of the body neutrality blueprint as your step-by-step guide from here to there; body image suffering to body neutral. Because each individual's journey will be unique and specific to them, I *can't* tell you the exact details of how your path will look, but I *can* tell you it will hit all the major points laid out in the blueprint. How you get from point to point is entirely up to you, though, and I encourage you to fit the blueprint to yourself, not the other way around. The blueprint is for *everyone*, but only because it's always pointing back to the *individual*; it should never replace your own self-knowledge and inner wisdom.

Ready to get started? Well, you already have!

By taking the body image avatar self-assessment and reading about each avatar, you've (hopefully) been able to conceptualize the world of body image suffering with more clarity, and started to locate yourself within it. Maybe you even have an inkling of your hidden body image purpose already! Next up you'll be working to identify the exact and specific problems your body image issues have been trying to solve for you so that you can figure out how to solve those problems another way.

The body neutrality blueprint is based on the simple premise that your body image issues will never disappear if any part of you still thinks you need them. The only way to let them go is to remove their *reason for existing*. Curious about how this might look? Here are a few examples!

- If you discover your body image issues exist to offer you a *feeling of control in an out-of-control world*, you might either find healthier ways to feel in control, or just learn to tolerate the feeling of not being in control all the time.

- If you discover your body image suffering exists to *distract you from the pain of your deep loneliness*, you might figure out how to build a life that feels more connected and less lonely.

- If you discover your obsession with your appearance *exists to "earn" you a romantic partner*, you might first dismantle your belief that partnership is based on self-objectification and then focus on more vulnerable and meaningful connections.

♦ If you discover you *take your feeling of confidence or self-worth from how you look*, you might cultivate other sources of feeling good about yourself.

♦ If you discover you're *waiting to live the life of your dreams* until you lose weight, you might identify your exact dream life, and then . . . go start living it.

Hopefully these examples demonstrate the importance of identifying the exact and specific reason your body image issues exist: your hidden body image purpose. That critical information will illuminate your entire path forward. And while the avatars are great at helping a person locate and understand themselves, they're far too broad to help us fully identify our individual, personal, and unique hidden body image purpose. Don't worry, though, that's what the next chapter is going to help us uncover!

CHAPTER 13

Identifying Your
Hidden Body Image Purpose

I F YOU DON'T YET KNOW WHAT SPECIFIC problems your body image issues are trying to solve for you, that's okay. Each avatar points you in a *general direction* for how to find this information, but now you need to try to understand your hidden body image purpose in a more specific, detailed, personal, and emotionally resonant way.

For example, if the outsider resonates with you, you might know that your body image issues have *something* to do with connection, acceptance, and belonging. But what, exactly? There's a huge difference between wanting to lose weight to earn yourself access to a supportive community of like-minded individuals and wanting to lose weight to avoid being humiliated by people talking about you behind your back, right? And even those categories are too broad. A person seeking connection might really be seeking close female friendships, a supportive community of fellow artists, the ability to be authentic with their family, or even just more relief from the burden of parenting. Each of those would require very different next steps, right? That's why the first step of the body neutrality blueprint is to find and name *your* specific hidden body image purpose, with clarity, specificity, and vulnerability.

Exactly what problems have your body image issues been trying to help you solve? Exactly what task, job, or responsibility have you assigned, consciously or subconsciously, to your body? What exactly are you hoping to "earn" by having the right kind of body, and what exactly are you afraid will happen if you don't?

Exploring these kinds of questions (as well as the exercises I give you later in this chapter) should help you start coming up with options and ideas for your hidden body image purpose. I recommend writing everything down now, even if it's not quite right yet. Just make a list of ideas and then see what feels the most true and powerful.

I, for example, am historically a runner as well as a self-objectifier, and I've learned that I fixate on my appearance when I'm feeling something I don't want to feel—usually anxiety, vulnerability, or grief. That right there would have been a perfectly valid way of stating my hidden body image purpose, because it's true and clear, and I also could have said, "My body image issues exist to protect me from my feelings." The phrasing that felt most visceral and powerful to me, however, was this: "My brain makes me obsess over my appearance when it thinks I need to be distracted or protected from pain."

You can phrase your own hidden body image purpose in any way that feels best for you, as you can see from my example. I think the simplest place to start is to try finishing the sentence "My hidden body image purpose is . . ." or "My body image issues exist to . . . ," but feel free to explore what feels right. You might get more specific about your body image experience, for example, "I hate my body because . . ." or "I can't stop body checking because . . . ," or you might prefer to frame your answer from your brain or body image issues' perspective, like "My brain is trying to . . ." or "My body image issues want to . . ." Any way you want to put it is valid, as long as it clearly identifies the *purpose* your body image issues are either serving or trying to serve. And don't underestimate the power of nuance and specificity in the language you use, because we're looking for something that you feel emotionally connected to, or even moved by. Try to phrase your hidden body image purpose in such a way that it hooks into a deep, visceral place inside you. This is how you know you're on the right path: when you name your hidden body image purpose in such a way that it rings true not only intellectually, but also deep down in your heart, soul, bones, or gut.

I once reflected to a client that it sounded like her body image issues were functioning to allow her to differentiate herself from her mother, whom she did not want to be like. She agreed, and we talked about how obsessively maintaining a superthin body felt like a way of proving to herself that she didn't have to be like her (large-bodied and also narcissistic) mother, and how her desire to be thin was about wanting a sort of visual and metaphorical boundary between them. Throughout the whole conversation, my client was steady, curious, and calm. But at one point she suddenly gasped and said with a shaking voice, "Oh my god, I've been chasing *freedom*! She wanted me to be like *her*, and I felt trapped. I think I've been hoping that if only I can get thin enough, I'll be free to be my own person. All this body hatred was just trying to liberate me!"

This particular statement wasn't altogether very different from what we'd already been talking about, but from the way she reacted, I knew we had just found her visceral hook. Her body image issues existed to protect her from an overbearing mother. Obsessively controlling her body was an unfortunate trade-off for what felt like the freedom to be herself. Being thin was her way of saying, "I'm not like you, Mom. I'm my own person." And while she had already known this intellectually for a while, it wasn't until it clicked on that deep visceral and intuitive level that we were able to move on to the next step.

And what *was* that next step? My client had to find another way of solving her problem, without relying on her body to do it for her. She worked to find other ways of establishing boundaries and differentiation from her mother, to affirm and express her freedom to be herself, to reinforce her independence, and to let go of the narrative that she was destined to live the same kind of life her mother did. Over time, as she made these changes, it seemed less and less important to be thin.

The subconscious meaning and significance she had assigned to her body (to "earn" her freedom) faded as she felt more free day to day, and eventually the size of her body became nothing more than a vague preference in the back of her mind.

This is the power of naming your hidden body image purpose with specificity and emotional resonance: doing so automatically illuminates your exact next steps to body neutrality, with precision and clarity.

A quick reminder: You might have multiple hidden purposes, because body image issues can crop up to try to solve so many different problems. Most people with multiple body image avatars will end up with multiple hidden purposes (though not always), and a person with only one avatar can sometimes still end up with multiple hidden purposes anyway. That's all okay!

Just start wherever you are today, and try to identify whichever hidden body image purpose feels the clearest, easiest, most relevant, or most interesting to you. You're free to try to identify all of your hidden purposes up front, *or* just work through the blueprint steps with one and then start the process again to find another. There is no right or wrong order for this work, and you don't need to know where it's all going as you get started. New layers, new hidden body image purposes, and even new avatars may reveal themselves over time as you do this work, and that's totally fine. My clients often say it's like peeling an onion; you start by peeling the most superficial layer, and once you've dealt with that, you're rewarded by having the next layer come into focus, and on and on. Plus, our bodies are constantly fluctuating, changing, and evolving, and so are our relationships to them. So don't worry if this all feels a bit overwhelming right now. Just start *anywhere*, and the rest will become clear as you go along.

Still not sure where to start? Try one or more of the following four exercises to come up with your own unique hidden body image purpose.

1. EXAMINE YOUR POSITIVE BODY IMAGE FANTASY.

What do you hope, imagine, wish for, or expect would be different in your life if you had the body or appearance of your dreams?

Your answer to this is what I call the *positive* body image fantasy, and each person's fantasy will be completely unique to them. By exploring your own positive body image fantasy, you can learn a lot of important information about what problem your body image issues might be trying to solve!

To help you explore and articulate your own fantasy, consider the questions below. Then describe your positive body image fantasy, with as much detail as you can. (Note: I highly recommend doing this as a written exercise.)

- What are the perks, rewards, or benefits that populate your fantasy for what life would be like if you suddenly fixed your perceived "flaws" and never had to worry about the shape, size, appearance, function, or ability of your body ever again?

- What are you hoping or expecting would be different in your life if you could wave a magic wand and have the "perfect" body? How do you imagine you would feel?

- What do you imagine you would earn, get, feel, experience, or have in the body of your dreams?

- What do you imagine you would be able to *do* or *be* in your dream body that you don't or aren't now?

- What do you imagine would be easier, better, or more abundant, if all your "flaws" were magically fixed?

- What emotional needs do you imagine would be automatically met?

- What risks would you feel comfortable taking in the "right body" that you don't in the one you have today?

- What would you feel worthy of in your ideal body that you don't right now?

Bear in mind this is an exercise in creative daydreaming, not planning or solving anything. Let yourself fully sink into the fantasy as you answer these questions, and don't worry about making sense or being logical. A client once told me that if she could fix all her flaws, then nobody could ever be mean to her ever again. Obviously that's not true or realistic, but by acknowledging that it was part of her body image fantasy, we were able to see how her body image issues were trying to protect her from the pain of other people's unkindness. That was an important insight!

After writing out your positive body image fantasy, consider what you've written as your actual "body goals." This fantasy represents what you're *subconsciously* hoping for, wanting, craving, or trying to get via your body. What can you learn from that, as you consider what you've written, about your hidden body image purpose? Is there a problem your body image issues are trying to solve for you? A need or desire they're trying to meet? An experience or emotion they're trying to earn you?

By considering your positive fantasy this way, your hidden body image purpose will often become clear. Here are a few examples from my coaching practice:

- Max imagined themself in their dream body feeling vibrant, alive, and full of energy and joy. So what they *really* wanted was to feel vibrant, alive, and full of energy and joy, not to actually have a "perfect body." Max's hidden body image purpose was to help them feel vibrant, alive, and full of energy and joy all the time.

- Camila imagined herself surrounded by friends and community, and everyone liking her, when she lost weight. Clearly, she was seeking *connection*, not weight loss. Her body image issues were trying to help her find friends, feel welcome, and build community.

♦ Mateo imagined that once he hit his body goals, he would have amazing sex with lots of beautiful women, get lots of positive feedback about his body, and feel super confident. This showed us that Mateo *really* wanted a more fulfilling sex life, affirmation that he was desirable, and confidence. His hidden body image purpose was to make women desire and affirm him, but even deeper than that, it was to finally *feel* worthy and desirable.

2. EXAMINE YOUR NEGATIVE BODY IMAGE FANTASY.

What are you trying to avoid or escape by having a different body? What scares you most about being stuck with the body you have? What scares you most about your body getting "worse"? Your answers to these questions are what I call your *negative* body image fantasy, and they contain just as much information as the positive fantasy, when it comes to identifying your own specific hidden body image purpose.

We normally associate the word "fantasy" with positive experiences, so this can be a little confusing, but I'm simply referring to the fact that the negative fantasy is a kind of imaginary vision that lives exclusively in an individual's imagination. It's unpleasant, sure, but people who suffer from body image issues will often have spent a ton of time and energy cultivating and living in it anyway.

To help you explore and articulate your own negative body image fantasy more clearly, consider the questions below, and then describe your negative body image fantasy with as much detail as you can. (Again, I recommend exploring this in writing!) Feel free to include any fears or projections based on the body you currently have, *and* any fears or projections based on your body getting "worse," whatever that means to you.

- What do you imagine having the "right" kind of body would protect you from needing to experience? Do? Have? Be? Feel?
- What is the most uncomfortable, scary, or painful part of having the "wrong" kind of body?
- What do you imagine a different body would help you avoid or escape?
- What does focusing on your body distract you from facing or feeling?
- What changes are you most afraid of happening to your body or appearance? Why?
- What do you imagine, expect, dread, or fear would happen if those changes occurred?
- What needs and desires do you imagine would go unmet if those changes occurred?
- How do you imagine you would feel if those changes occurred?
- What do you imagine would become harder or worse in your life if those changes occurred?
- What kind of life would you feel worthy of if those changes occurred?

Again, let your mind run free as you answer these questions. After writing out your negative body image fantasy, consider what you've written. What can you learn about your hidden body image purpose from your answers? Are your body image issues trying to help you avoid something, escape something, or cope with something? Is there a fear your body image issues are trying to protect you from? A need or desire they're trying to keep from going unmet?

By considering your negative fantasy this way, your hidden body image purpose might be able to come into focus. Here are a few examples from my coaching practice:

+ Maya was terrified her partner would stop being attracted to her as she aged and got bigger, softer, flabbier, and wrinklier. Her hidden body image purpose was to protect the security of her relationship, and keep her partner from abandoning her.

+ Jamal was afraid of gaining weight, because he imagined it would lead to the loss of respect from people, people seeing him as less masculine, and possibly the loss of opportunities in his career. His hidden body image purpose was to maintain his current level of social privilege and keep his career options open.

+ Angel felt dread and panic when they thought about the changes their body would go through if they gave up their rigid eating and exercising habits, because they imagined they would constantly be misgendered, misunderstood, and invisible without a curve-free "androgenous" body. Angel's hidden body image purpose was to clearly express their gender identity to others so Angel didn't have to.

It has to be said here that both the positive and negative body image fantasies can represent either true and realistic views of reality, *or* completely nonsensical make-believe. For example, a person might imagine that having a thinner body would protect them from ever being lonely (false), or they might imagine that having a thinner body would help them avoid weight discrimination (true).

Often, however, the positive fantasy centers on wanting to *gain* social status, privilege, and power—and the negative fantasy centers on a *fear of losing* one's social status, privilege, and power. And because we live in a world where a person's body actually does affect those things,[1] some of this is appropriate, objective, and even neutral. But other times, we use status, privilege, and power as a stand-in for, or indirect path toward, our deeper and more specific needs and desires.

The purpose of these exercises is to get to our deepest truths, so I encourage you to stay open and curious about the role social privilege and status play in your own fantasies, and to consider whether or not they're covering up something deeper or truer.

I once worked with a man who struggled with insecurity about his penis size, and in his positive body image fantasy he was rich, successful, and highly sought after. He imagined himself partying with Victoria's Secret models on Leonardo DiCaprio's boat, because of the confidence-boosting power of "big dick energy." But that fantasy was obscuring his deeper truth. When I asked how he imagined partying with models on a boat would make him *feel*—what the underlying purpose or benefit of "big dick energy" was—he admitted that he just wanted to feel confident, happy, and worthy.

Given all of the messages we receive about who is worthy of what, and how to be happy, it makes sense that status and privilege *seem* like the key to everything we want (like confidence, self-worth, and happiness), but it's a red herring. Be honest and specific about what you're hoping these privileges will actually do for you, and what you might be subconsciously seeking by pursuing them.

Likewise, if your hidden body image purpose is to avoid marginalization and oppression, that's worth exploring. Of course, nobody wants to be marginalized or oppressed, but there's something darkly uncomfortable lurking within this plan. It's a little like trying to avoid getting squished by climbing to the top of a pile of bodies; you know *someone* is going to be hurt, and you're just desperately trying to make sure it's not *you*.

Trying to lose weight to avoid weight discrimination is completely understandable, but it can also be a way of shutting your eyes to the system of oppression that disadvantages, hurts, and kills people based on their body size. It can be a way of saying, "This system is okay, as long as it doesn't affect me, and I don't mind if other people suffer, as long as I don't."

To be clear, there is no right or wrong way for a person to deal with their own oppression or marginalization, and I believe in complete and total bodily autonomy, which means every individual has the right to do whatever the hell they want with their own bodies without judgment. Not only that, but due to the challenges and disadvantages facing folks with marginalized bodies, sometimes "playing the game" is the right choice. It doesn't make a person any less feminist or body neutral to try to escape their own marginalization.

I had a client who got a gastric bypass, for example, because her thin coworker had gotten the promotion my client was significantly more qualified for, and she refused to let that happen again. Her career was very important to her, and she did what she needed to do to protect and advance it, even though she knew the surgery was associated with some scary side effects and serious health issues and was unlikely to keep the weight off long term. Rather than judge her decision as anti–body neutral or catering to oppression beauty and body ideals, I commended her for making such a brave and mindful decision. She did it from a place of clear and neutral vision; she knew a smaller body wouldn't make her more worthy of a promotion, just that it would make her more likely to get one, given her boss's fatphobia. I'm furious that she was put in such an unjust position, but I respect the fact that she knew what she wanted and was willing to make it happen. Frankly, I would wish my client's level of clearheaded neutrality upon anyone who finds themselves in a similarly unjust position, and support any decision they made.

All of this is to say that every individual gets to decide what's right for them and their body, but be careful you're not pursuing social privilege for privilege's sake, or trying to avoid facing an unjust system by just rising to the top of it. I recommend spending a few minutes considering the role privilege and oppression might be playing in the body image fantasies you've written out, and by extension, what role they might be playing in your hidden body image purpose.

3. EXAMINE YOUR BODY IMAGE *BEHAVIORS*.

Exploring the specific behaviors you engage in around your body and body image, and why you do them, can lead to clarity around your hidden body image purpose too. This exercise starts by brainstorming a big list of any and all behaviors you do (or don't do) with regard to your body or appearance, or because of how you *feel* about your body or appearance.

Include behaviors around food and exercise on your list (counting calories, tracking steps, making yourself exercise on a specific schedule, restricting certain foods or food groups, following a diet or other weight-loss-focused behaviors), as well as body checking (weighing or measuring yourself, taking "progress pictures," picking yourself apart in the mirror, grabbing certain body parts to see how big or small they feel), or beauty work (makeup, hair, skin, teeth, nails, clothing, injections, treatments, or surgery) that exist in any way because of your body image issues.

Also include any events you skip, dreams you don't chase, actions you don't do, or risks you don't take based on how you feel about your body or appearance. According to the findings of the 2005 Dove Global Study, two thirds of women globally have skipped an event or activity because they felt bad about how they looked, including many who opted out of important identity-affirming activities like going to school, work, or a job interview.[2] Have you ever avoided an activity, skipped an event, or not fully participated in something because of how you felt about your body or appearance? Write that down!

Don't worry about making this list perfect; just write down anything you can think of. Food rules, clothing rules, exercise rules, and other body rules are a good place to start. Any thought about your body that starts with "I can't" or "I have to" should probably go on the list, like "I can't eat sugar because I'll blow up like a balloon," or "I have to wear high-waisted jeans because my legs are so short." If

picking up a particular behavior would make you feel incredibly insecure about your body, or if not doing a behavior that you normally do
would make you feel that way, put it on the list.

Do you weigh yourself every morning, grab your back fat in disgust
on a regular basis, critique your body in the mirror, trash-talk your
body with friends, avoid photos, or obsessively shop for antiaging
products online? Do you refuse to wear shorts, or ask someone out, because your body makes you too insecure? Write it all down!

Then, once you have a pretty good list, consider how each *individual
behavior* might be serving a purpose, trying to help you, or trying to
solve a problem. What might obsessing over calories be distracting you
from? How might constant body checking be protecting you? What
might overexercising be trying to help you cope with?

It's okay if you don't have super-specific answers for each behavior,
but I recommend going through your list and at least considering each
behavior individually to see if anything jumps out at you. The purpose
of this exercise is to identify your overall hidden body image purpose,
though, so after exploring each behavior on its own, pull back to see
whether there are any patterns or insights you can glean from what
you've written. What can your behaviors tell you about the purpose of
your body image issues?

Here are a few examples from my coaching practice:

- Catalina regularly engaged in body-bashing conversations with
  other women, where they stood around and talked about how
  much they hated their bodies. The purpose of that behavior
  was to relieve her feelings of social anxiety and vulnerability
  when she didn't know someone very well. This shed some
  light on her hidden body image purpose as an outsider, which
  was to keep people from rejecting or humiliating her.

- Talia was obsessed with her twice-a-day skin care routine, and
  felt terribly anxious, guilty, and out of control if she skipped
  any part of it. The behavior existed to calm her down, relieve

her anxiety, and give her a feeling of control over her life. All of her behaviors served a similar function, in fact, because her hidden body image purpose was to be perfect enough that bad things didn't happen to her.

4. EXPLORE YOUR BODY IMAGE *SUFFERING* ITSELF.

In this last exercise, you'll be exploring the purpose of your actual body image pain and suffering, because sometimes it is that pain and suffering itself that exists to solve a problem or meet a need for you.

Some people's body image suffering provides them with a valid excuse to withdraw, shrink themselves, dim their light, avoid doing scary things, or just stay busy. Some suffering is a person's way of screaming to the world, "I am not okay!" and some is a person's brain screaming to them, "Something is wrong!" when they don't want to listen. Sometimes being upset about how we look protects us from facing our feelings, and sometimes it protects us from taking up space, going after our dreams, or making ourselves vulnerable. Sometimes we would rather hurt ourselves than let someone else hurt us. Sometimes hating our bodies is easier than hating our lives, or our circumstances, or ourselves. Body image suffering is painful, yes, but sometimes being in pain is the whole point.

For this exercise, write down a list of ways your body or body image causes you pain or suffering, and what that experience feels like. Consider the moments your body image makes you miserable, upsets you, stresses you out, or ruins your day, and how it affects you. You can be as detailed or specific as you like, and write down as many or as few statements as come to you. Some examples would be "thinking about my body makes me feel disgusted and like I want to run away," or "looking in the mirror fills my chest and belly with a heavy, achy kind of shame." If nothing specific is coming to you, it's also fine to write more general statements like "when I think about my body staying the

way it is, I feel like I'll die," or "hating my body feels like being in excruciating pain, but nobody else can see it."

Once you have at least a few descriptions of how your body image
causes you pain or suffering, and what that experience feels like, consider how that experience of pain and suffering might have actually
been trying to help, serve, or protect you. For each statement on your
list, try to answer any of the following questions that feel relevant, or
just come up with your own ideas for how that experience might be
helping (or trying to help) you.

- What has being upset about your body led to your doing, or
  not doing?

- What might being in pain communicate to others that you
  can't?

- What might your body insecurities be protecting you from?

- What needs or desires are being met (or *trying* to be met)
  through your pain or suffering?

- What problems are solved by hating your body so much?

- What does your body image suffering distract you from, or
  help you avoid?

- In what way might your body image suffering be a form of
  self-harm: a way in which you cause yourself pain, because
  pain is more tolerable than other kinds of pain or because it
  provides you with a sense of agency, autonomy, power, or
  control?

- Why might your brain not want to give up its body image suffering?

- What's the hidden purpose of your body image suffering?
  How is it serving you?

Once you've answered these questions, go back through what you've
written and see what you can learn about your underlying hidden

body image purpose. Here are a few examples from my coaching practice:

- Rachel had been telling herself for decades that once she lost weight, her "real life" would begin: she would quit her job, take a year to travel, and then transition into a more fulfilling career and start dating. And while she did genuinely *want* those things, she was also very scared of them. Hating her body (and constantly chasing weight loss) kept her life small and safe, because she couldn't imagine doing any of those things while still hating her body so much. Her hidden body image purpose was to protect her from the vulnerability of daring to pursue a big, juicy life.

- Luca had done a lot of body image healing work by the time we met. He intellectually understood that there was nothing whatsoever wrong with his body, he had stopped dieting, and he listened to his body whenever it needed rest. But he still couldn't seem to get over the hatred and disgust he felt when he looked in the mirror. This exercise helped him discover his brain didn't want to give up this last bit of suffering because it felt like "proof" of the hardships he'd been through. "Proof to whom?" I asked. "To my mom, I think," he responded. "I feel like if I get over this, like actually get over it and move on, my mom will think I turned out okay, and she didn't make any mistakes." Luca's body image suffering existed to communicate his pain to others, and to hold his mother accountable for her mistakes. His hidden body image purpose was ultimately to get enough validation from others that he would finally feel valid in and of himself.

If you've actually been tackling these four exercises with me in real time, your hidden body image purpose should be coming into focus.

Again, you can state it any way that feels good for you, but I recommend first trying to finish the following sentences:

- "My hidden body image purpose is to . . ."
- "My body image issues exist to . . ."

If neither of those resonate with you, you can make up your own, or try one of these:

- "My body anxiety (or obsession, dysmorphia, insecurities, or hatred) exists to . . ."
- "The problem my body negativity is trying to solve for me is . . ."
- "The need or desire I'm trying to get met with my body is . . ."
- "My body image issues are trying to motivate me to . . ."
- "My body image issues are trying to help me . . ."
- "My body image issues are trying to earn . . ."
- "My body image issues are trying to protect me from . . ."
- "My brain wants to . . ."

Feel free to play with this, restating your hidden purposes in different ways, meditating on them, journaling about them, bouncing them around with others, and letting them evolve, until you find a version that feels both intellectually honest and emotionally powerful and resonant. It should be relatively concise and concentrated—able to be explained in one or two sentences—or else you might not have quite gotten to the core of it yet. And while it's very common for one person to have two, three, or even four different hidden purposes, if you find yourself with closer to ten or fifteen, you might not have gone deep enough either.

CHAPTER *14*

Creating a Vision for a Body Neutral Future

O NCE YOU'VE IDENTIFIED EXACTLY WHY your body image issues exist, the next step is to figure out what it would take to remove that reason from existence.

Remember that our body image issues exist to solve a problem, and they're not going anywhere if we still believe we need them, on any level. Our behaviors, coping mechanisms, fixations, and suffering all serve a purpose, and it's only when *we no longer need them* that they go away.[1] That's why the next stage of the body neutrality blueprint is to figure out what would actually need to happen for your body image issues to become obsolete.

Given your unique and specific hidden body image purpose, what would need to be true in your life for you to no longer need your body image issues? What would you need to feel, do, have, be, or experience for your body image issues to serve no purpose, and have no job? I call this step of the blueprint creating a vision for a body neutral future, because you're literally trying to imagine a possible future in which your body image issues simply have no reason to exist. This step can be challenging, but it's also critical, because your vision of this future will shape and anchor all the body neutrality work you do from here on, as well as provide motivation and a sense of your own efficacy and self-determination along the way.

Before we go any further, I want to be clear that there is no right or wrong answer when it comes to your vision of a body neutral future. In fact, there are often many different answers and details that would all function, sometimes individually, and sometimes all together, to make a vision work. Imagine an outsider, for example, whose body image issues existed to "earn" them permission to express themselves more authentically so they can feel seen, known, and able to connect deeply with others. What would have to be true in their future for them to no longer need their body image issues? They might just need to give themselves permission to express themselves freely and authentically on a regular basis. Or maybe they would also need to cultivate the deep and nourishing relationships that make them feel seen and known. And perhaps they'd also have to cultivate resilience in the face of rejection so they are no longer scared of rejection.

Can you see how each of the details of this vision helps get to the root cause of the outsider's body image suffering and puts their body image issues out of a job? One person might have stopped with just the first one, if that felt complete to them, and another might need to continue adding details until they create a vision that would *totally* negate their hidden body image purpose. Everyone is different, and the only person who can say whether a particular vision would effectively nullify your body image issues is *you*.

To start creating your own vision of a body neutral future, try answering the following questions. (As always, I recommend doing this in writing!)

- What would need to be true for your body image issues to no longer serve any purpose whatsoever?
- What would need to be different for you to stop placing so much importance, significance, meaning, or power on your body?

- What problems would need to be solved for your hidden body image purpose to become useless?

- What needs could be met to make your body image issues pointless?

- What would you have to believe, feel, know, do, have, let go of, or overcome for you to really and truly believe you didn't need the help your body image issues are trying to offer?

Write down as many ideas or details for how to put your body image issues out of business as you can. Feel free to get creative and think outside the box as you jot things down—just remember you ultimately want this vision to be something that could actually happen.

When I asked my client Jules what would need to be true for their body image issues to become obsolete and pointless, for example, they first said, "I would need to be thinner." This is a tempting answer, of course, because it's exactly what we've all been taught to think about our bodies and the world, but it's both unrealistic for most folks, and frankly, kind of a cop-out. After all, even if Jules had successfully been able to sustain long-term weight loss, their real issue (the constant avoiding and numbing of emotions) still would have been there, and their real need (to feel safe in their own body) would still have gone unmet. When I prompted Jules to consider both a more attainable scope of reality and the deeper reasons they wanted to be thinner, they wrote down some way more potent (and vulnerable) ideas, like:

- I'd be better at identifying, facing, and feeling my emotions so I didn't have a reason to numb or avoid them.

- I'd know how to communicate my needs to others, set boundaries, and stand up for myself so that more of my needs get met, and feel safer in my relationships.

- I'd be better at handling pain and discomfort so I wouldn't feel so anxious all the time.

Now *those* are some powerful and specific visions for a body neutral future; each one addresses the deeper issues at play *and* offers an attainable possibility that Jules could work toward. They actually ended up combining the ideas into one single vision, because all three details seemed to play an equally important role in making their body image obsolete.

If you find it difficult to come up with a vision that is both effective and realistic, you're not alone. When that happens for my clients, it's usually because they haven't yet gotten specific enough about what *meaning* they're assigning to things, or the deeper purpose for their goal. My client Anthony, for example, whose hidden body image purpose was to "earn himself a husband," tried to tell me that the only possibility in which he would no longer need to obsess over his appearance was if "all gay men stopped being so superficial." Not particularly realistic, right? But what would the point of this even be? He told me the point would be that then he could find his husband—that was the real desired outcome. But even that wasn't particularly realistic, insofar as none of us can predict or control when (or if) the One will walk into our lives. So I pushed him to go even deeper.

"What is it that you're hoping a husband will bring you?" I asked Anthony. "What needs do you imagine being met, or problems being solved, by finding and marrying your dream man?"

This question led to us making a list of all the things Anthony had subconsciously associated with finding a husband: feeling chosen and special, feeling validated and "good enough," showing his family that he was a legitimate grown-up, companionship and the ability to travel, having access to regular sex and intimacy, and finally feeling free to be his true self.

With this list in hand, Anthony went back to trying to come up with an effective and realistic vision of a body neutral future, and it just poured out of him. He envisioned a future in which he had a stronger sense of self-worth (and no longer needed to prove to anyone that he was good enough), he had cultivated strong and meaningful friendships with people with whom he could travel often, he got his needs for sex and intimacy met more casually (without guilt or self-criticism), and he no longer let the fear of rejection keep him from being his authentic self. Whew! All these details came together to effectively address Anthony's hidden body image purpose, and while each one was a serious undertaking, each one was possible. For the first time in our coaching together, Anthony was able to imagine a future in which he didn't *need* to obsess over his body, and it changed everything. This was the first moment I saw him fully buy into the body neutrality blueprint and believe it could work for him; it was the first moment I saw him feel hope.

As you brainstorm your own list of ideas for a body neutral future, I encourage you to think small, be specific, and get granular about the purpose and meaning attached to each goal. If you want to be married, what do you think would be different if you were married? If you want to be rich and famous, what associations or meanings are connected to money and fame in your mind? Try this if you get stuck, and see how many new ideas pour in.

Essentially, the process of envisioning a body neutral future is about finding attainable ways to solve your problems and meet your needs directly so that your body doesn't have to play any role. If your body image issues exist to protect you from people's judgment and criticism, for example, you might get stuck imagining an impossible vision of the future, in which nobody ever judged or criticized you ever again. But because that's not within your control (and therefore not attainable), you'll need to solve the problem of other people's judgment and criticism another way. What would have to be true for you to no longer need protection from judgment and criticism? Certainly you could try to prevent it from happening for the rest of your life, but you might be better served trying to find a way to be *okay* with it happening. If other peoples' judgment and criticism had no effect on you, you would no longer require protection from it, right? Bam: body neutral vision created. And don't worry, you don't need to know how you'll get there yet!

Right now you just need to identify what would need to be true for your body image issues to become obsolete.

That said, you might also decide to dig deeper into the specific meaning you've attached to being judged and criticized. What do you imagine would be different in your life if nobody ever judged or criticized you again? Would you feel less anxious and take more risks? If so, maybe your vision should include you having gotten your anxiety under control and doing big things with your big life. The more you explore, the more information you're likely to find, and you can use that information to fine-tune your vision of a body neutral future.

After you have your list of ideas and details, pull back and consider what you've written. Does your vision need to include multiple details, or is there one that gets the job done alone? Are there multiple details that all accomplish the same goal? If so, which one feels like the best fit for you? Which ones help you achieve the most effective and attainable vision?

You can describe your vision any way you like, and it can be as simple or complicated as feels right. A self-objectifier whose body image issues were trying to earn them intimacy, for example, envisioned a future in which *either* they got their needs for intimacy met *or* they made peace with the fact that they can't. Having an either/or vision like this is totally fine! And a runner whose body image issues existed to protect them from all of their emotions and vulnerabilities ended up writing out a list of twenty-five details that would all need to be true for their vision to work. There is no right or wrong way to create this vision.

I also want to point out that you may not ever actually "arrive" at this future, and that's okay. As my dad likes to say: life is a journey, not a parking lot. You're never going to arrive anywhere, really, so instead of thinking about your vision for a body neutral future as an end point you need to eventually arrive at, think of it more as a compass: a tool designed to always keep you pointed north on the journey. Ultimately, this part of the body neutrality blueprint is designed to clarify exactly what you're aiming for, provide you with hope and motivation, and make it possible to come up with an effective action plan.

CHAPTER 15

Creating a Body Neutrality
Action Plan

AFTER YOU HAVE A CLEAR VISION FOR A body neutral future, it's time to figure out how to actually get there! The third step of the body neutrality blueprint is to create what I call the body neutrality action plan, which is a set of specific action steps that help an individual continuously move down the path toward the future they've envisioned.

An individual's action plan is unique and specific to them, and completely responsive to their lived experiences. For that reason, a good action plan is fluid, flexible, and ever evolving, not strict, rigid, or permanent. Think of it more like a tool for self-coaching than a magic formula; be prepared for the path to be continually shifting and unfolding as you walk it. This is how it *should* be, because every step you take will bring you more information, insight, and clarity, with which you can then edit and improve your plan. You might come up with ten action steps you plan to do in order, for example, but then discover upon doing the *first* step that the next nine steps don't actually make sense anymore. That's okay, and actually an important part of the process!

Before diving into the process of creating a body neutrality action plan, let's see a few examples of it in action.

Kelsey, a high achiever who desperately wanted to become a mom, had been struggling for years to get pregnant. In the process of trying to "do everything right," she had become obsessed with purifying and perfecting her body in the hopes that an über-healthy body powered by celery juice and chia seeds would give her a baby. Her body anxiety, shame, and disgust existed to try to "earn" her what she most desired: a baby.

When Kelsey tried to envision a body neutral future for herself, she was able to write only one thing down: "I would be a mother." Getting pregnant wasn't a possibility for her, so at first we explored what meaning she had attached to motherhood to see what she was really seeking: The intense bonding with a child? The leaving of a legacy? The ability to express her nurturing side? Through our conversation, it became clear that the thing Kelsey wanted most was the experience of *being a mother*. Having defined that as a different thing from *having a baby*, we decided it actually could be attainable if we were willing to get creative.

With *being a mother* as Kelsey's vision for her future, we explored her definition of "mother," and brainstormed every imaginable way a person could become one, other than getting pregnant.

"What are some ways you could realistically get from here to there?" I asked her.

"I could always try to adopt a baby," she told me. "Or hire a surrogate."

At this point we were just exploring the possibilities, so we didn't stop to critique or consider the details of either option. Instead, we kept brainstorming, trying to come up with as many creative, unusual, or undervalued ways to become a mother as we could. By the end, Kelsey's list of possible pathways included fostering older kids, seeking out a parental role in a polyamorous or communal-living setup, and even opening a childcare facility (which had always been a sort of daydream for her).

After we had come up with all the ideas we could, Kelsey started to play out each pathway in her mind, to see how it felt. She did some research about what action steps would be required for each one, considered which ones made sense for her logistically and financially, and which ones would best honor and meet her desire to be a mother. She chose several options to pursue simultaneously and identified a few action steps she could take for each, like researching organizations, reaching out to people who had gone through the experience, and making phone calls.

Within a year, Kelsey was on two separate adoption lists, and still considering moving forward with surrogacy in the meantime. And in that time—with her path to motherhood feeling more and more within her grasp—Kelsey's obsessive body habits had faded significantly in both frequency and intensity, only hitting their old fever pitch when one of her grief triggers got hit, like a friend getting pregnant or having a baby.

Brainstorming various pathways for getting to the future you've envisioned for yourself tends to require some creative problem-solving and out-of-the-box thinking, as it did for Kelsey. You may end up with an overwhelming number of possibilities to choose from, or with very few, but don't put too much pressure on yourself to choose "correctly," as there is no right or wrong choice here. Thanks to the clarity and specificity gained by first identifying your hidden body image purpose and envisioning the details of your body neutral future, the action plan should always be precisely focused on the heart of your body image issues. So no matter which pathway you choose, or how many times you rewrite the steps, you will always be moving toward a more body neutral future.

Plus, you don't have to be able to see the whole plan to begin. Because she didn't know anything about the process of adoption or surrogacy before she started, Kelsey didn't know what actions she would need to take to get from here to there, but that didn't matter. All you ever need is the *next* step, so while it can be very satisfying and motivating to identify a complete list of action steps for reaching your goal, it's also completely valid to have a list with only one item on it, saying something like "find out more about _____," or "call ____ and ask what the next steps are." The purpose of creating an action plan is to put you into action immediately, so as long as you've set your sights on the right goal (i.e., your vision for a body neutral future), *any* action step you can take is a good one. Undoubtedly, as you take action, you'll gain information and clarity about the specific steps required, and your action plan—which is fluid, flexible, and ever evolving—will fill out.

I also want to mention here that Kelsey's story may sound pretty straightforward, but it was also emotionally intense. After all, none of the pathways she came up with felt perfect, because the only perfect plan was an impossible one: getting pregnant. So while clarifying, adding to, and carrying out her realistic body neutrality action plan, Kelsey was also moving through a lot of pain and grief over not being able to get pregnant on her own, and letting go of her attachment to how she thought the process of becoming a mother would and should have gone.

This is a very common experience, and an item that a lot of people have to add to their action plan to-do list: Grieving the loss of the life they *imagined* so they can embrace the life they *have*. Releasing their attachment to how they want reality to be so they can accept it as it is. Not an easy task, to be sure, but one that aligns beautifully with the rest of the work you've been doing, as it's focused on acknowledging and accepting the truth of reality without adding layers of meaning, significance, or interpretation.

Another example was Ali, an introverted nonbinary outsider with social anxiety, whose body anxiety existed to earn them connection and belonging, so they didn't feel so alone all the time. When they envisioned a body neutral future, it was full of deep friendships, a feeling of belonging in multiple spaces, and a tight-knit community of artists and other creatives. I asked them to brainstorm all the different ways they might be able to get from here to there, and they wrote down about thirty ideas for building community and meeting like-minded people: enrolling in classes and clubs that interested them, going to relevant meetups or events, and spending one day per week working from a coffee shop instead of from home, for example. Not feeling a strong connection to any particular option, Ali just chose from their list at random to get started, and joined a local book club.

Ali came to the first session after the first book club meeting utterly deflated. They reported hating everyone there, feeling incredibly anxious and defensive, and having a terrible time. We unpacked the experience and discovered that they had gone into the night with a negative and critical mindset, as they go into most things, because it feels less vulnerable to expect things to suck from the beginning than to get their hopes up and be disappointed. We also recognized how Ali's anxiety sometimes made them come off as cold or awkward, which made connecting with people exceptionally difficult.

Ali was bummed to find all this out, but I was *excited*. This is how a body neutrality action plan is made—through action! By choosing one random pathway and taking action toward it, Ali had given us all the information we needed to identify the next step!

From there, Ali went back into brainstorming mode, coming up with potential pathways toward their newly found "micro-goals": the smaller and more specific goals which are required for a person to continue progressing toward their overall vision of a body neutral future, and therefore must temporarily take precedence. Most often, micro-goals are discovered as a person takes action, and runs into obstacles or setbacks. My vision for a body neutral future as a runner, for example, was one in which I felt safe and calm, and my body's default was to be soft and relaxed. I first decided to try meditation as a way of calming and relaxing my mind and body, but found that sitting still and focusing on my breath led to panic attacks instead. Rather than getting frustrated or blaming myself for not being able to meditate properly, however, I got curious about what would need to be true for me to access the calming benefits of meditation. This spawned a new list of micro-goals: explore other types of meditation (like walking and mindful movement); work with a therapist to safely explore the source of my panic; do exercises to make slow, deep belly breathing easier; find other ways of relaxing and releasing physical tension; and work on my hip and spine mobility to make sitting more comfortable. It might seem a little overwhelming, but ultimately that list led me exactly where I needed to go.

Ali's brave action had revealed an obstacle too: they didn't yet have the skills, mindset, or practice needed to genuinely connect with people! This presented a major hurdle to Ali's ability to move forward with their plan, so handling that obstacle became the immediate focus and priority, in service of the ultimate body neutral future Ali envisioned.

"What might have to be true in your life for you to have a more open and positive mindset going into social situations?" I asked. "And what might have to be true for people to have an easier time connecting with you?"

Ali brainstormed a big list of possible action steps they could take, including journaling to better understand their negative assumptions about people, learning more about friendly and connective body language, role-playing small-talk with me for practice, and working with a therapist on their fear of vulnerability. They chose a handful of action steps to move toward immediately, reading books on how people connect and how to have a positive mindset, watching videos about body language and nonverbal communication, role-playing meeting people, and then exploring what parts felt hard, and why. They eventually practiced facing their fear of rejection and vulnerability in low-stakes environments, because they had discovered their negative attitude toward others was a sort of offense-is-the-best-defense policy to avoid being rejected. And after a few months of working on these kinds of skills, Ali was able to step back into a social space (a hiking club this time) with more social competence, self-awareness, openness, and confidence, and found it *much* easier to connect with people. They even ended up making a friend from the hiking club, which gave Ali more opportunities to continue practicing and improving their connection skills.

Hopefully these examples have demonstrated what the body neutrality action plan can do: encourage creative problem-solving, put you into action, uncover obstacles, and make sure you're always moving in the right direction (i.e., toward a body neutral future). In this way, the body neutrality path is *made by walking*. Each step will be informed and illuminated by the last step, so as long as you continue to take action (and are willing to get curious about the results), you'll stay on the right path.

Ready to create your own body neutrality action plan? Follow the step-by-step exercises below!

1. BRAINSTORM POTENTIAL PATHWAYS FOR GETTING FROM *HERE* TO *THERE*.

Consider all the possible ways you might be able to go from here (i.e., your current life, and your current relationship to your body), to there (i.e., the body neutral future you've envisioned for yourself).

Try using your body neutral vision to fill in the blank, and ask yourself the question, "What are all the possible ways I could _____?" Then just write down as many realistic and attainable ideas as you can!

Depending on the specifics of your body neutral future, you may have more than one relevant question to ask, and therefore more than one brainstorming session to do. For example, in Kelsey's vision of a body neutral future, she was a mother, so the question became simply "What are all the possible ways I could become a mom?" In Ali's case, however, they had a handful of close friends *and* one or two communities in which they felt a sense of belonging, so they came up with two questions to answer: "What are all the possible ways I could make friends?" and "What are all the possible ways I could join or build a community?"

If your vision of a body neutral future includes many details or stipulations, you might want to separate each stipulation into its own category and do a brainstorming session for each. I do this by asking each question at the top of a clean page and then filling out the page with answers to that question only, but I've also had clients who prefer to do it all together. You're welcome to do whatever works best for you, but one benefit to separating each question this way is that you can always go back and add to each list as ideas occur to you over time.

If you're having a hard time coming up with ideas for how to get from here to there, try bouncing ideas around with a trusted member of your inner circle, doing a little googling, or journaling your answers to the questions below. You can also try breaking your goal down into one of three categories: *skills* you'd need to learn or improve, *fears* you'd need to overcome, and *shame* you would have to release in order for you to get where you want to go. (Note: I'll be sharing more about these three categories at the end of the chapter!)

However you do it, be creative and think outside the box! This is not the time to worry about the details of each pathway, it's a time to write down every possibility you can think of—no matter how big or small, no matter how difficult or easy, and no matter how well they seem to suit you—for how a person could possibly move from *here* to *there*.

Questions to get your creative juices flowing:

- What's keeping you from already being in, or standing in your way of getting to, your vision of a body neutral future?

- What skills would you need to practice or improve to end up in this future? And how could you make that happen?

- What needs would you have to meet to end up in this future? And how could you get them met?

- What problems would you need to solve to end up in this future? And how could you solve them?

- What changes would have to happen in your life for you to end up *there*?

♦ What would you need to have, do, accept, release, or face to go from *here* to *there?*

2. PICK A PATHWAY, AND BREAK IT DOWN INTO MICRO-GOALS IF NEEDED.

Consider your list of potential pathways. Is there one or more that seems to call to you most, as with Kelsey? Or do all the ideas feel kind of equal, like they did to Ali? Are there some pathways that lend themselves immediately to clear and actionable steps, and some that don't? Do you want to do them all? Choose at least one or two pathways to start with, either at random, or through careful consideration. (And yes, you can totally do the following steps for every single one, if you like. Just know that you don't need to, because you can always return to this part.)

Once you've chosen a pathway, start thinking about what would need to actually happen for you to move along it. If your pathway is particularly broad or complex, you might want to first break it down into micro-goals before coming up with action steps for each micro-goal, and if it's pretty straightforward, you can just skip straight to the action steps. For example, if you decide an important pathway to your body neutral vision is to cultivate a strong and resilient sense of self-worth, that's a huge and complex goal, and coming up with action steps might feel overwhelming. To make it more manageable, you might want to break it down into micro-goals that will help you get there. Identify why your self-worth is so negative, fragile, or weak in the first place, and use that information to create micro-goals. For example, if your self-worth is low in part because of your financial or career situation, you might make "financial security" or "switch careers" a micro-goal. If it's fragile in part because you feel socially awkward or have very few close connections, you might add "improve social skills" or "cultivate more close connections" to your micro-goal list. Then you can break each micro-goal into actionable steps, instead of trying to break the whole big pathway down.

That said, sometimes a pathway is already pretty straightforward and manageable, and you can skip the micro-goal part altogether. Ali's pathway was to meet more people, for example, which lent itself easily to a long list of possible action steps. While we did discover some micro-steps later on, there was no need in the beginning to break their pathway down into micro-goals.

3. BREAK EACH PATHWAY (OR MICRO-GOAL) DOWN INTO POTENTIAL ACTION STEPS.

Back to brainstorming! For this step, you'll be coming up with any and all action steps that could move you down your pathway, or toward your micro-goal. It's important to write this part down, because this will become the first draft of your body neutrality action plan! Personally, I like to write each pathway or micro-goal at the top of a blank piece of paper, and then write down all the potential action steps I can think of underneath it, because this makes it easier to conceptualize (and track) my action plan, and also because it's nice to have space to go back and add ideas to the page later.

For some pathways or micro-goals, you might not come up with many action ideas, and that's okay; all you need to identify is the *first* action step you can take. (For example, Kelsey didn't know anything about the process of adoption, so her first step was simply to do some research about that process, and the next action steps required were illuminated bit by bit from there.) Other times you'll have tons of ideas to write down, either as a step-by-step list, or as a random collection of possibilities. All of this is totally okay!

Recently I worked with someone who made two lists: one for having better sex, and one for improving her ability to advocate for her needs.

The sex list was full of random ideas, like reading a book, taking a course, going to a kink party, buying sex toys, creating a daily self-pleasure ritual, reading (or writing) erotica, keeping a pleasure journal, practicing mindfulness, working through her specific anxieties, and tuning in to small pleasures throughout her day. Her other list, however, was very short, containing only one line: "Google how people work on self-advocacy." Both lists were perfect, because she was able to choose one item from each list to move forward with immediately.

Don't stress about getting these lists perfect or "right," because you'll be coming back to add, remove, or rewrite them as you move forward! Their purpose is to put you into action immediately, as well as to keep you moving in the right direction long term.

4. CHOOSE AN ACTION STEP AND DO IT!

Choose an action step that you can do immediately (doing a Google search, joining a book club, signing up for a class, going to a kink party, learning about intuitive eating, etc.), and go do it! You're welcome to choose more than one action step at a time, depending on what you feel available for. For example, you might choose one action step from each of your lists, or you might prefer to choose several action steps all from one list. There's no right or wrong way to do this, as long as you *actually take the action!*

5. CONSIDER THE EXPERIENCE, REASSESS AS NEEDED, AND CHOOSE ANOTHER ACTION STEP.

Consider how your action step went. How did it feel? What did you learn? Did it bring your attention to any obstacles, weaknesses, fears, or lack of information that might need to be addressed to get where you want to go? Did it spark any new action step ideas, make any you have written down seem unnecessary, or alter your understanding of the best order or approach to take?

If so, return to your lists (either pathways or action steps), and add, edit, or alter as needed. Once Ali attended their first book club meeting, for example, they discovered that they needed to add some specific new micro-goals to their plan for making friends: adopt a more open and accepting mindset, get more comfortable with vulnerability, develop welcoming body language, and improve their small talk skills. So they went back and created a new page for each micro-goal, and spent a little time jotting down possible action steps for each.

Maybe your first action step toward the micro-goal of buying a house was to look into your finances, and having done that, you now realize buying a house won't be possible until you pay off your student loans and get a better job. Great! Those two things can become their own micro-goals, and you can start taking action toward them both, while putting the whole house idea on a back burner.

Feel free to change directions in any way that you like. As long as your lists and actions are still moving you in the direction of your vision for a body neutral future, you can't go wrong. You can switch lists and tackle an entirely different pathway if you want, either because you feel stuck about the next steps for one, or because the action required is moving so slow. If you're working to pay off your student loans, for example, you might automatically send a chunk of your paycheck toward your loans every week, for years. And while you're technically taking action toward your goal during that time, if you want to take on some more active work as well, you could return to your original list of pathways, choose a brand-new one, break it into steps, and start taking action. Sometimes you'll need to choose a new list because you finished the one you were working on (yay!), or because you just feel bored, burned out, stuck, tired, frustrated, or unavailable for the one you were working on. I've had clients bounce between lists depending on their mood, schedule, environment, resources, and even their menstrual cycles! This is why the body neutrality action plan is so flexible. It ensures you can always be moving forward, no matter what. The important thing isn't that you follow any one list perfectly, but rather that you're using your lists to generate *consistent action toward your goal over the long term.*

Then, whether or not you did any shifting or altering to your lists, the next step in the action plan is always the same: choose *another* action step, and get back out into the world to do it!

6. RINSE AND REPEAT!

That's it! From here on, you just continue moving forward in this way: Choose an action from your list and go do it. Then consider what you learned from that experience, reassess or alter your list as needed, choose another action, and go do it. If you stay accountable to your plan and stick to it consistently, your body image issues will naturally lose power over time, and body neutrality will feel more and more possible.

How slowly or quickly you move through your action plan is entirely up to you. Some people choose one action item each month so that they're slowly moving in the right direction while also managing an otherwise full plate, and that's perfect. Others blast full speed ahead, tackling five to ten items each week, because they have the time, motivation, and resources to do so, and that's also perfect. Most people go through some stretches of time when their action plan is a priority and they're able to put a lot of time and energy into it and others when they have only the absolute bare minimum to put into it. All of that is normal and valid and fine, but I do encourage you to temper your expectations accordingly. If you can put only a tiny amount of time and energy into this plan, expect it to move very slowly and take a long time to see progress. If you can put a ton of time and energy into it, you will probably see much more significant progress on a faster timeline. I'd say two small action steps per week is probably what I see on average among my clients, but it's important to be realistic (and self-compassionate) about what you can actually get done.

As a final note, it can be incredibly helpful to have support and accountability for sticking to your action plan over the long term, whether that means finding a body neutrality blueprint buddy, working with a coach or therapist, or sharing your journey on social media.

Whew! Now that you understand the makeup of a body neutrality action plan, I want to go back to the three big categories I mentioned before—skill building, fear facing, and shame busting—and demonstrate what valuable resources they can be in the process of creating an action plan.

Many of my clients struggle to come up with pathway ideas (or break a goal down into achievable steps) out of thin air, because doing so goes directly against their habitual thought patterns. It's normal to have a hard time imagining how to go about doing something we always thought was impossible, or that we've been blocking out of our consciousness. For example, if we're used to thinking of our marriage as a miserable-but-permanent thing that we can never change or escape, it might feel nearly impossible to suddenly try coming up with ways to change or escape it. In such moments, my clients report drawing a blank, being unable to come up with anything tangible or specific, or feeling like the thing they want is just impossible.

For these moments (and actually, for *any* time during the action plan process!), I suggest using these three powerful categories to generate ideas. Instead of asking yourself the very general question, "What would need to be true for me to get from *here* to *there*?" you can ask yourself a more specific question from one of these three categories:

+ **Skill building.** "Where might a lack of skill, talent, practice, experience, or information be standing in the way of my getting from here to there?"

- ◆ **Fear facing.** "Where might fear be standing in the way of my getting from here to there?"
- ◆ **Shame busting.** "Where might shame be standing in the way of my getting from here to there?"

Each category can help generate new, specific, and tangible ideas for both pathways and action steps, so I encourage you to use them in your own body neutrality action plan, either weaving them into your plan right from the beginning, or just employing them anytime you feel stuck, out of ideas, or like something is impossible.

SKILL BUILDING

Think about the body neutral future you envisioned for yourself. What might the *you* in that future be good at that you're not currently good at? What skills, traits, talents, or abilities might future you have that current you doesn't? What knowledge, wisdom, information, or education might they have that you don't? And more important, what would you need to start doing, learning, practicing, or developing now to get to that place?

Skill building is a powerful strategy to use in your body neutrality action plan, because our body image issues so often exist to solve a problem that we don't have another way of solving. In such cases, our body image issues are just a workaround, a sort of "strategy B" that kicks in because we don't know how to implement "strategy A." In order to *no longer require* strategy B, therefore, we'll have to cultivate the specific skills, traits, education, or experiences that allow us to effectively implement strategy A! Luckily, modern neuroscience shows us that our brains are highly adaptive throughout our entire lives, which means we can get better at pretty much anything and everything, if we practice![1] That includes tangible skills like learning a new instrument or speaking a new language, as well as less tangible skills we might not normally think of, like being vulnerable, setting boundaries, connecting with our bodies, or cultivating self-worth. So by identifying the specific skills and abilities that stand in the way of your body neutral future, you can come up with a whole bunch of new micro-goals or action steps to add to your list!

Think about your hidden body image purpose and what problem it's trying to solve. What would you need to be better at to solve that problem yourself? If your body image issues exist to protect you from conflict, for example, then improving your ability to handle conflict would naturally move you toward neutrality. If they exist to earn you enough external validation that you finally feel good enough, then cultivating a strong and positive sense of self-worth would eventually render them useless. And if your body image issues protect you from facing your feelings, then developing your emotional intelligence, increasing your capacity for discomfort, and cultivating a positive relationship with your feelings would help put them out of business.

Identify each skill, quality, or area you want to learn more about, practice, cultivate, or improve, and then break it down into possible action steps. Want to improve your relationships? You might need to cultivate your tolerance for vulnerability, improve your communication skills, overcome your fear of rejection, get better at active listening, and practice speaking other people's love languages. Each of these might actually be best treated as a micro-goal at this point, so you could brainstorm actionable steps for each one individually, *or* if your list is already specific enough, you can be done. Either way, these ideas and lists will now be included in your action plan so that you can call upon them as desired over time.

As you start putting your body neutrality action plan into motion, you will most likely bump into new and different areas that need cultivation, so be prepared for this to be very fluid. Maybe you decide to join Toastmasters because you want to improve your public speaking ability, for example, but being at Toastmasters reveals a habit of involuntarily shrinking, both physically and vocally, when people are looking at you.

Cool! You could brainstorm a few action steps for improving *that* (e.g., researching how to adopt powerful body language, doing some posture exercises, taking a movement class, practicing yelling and taking up space), and then either leave those ideas in your lists to pick back up later or just take action on one of them immediately.

The more you learn, cultivate, and develop your skills, knowledge, and experience in this way, the less you'll *need* body image issues, and the easier body neutrality will be. Plus, the more you improve, the more empowered and confident you'll feel, the more you'll trust yourself, the more needs you'll get met, the stronger your self-worth will be, and the better your life will become overall.

FEAR FACING

Where does fear show up in your hidden body image plan? What fears do your body image issues help you avoid? Which fears have the power to keep you from taking certain action steps? Where might fear make you feel stuck or paralyzed in your action plan? And which fears would you need to face or overcome to arrive at your body neutral future?

Brin, an advertising intern in her early twenties, hadn't worn a swimsuit since she was thirteen, because the thought of wearing one always sent her into a body image panic. When I asked her what skills she would need to practice or develop to wear one in public, she couldn't come up with an answer other than "I would just need to not be so uncomfortable." Right away, I knew we needed to employ the power of strategic fear facing.

Fear facing is the practice of gradually exposing yourself to the thing you are most afraid of (or uncomfortable with), taking small and incremental action steps over time, until the fear loses its power over you. You can think of fear-facing work as a form of self-directed exposure therapy, because it kind of is. Exposure therapy is a psychological treatment technique therapists use that is designed to help people break the fear-and-avoidance cycle and overcome fears, anxieties, and phobias. The person essentially just confronts the thing that triggers their fear, in a safe and controlled environment, over and over under the therapist's guidance, until they no longer feel a fear response to it. It's thought that exposure therapy facilitates four effects to accomplish this goal: "habituation," which is the fear lessening over time as the person gets used to it; "extinction," which is the gradual weakening of the associations between fear and that trigger; "self-efficacy," which is where the person becomes more confident in their ability to safely face their fear; and "emotional processing," which means new associations are created with the fear trigger, and also that the person becomes more tolerant to the experience of fear.[2]

To be clear, the kind of self-guided fear-facing work I'm talking about here is in no way a replacement for the skilled guidance and applied technique of a qualified therapist, but it *is* something that most people will find accessible and effective, and it can lead to similar outcomes. By identifying a fear and then consistently taking incrementally bigger and bigger action steps to confront it over time, you will slowly build the resilience, tolerance, self-trust, emotional skill, and confidence that make the scary thing stop seeming so scary. Plus, including fear facing in your body neutrality action plan serves two other powerful purposes: getting you unstuck, and giving you information that you need.

Brin decided the first little baby step she could take toward facing her fear of swimsuits was to buy one and start wearing it around the house when she was alone. This immediately gave her some important information, because the first time she did this, she reported having a lot of anxiety about sexual assault, even though she was home alone. This insight clarified why she was so afraid of swimsuits, allowed her to be more compassionate toward herself for struggling, and encouraged her to talk about her history of sexual abuse with her therapist. While it didn't magically give Brin the ability to wear a swimsuit in public, this insight was like rocket fuel for her body image healing, and fear facing is what got her there.

That's the beautiful thing about fear facing: it immediately gives you a whole bunch of information you can't usually get without it. After all, if you always avoid the stuff that scares you, then you never have the opportunity to figure out why it scares you so much, what's underneath that fear, or what it would take to overcome it.

In this way, a lot of my clients end up moving back and forth between skill building and fear facing as they undertake their body neutrality action plan. Each type of action supports and leads back to the other. Whether you want to weave this strategy into your action plan from the beginning or employ it only when you run into a fear that's keeping you stuck, just break each fear down into scary-but-doable action steps for confronting it that you can do consistently over time. Start with an action step that makes you uncomfortable but also feels doable and safe, and then repeat that action over and over until it no longer makes you uncomfortable. Then choose a step that feels even more uncomfortable, but still doable, and repeat. Do this for as long as it takes—days, weeks, months, or years—until you've faced your fear in its entirety and it no longer has any power over you. You'll know your fear-facing strategy worked when you can look back at the action steps that once felt super scary but now seem silly, easy, or mundane.

When Brin first started wearing her swimsuit around the house alone, she described her heart racing, her palms sweating, and an anxious, jumpy, hot-in-the-face feeling. After dealing with her trauma in therapy for a while, however, she tried wearing her swimsuit at home again, and reported it felt like *nothing*. So she challenged herself a bit more by asking her boyfriend to help her continue her fear-facing practice. First they wore swimsuits in the bath together, then he joined her at a public pool, where she wore her swimsuit under a full-body cover-up. Eventually that became easy, so she progressed to a smaller and more sheer cover-up, and then eventually just her suit! This was *months* of work, but when I asked Brin to reflect on those first few action steps (buying the suit and wearing it alone at home), she laughed and shook her head, like she couldn't believe she had ever been afraid of something so silly.

And while fear facing can work great on straightforward and tangible fears like Brin's, the same strategy applies to complex or intangible fears too. If you're willing to get creative, you can find ways to gradually and progressively face fears like vulnerability, rejection, criticism, heartbreak, conflict, and abandonment too.

The more fear-facing work you do, the less your fears will have power over you, and the easier body neutrality will become. Plus, as an added bonus, regular fear facing will help you cultivate a sense of your own capacity to do hard and scary things, which is a huge booster for self-worth, self-trust, and self-confidence. After all, courage is a skill, too, and fear facing helps to develop and cultivate it. Many of my clients who throw themselves into fear-facing work have even ended up taking their sense of identity and worth from it, identifying as brave, strong, resilient, or powerful, which allowed them to stop taking their identity and worth from being attractive, thin, good, perfect, disciplined, or likable!

SHAME BUSTING

What role does shame play in your relationship to your body, your relationship to yourself, and your hidden body image purpose? What would you need to no longer feel shame about in order to let go of your body image issues and to fully accept and approve of yourself?

My client Dani's hidden body image purpose was to look good enough to make people love them, despite feeling fundamentally broken and "too much" deep down. Dani spent a lot of time and energy trying to monitor themself, their body, and their behaviors to hide the parts of themself they had learned in childhood were wrong, bad, or a burden on others. Dani's body neutrality action plan had them spend months developing self-awareness, improving communication skills, getting better at handling conflict, and facing the fear of abandonment, but eventually we hit a wall, and Dani's body image issues weren't budging. That was when we shifted gears and adopted the last of the three strategies: shame busting.

According to shame researcher and author Brené Brown, shame is the "intensely painful feeling or experience of believing that we are flawed and therefore unworthy of love and belonging—[that] something we've experienced, done, or failed to do makes us unworthy of connection."[3]

Shame makes us believe other people would reject or abandon us if they discovered the thing we feel shame about, so we naturally try to hide those parts of ourselves from others. We can feel shame about any part of ourselves, including our thoughts, feelings, behaviors, and personality, but in our racist, sexist, ableist, patriarchal, anti-fat, and sex-negative culture, shame *very* often shows up around our bodies. And as true as our shame belief might feel to us, it's almost always a lie born out of systems of oppression, trauma, and pain. Almost always a false interpretation, a projection of false meaning or significance onto ourselves and our bodies. Which means shame is not only just a whole bunch of smoke and mirrors, but also a whole bunch of smoke and mirrors that prevent us from accessing body neutrality.

Luckily, the antidote to shame is pretty simple, if not easy. We basically just have to drag the shame out of the dark and isolation that help it thrive, and share it with someone who can hold it with kindness and acceptance. As Brené Brown says, "If we can share our story with someone who responds with empathy and understanding, shame can't survive."[4] In other words, while we keep our shame a secret, it has power over us. It can make us believe that something about us is so bad and broken, so unworthy and unlovable, that if anyone ever found out, we would certainly end up miserable and alone. But when we drag our shame into the daylight and connectedness, it starts to wither. By sharing the parts of ourselves we're ashamed of with people who will still love and accept us after seeing it, we prove our shame to be a pathetic little con artist, and its power weakens. *This* is shame busting.

Shame busting is the practice of stripping our shame of power by sharing the parts of ourselves we feel shame about with others. Just like the practice of fear facing, this practice starts with very small and safe action steps—like sharing a not-too-vulnerable bit of shame with a person we know will meet it with empathy, understanding, love, compassion, and acceptance—and can increase incrementally over time as needed. This allows you to build tolerance, self-trust, confidence, and resilience to keep going down the shame-busting path, which is important, because this can be a lifelong practice.

In some ways, shame busting is just another type of fear facing. Our shame has convinced us that sharing these parts of ourselves will lead to rejection, attack, humiliation, or abandonment, and it takes a ton of courage to face those fears.

Dani told me during a coaching session that they were afraid I would hate them and stop wanting to work together if they told me everything going on in their head. I assured them that I didn't think this was true, but also didn't push. (Shame is not only emotional but also very much physiological; forcing someone to face it before they're ready can be dangerous.) A few weeks later, though, Dani asked to share a list of things they were sure would shock and revolt me. I agreed, and they started with "sometimes I think about mean or cruel stuff, like if someone is rude to me, I imagine them dying some kind of horrible death." I paused, waiting to see when the shocking part would come, but that was it.

I told Dani that these kinds of intrusive thoughts were normal, and that I've even experienced them myself. I asked about the rest of the list. "I don't know if I actually even love my parents!" they said. "And sometimes I hate being a parent! And the fastest way for me to reach orgasm is to play out a rape fantasy! Oh, and I think I might be trans-gender or nonbinary!" (At the time they were using she/her pronouns.) Dani seemed exhilarated, having said all these terrible things out loud for the first time and realizing the world hadn't exploded.

I thanked them for sharing, validated and normalized each one, and reassured Dani that not only did I still like them, but I actually thought *even more highly* of them after hearing all that, because I was able to connect more deeply to who they were as a person. I was honored that Dani had trusted me, I marveled at their courage and dedication to healing, and I recommended some resources to help them better un-derstand and normalize some of their concerns.

This session ended up being a massive turning point in Dani's body neutrality journey; something in them shifted after that forever. Hav-ing been met with understanding by one person, Dani's shame had lost a significant amount of its power, and they found themselves newly able to open up to people in their life about these topics, which led to some incredible discoveries. Dani learned about how normal their sex-ual fantasies were and told their partner they wanted to start playing with some light BDSM, which led to huge leaps forward in their mar-riage and sex life. They joined a few discussion and support groups on parenting and family dynamics, which made them feel validated and less alone in their struggles, and they started to explore their gender identity, which led to a much more authentic way of expressing them-self in the world.

All this shame-busting work, interwoven with skill-building and fear-facing action steps, led to Dani's finally feeling *worthy* of love as their whole self, and no longer needing their body to play a role in that. By the end of our work together, Dani said they hardly ever even thought about their body anymore, because it just seemed completely irrelevant.

When I asked Dani if they still worried about being "too much" for people, they said no.

"Why not, do you think?" I asked.

They just shrugged, and said, "I don't know, maybe because I'm no longer too much for myself."

Ready to bust some shame? Consider these questions to explore and identify any sources of shame you might want to strip of their power:

+ What parts of yourself do you feel ashamed of?

+ What aspects of yourself do you consider unlovable, bad, wrong, broken, or proof that you're unworthy of love, acceptance, or belonging?

+ What are you afraid would make people hate you, leave you, or ridicule you, if they ever found out?

+ What parts of yourself are you hiding, suppressing, or rejecting?

+ What secrets are you keeping, from others or even from yourself, in order to maintain an appearance of being good, right, worthy, or lovable?

+ What shame might you be projecting onto your body?

+ What shame might you be using body image issues to avoid, distract yourself from, numb, or cope with?

+ And of course, what about your actual *body* makes you feel ashamed?

Once you have your list—or if you don't feel like making a list, then once you stumble upon a new source of shame in the wild—the next step is to break down each individual source of shame into actions that will strip it of power. This action can be as simple as telling a secret to a trusted friend, or showing your partner your cellulite under bright light, but don't forget the shame-busting power of education and normalization too! Sometimes the best shame-busting action step is to read or listen to the stories of other people who have experienced what you're experiencing, to normalize it and feel less alone. Other times, shame comes from either misinformation or a legitimate lack of information (think feeling ashamed of your sexuality because you grew up in purity culture), in which case the best way to strip it of power might be to get properly educated. Consider the following questions if you need help coming up with shame-busting action step ideas:

- Whom in your life do you trust to meet you with empathy and understanding if you *tell* them about your source of shame?

- How might you be able to break this source of shame into incremental steps or stages for telling them?

- Whom in your life do you trust to meet you with empathy and understanding if you *show* them your source of shame?

- How might you be able to break this source of shame into incremental steps or stages for showing them?

- Can you identify any aspects of your shame that are based on misinformation, or a lack of information, which could be remedied by getting educated or relearning about a topic?

- How might you be able to connect with other people who have experienced the same thing, or otherwise normalize it to yourself?

- What are your options, if you don't already have someone like that in your life? Can you hire someone, like a therapist, coach, or sex worker? Can you share it with your dog? Can you post it on an anonymous forum for like-minded people? Can you tell an anonymous stranger?

It's important, especially at first, to approach shame busting very slowly, gently, and cautiously, to keep your system from getting overwhelmed. But as you build tolerance, confidence, and self-trust, you might find yourself wanting to go bigger and get more daring, which is great! Maybe you start by telling your partner, then a few friends, then everyone at work, and then you just post it on social media. Maybe you first "come out" in an anonymous forum, then you tell your family, and then you start living your truth publicly. Some shame busting is about getting a secret off your chest, some is about living your whole truth, and some is just about making it public so you no longer have to carry the burden of hiding it.

Some of my clients create ongoing or even preventive shame-busting practices for this purpose. Wearing a T-shirt that reads "fat & fabulous," or a pin that reads "they/them" might help a person fight back against the shame that whispers, "These parts of you are bad and should be kept hidden," on a daily basis.

For a similar reason, I sometimes encourage clients to introduce themselves *with their shame* at parties or on dates, like "it's nice to meet you, I have a learning disability!" or "hi, I'm ___, and I have extreme social anxiety." It may sound silly and awkward, but it instantly erases the feeling that you have a secret so that you can actually *enjoy* interacting with other people (assuming they stick around), instead of wondering how they'd react if they found out.

It might sound like a nightmare right now, but it's actually incredibly liberating when everyone in your life is fully aware of (and cool with) the stuff you've been ashamed of. Personally, while in the depths of depression, I would always talk about my depression to people as openly and honestly as possible—even people I didn't know very well! It made *some* people uncomfortable, sure, but it made other people immediately open up and take our connection to a deeper and more vulnerable place, which I loved.

Most important, though, talking openly about my depression kept it from ever feeling like a shameful secret. I'd say something like "I'd love to see you on Saturday, but to be perfectly honest, I'm in the throes of a debilitating depressive episode, and as such I may be in a very raw place when we meet, or even need to cancel at the last minute. If that would be too disruptive for you, I completely understand, but if you're okay with that, let's make a plan!"

Take *that*, shame!

Along these same lines, I've had clients make posters to hang on their wall declaring their most shameful secrets, or print them on a hat and wear it, or buy a little ad space in a local newspaper to announce them. Many have put things like "extremely anxious and needy," "sexually inexperienced," "self-conscious about my cellulite," or even "fatter than I look in pictures" in their dating app profiles, both to enjoy the freedom of its being out there, and also to vet their potential matches. One woman with a prestigious job even wrote, "I am not smart enough," in a fancy bold font and hung it on her office wall in a gorgeous frame so that anyone walking in would see it. It became a wonderfully connective icebreaker with both her prestigious clients and her coworkers! So be sure to build shame-busting skill slowly and incrementally, but eventually you can feel free to get creative and do *anything* that strips your shame (and therefore body image issues) of their power.

Congratulations, that's the entire body image blueprint! While it might take months or years to execute all the various elements, you now know the exact steps and tools needed for *you* to access body neutrality. I realize the blueprint can feel a bit complicated or overwhelming when written out like this, but I've found most people do best when they can see each element broken down microscopically. Ultimately, though, the blueprint is just a framework—a process and a set of tools—to help you do something pretty intuitive: figure out what you need, and then go get it.

Most of my clients find it's best to start out by following the body neutrality blueprint exactly, going through it in writing, and using every single step and tool. But with enough time and practice, many start making it their own, skipping parts that don't feel relevant, adding tools of their own, or moving the process from the page to the mind as it becomes second nature. You can feel free to do the same! I recommend going through everything in written detail at least once so that you have the fullest understanding of both the blueprint and of your own journey, but after that it's up to you. The exercises and tools will always be there for you to return to if you get stuck, start working on a new avatar, or decide to do some dedicated work on a specific body insecurity. Personally, I haven't sat down to journal about my body image in nearly a decade, but I still go through a shorter version of this process in my head whenever I run into a new bit of old conditioning about what bodies mean.

In the next chapter, I'll be putting all these steps and tools together, so you can see the body neutrality blueprint in action from beginning to end, using case studies from my own coaching practices. You'll see how individual tools and steps can be adapted to the person, but the beats are always the same: identify the root cause of body image suffering, identify what would need to be true for that root cause to no longer exist, and then go make that happen.

CHAPTER 16

Putting It All Together

TO DEMONSTRATE HOW THE BODY neutrality blueprint looks when strung together from beginning to end, I'd like to introduce you to my client Elle.

Elle was a single woman who found herself constantly insecure about, critical of, and preoccupied with her appearance—especially when it came to dating, sex, and men. She immediately recognized herself in the self-objectifier, who assigns an inappropriate amount of importance to being attractive, and admitted to feeling like she wasn't attractive enough to get any of the things she wanted and needed in life.

To get a clearer picture of all the things Elle believed she could only "earn" by being more attractive, I asked her to describe the life she thought she'd have if she were more conventionally attractive (her positive body image fantasy). She imagined she would be married to a fabulous, sexy guy, they would have kids, and she would feel confident and happy. And what about the opposite, her negative body image fantasy? I asked Elle what she was most afraid would happen, if she continued to look like herself, or even (God forbid!) became *less* conventionally attractive? Her chest and shoulders sank as she described her fear of becoming a desperately lonely old maid who dies alone, having missed her chance to find a partner or have a family.

From those exercises, we learned that what Elle wanted wasn't really to be more attractive, but rather to feel more confident and happy overall, and to find a partner and start a family. Interestingly, though, Elle was so insecure about her appearance (so sure that nobody would ever love or desire her) that she never pursued anyone sexually or romantically, she refused to use dating apps, and she rarely spent time in spaces where she could meet people. When I asked how it would feel to start putting herself out there more, Elle stumbled onto a long-held subconscious belief that if a person is attractive enough, they will just *automatically* be found and chosen by someone amazing. Bingo. We had found the clever way Elle's negative body image thoughts, feelings, and behaviors were protecting her. They helped her avoid the terrifying vulnerability of putting herself out there, risking rejection, and being an active participant in finding and cultivating a great partnership.

Elle decided her body image issues existed to help her "earn" a partner without making herself vulnerable, as well as to keep her from needing to do the hard and scary parts of partnership building (her hidden body image purpose). At one point she even said, while laughing at how silly it sounded to say aloud, that some part of her genuinely believed "hot people get a sort of free pass—they don't have to do all that scary shit!"

Using this information, I had Elle try envisioning a body neutral future, in which she no longer needed to be protected or given a free pass (her vision for a body neutral future). At first, she could only imagine a future in which she was either more attractive or had magically been chosen by a partner—two pathways that felt unattainable and out of her control. To generate more ideas, I asked Elle what fears she might have to face or overcome to no longer need protection from the hard, scary, and vulnerable aspects of finding and cultivating partnership (fear facing). This seemed a lot easier to answer.

"Oh god, I'd need to overcome the fear of putting myself out there, being vulnerable, and being rejected, for sure. I'm terrified that men are only into women who uphold a certain level of attractiveness, so nobody will ever choose me . . . and also that I'll never feel happy or confident until I find a partner. So I'm terrified of putting myself out there, and also terrified of ending up alone."

After also exploring what skills she'd need to improve (skill building) and shame she'd need to release (shame busting), Elle's vision of a body neutral future started to come together. She imagined a world in which she had cultivated better dating and relationship skills, become more comfortable with vulnerability and rejection, unlearned the belief that objectification and love go hand in hand, and stopped measuring her worthiness by her relationship status.

I should mention that Elle wanted to include a partner in her future vision, but to make sure this plan was completely achievable and within her scope of control, I had her leave that part out. After all, we can't control who shows up in our lives, or when. All Elle could do was create a life in which her odds of finding a great partner were higher (e.g., by seeking out dates, learning what she liked and didn't like, working on her mindset and body language, building her confidence) and build a life that felt good even if she didn't. So her body neutral future vision was one in which she had both created a fertile environment for partnership to spark and flourish instead of "waiting to be chosen," *and* had cultivated such a richly fulfilling and abundant life for herself that she didn't suffer while waiting to meet the One. Elle's body neutrality action plan pretty much wrote itself from there! We broke each detail from her vision down into possible action steps (including many skills to learn and fears to face!) and picked a few at random to start with.

Elle started putting herself out there by signing up for a few dating apps, telling her friends she was looking for someone, and signing up for local classes and events on things she was interested in, to meet people and expand her social circle. Through these actions, Elle was rapidly learning about herself and discovering more skills she wanted to improve, like how to chat with potential dates, how to figure out (and then tell people) what she was looking for, how to ask men out, how to stay focused on her own feelings instead of focusing on what someone else feels about her, and how to show up authentically on a first date. She identified some qualities she wanted to develop, like assertiveness and trusting people, became interested in learning more about queer, kinky, and ethically nonmonogamous relationships, and set new boundaries and standards for what she would tolerate. She also discovered some fears she needed to face, like the fear of expressing her needs and the fear of being a burden, and some shame she felt about being "too much" for men: too emotional, too needy, too feminine, and just generally not what men want. Every week or so, Elle would revisit her original body neutrality action plan lists to add, update, assess, and choose her next action items.

The path was made by walking, as you can see. Each experience informed the next, and Elle just kept moving forward until she felt like an active and empowered participant in her love life, instead of a disempowered fairy-tale princess wishing to become so attractive that Prince Charming would pluck her out of her misery and make her live happily ever after.

After about a year and a half of working together, Elle had opened up considerably, knew a lot more about what she actually wanted, found it much easier to be vulnerable, found her life significantly more joyful and satisfying, and knew her worth as a partner (outside of her appearance). By that point, our sessions had become more focused on the evolution of her action plan than on her body image; we focused on supporting her skill building, processing her feelings, identifying her needs and coming up with ways to get them met, encouraging her fear facing, tapping into her intuition, and unpacking her relationship to sex and partnership.

When I checked back in about body image at this point, Elle paused for a moment, a look of bewilderment on her face. She told me it had been a long time since she'd had a bad body image day, and that it was actually bizarre to realize how little she thought about her weight or her skin (her two big body image triggers, previously) anymore.

More important (in my eyes at least), Elle reflected that she now understood the direct connection between her body insecurities and her feelings of intense vulnerability and fear of rejection, so even when she *did* have a bad body image day, she didn't freak out. Instead, she would just notice, acknowledge that her brain was trying to protect her from something, look inward to figure out what it was, and come up with a plan to deal with it. Once, for example, Elle got hit with a big tornado of body insecurities after seeing her friend get married. Her friend's relationship seemed to be so perfect and so easy, and she found herself desperately wishing she were thin and hot enough to have a relationship like *that*. But instead of believing her body image issues, Elle recognized that her brain was lying to her. She couldn't know how her friend's relationship was behind closed doors, but it was undoubtedly imperfect. *Nobody* gets to skip the hard and scary parts of relationship building. Luckily, even though it was scary and hard, Elle now knew she was up for the task and didn't need a free pass to get out of it. Having reminded herself of this, Elle was able to just move on, and by the next day her body image issues had faded again.

The details of Elle's body neutrality journey were specific and unique to her, of course, but the story-beats of the body neutrality blueprint will always be the same. She found the root cause of her body image suffering, she figured out what would need to happen for that root cause to no longer exist, and then she made that happen.

Now let's look at another case study, to see those same story-beats play out again, but in a completely different context.

Cody had struggled growing up, due to a debilitating case of ADHD and dyslexia. He was often called lazy, stubborn, stupid, difficult, and a "troublemaker" by teachers and other adults, and he knew he could come off as weird, annoying, or rude to his peers. He often felt like nobody understood him, and that everyone—including his family— considered him a crushing disappointment. When it came to sports however, Cody thrived. He loved being in motion because he got too restless sitting still, and he found the only time he could actually focus was on the field. His coaches were the only adults who didn't seem to think he was a failure, he received praise for his athletic skill, and his teammates made him feel like he actually *belonged* with them. When Cody told me this story, he had tears in his eyes.

"It was the only time I felt like I made *sense*," he said. "It was the only time I felt like I was worth anything."

After college, Cody stopped playing sports, and settled into a nine-to-five office job. He tried to work out for a while, but found it too difficult to stick to a routine. Going for a run or lifting weights alone just wasn't the same as being on a team, and over the years he became sedentary, gained weight, and felt absolutely miserable about his body. When we met, Cody was disgusted by his body, and angry that he had let himself get this way. He hated feeling out of shape, he hated being fat, and he was ashamed about being too lazy to do anything about it.

I asked Cody what he imagined would be different if he were lean, athletic, and strong, and had abs again. He described a life full of community, bonding, friendships, and a feeling of belonging, as well as a feeling that he was "no longer such a piece of shit." When I asked what the last part meant, he admitted to feeling like a failure all the time, like he couldn't do *anything* right, and like everyone was right about him: he was just completely worthless.

His answers immediately made me think of the outsider, whose body image issues are often about being what they think people want them to be, in order to secure connection and belonging. Cody missed having a body whose athleticism made people happy, because he missed the connection and belonging that afforded him. There was a whisper of the high achiever in his story, too, because Cody also missed having a body that made people celebrate him for being exceptional. But even though Cody might have been hoping the external validation of athleticism would translate into internal self-worth, his core issue was heartbreakingly outsiderish. Being neurodivergent in a neurotypical world had taught Cody that he was too different, that he didn't belong, and that he had nothing much of value to offer.

While trying to name his hidden body image purpose, Cody was able to acknowledge that he had been subconsciously hoping his body would solve two separate problems: how lonely and disconnected he felt in general, and how much he hated himself. We held each of these as separate hidden body image purposes for clarity. His body image issues existed to both earn him the attention, approval, connection, and belonging of others, and earn him self-acceptance, self-worth, and self-approval.

When I asked Cody what would need to be different in his life to no longer need his body hatred and disgust, he answered for each hidden purpose separately.

"I would need to feel more connected to people who like me. And I would need to believe I was worth something."

The first one was pretty easy to break into pathways and action steps, but the second one was more challenging, because he had no reference point for how a person could start believing something like that, or what it would even feel like. Given how similar and interconnected self-loathing and shame can be, I asked Cody to tell me why he felt so worthless in the first place, in the hopes of identifying the shame that needed busting. This got things moving! As he listed the reasons for his violently low self-worth, it became clear that his neurodivergence had played a catastrophic and horrifying role. Cody hadn't actually been stupid, lazy, or difficult, but his ADHD and dyslexia had made people *treat* him as if he were, and he had believed them. He had come to see himself as broken and worthless because that's how the world had treated him. Clearly Cody's neurodivergence was a deep source of shame, isolation, and disconnection, so we named some ways to strip that shame of its power, and he decided to start by both getting better educated on ADHD and dyslexia, and forging some connections with other neurodivergent folks.

The more Cody learned, and the more stories he heard that echoed his own, the more self-compassion he felt, and the more he came to understand himself as *different*, but not *broken*. This release of shame was transformative: his energy shifted, his posture improved, and ideas were flowing. He suddenly found himself able to come up with skills he wanted to cultivate and things he wanted to do, like get better at expressing himself, start a blog or YouTube channel about living with ADHD, change careers to something that felt meaningful, and make more friends. Each of these new micro-goals generated their own lists of action steps, and Cody was always working on two or three of them at a time. At some point, he discovered that he was still feeling a lot of anger and disgust, but now it was aimed at a society that made neurodivergent folks like him feel so excluded and broken, instead of at his body.

Eventually, he got involved in some advocacy groups that fight for the rights, accessibility, dignity, and justice of what he now calls "his people," and started developing some incredible friendships, as well as a sense of purpose and meaning in his life. After about eight months, Cody's life was nearly unrecognizable. He felt deeply understood and accepted by his new neurodivergent peers and friends, he felt a real sense of belonging in the social justice circles he spent time in, and he was working toward a career change that excited him. But the biggest difference was how he felt about *himself*. By fully understanding the systemic injustice facing folks with cognitive differences, Cody was able to stop blaming himself for being a failure, and start making space for self-compassion, self-forgiveness, and even pride in his cognitive differences.

The more positively Cody felt about himself as a person, the less negatively he felt toward his body. He no longer felt any strong feelings toward or about his body, and no longer spent much time thinking about it at all. Without all the shame, disgust, and hatred clouding his vision, Cody could also see that he actually just missed playing team sports. He decided to sign up for a recreational soccer league, and joined a weekly Frisbee golf group—not because he felt like a "piece of shit" who needed to get in shape, but because he finally felt like he deserved to be happy and feel good.

Are you getting the hang of this yet? Cody's story was obviously very different from Elle's, but he still hit all the same blueprint storybeats: identifying the root cause of his body hatred, figuring out what it would take to make that root cause useless, and then making that happen. So far, however, the stories you've heard have been pretty straightforward and simple. To show you what happens when they get more complex (think multiple avatars and multiple hidden purposes), I'd like to introduce you to my client Beth.

When I first met Beth, she was fighting her way out of an eating disorder. She had a team of support (including an eating disorder nutritionist, therapist, and doctor) to help her manage and heal her relationship with food, but she found herself stuck when it came to her relationship with her actual body. On her therapist's recommendation, she started coaching with me.

Beth liked the idea of body neutrality, because she was, in her words, "sick and tired of thinking about my body." She admitted to being hypercritical of other people's bodies in her own mind, too, and to feeling a judgmental mixture of pity and superiority when she saw fat people. She loved being the thinnest or leanest person in a room—it made her feel empowered and almost euphoric—but the presence of a thinner or leaner person could send her into a complete spiral of panic, shame, and self-loathing. Beth was constantly seeking external validation, she compared herself with everyone else to see who was more impressive, she associated her worth with her discipline and self-control, and she was a total perfectionist.

When Beth took the avatar self-assessment, the high achiever won by a landslide, with just a handful of points showing up in each of the other three. Right away, I asked her to consider the underlying *purpose* of being thinner and leaner than everyone else, and the underlying *purpose* of everyone knowing she was disciplined, self-controlled, or impressive. She had a hard time answering, other than to say that these things just "make her feel good," so I asked her to describe her positive body image fantasy. Again, she couldn't name many details, just that she would feel confident, secure, and good enough.

It sounded to me like Beth had attached her self-worth to her ability to be superior in some way, and that she had developed a violently anti-fat bias, all of which were leading her to pursue exceptionalism via thinness. This was classic high achiever so far, but when we started to talk about her body image behaviors and suffering, something else showed up. Beth's list of compulsive or repetitive behaviors relating to her body was a mile long: weighing herself, trying clothes on over and over, picking her body apart in the mirror, comparing herself with old photos of herself, endless scrolling on social media to compare bodies and lives, following a very rigid and specific set of food rules, overexercising, and picking apart all of her decisions. Most of these behaviors were clearly intended to make Beth feel better—she was seeking temporary relief from her constant body anxiety—but the overall effect was that she constantly felt miserable.

I started to wonder why Beth's brain might be working so hard to keep her distracted and miserable; what was it all protecting her from? I suspected that, despite what her self-assessment had said, Beth's high achiever tendencies existed alongside, or even in an effort to disguise, a runner core. I wanted to understand how all this distraction and suffering might have been serving or protecting her, so I asked Beth to tell me about the time in her life when she *first* developed food and body issues, to look for clues.

Beth was thirteen years old when she developed a preoccupation with her weight. Her older brother had been born with a severe disability, so her parents spent a lot of time and attention taking care of him, which meant Beth was often left alone to take care of herself growing up. Her parents always seemed stressed and exhausted, and they tended to either praise Beth for being such a good, easy, and self-sufficient child, or yell at her for being "difficult" or "attention seeking" when she got upset. Eventually, Beth internalized the belief that she wasn't allowed to have needs or desires of her own, and that her job was just to make things easier on her parents. By thirteen, she was proud of the fact that she could be so independent and "good," never require anything from them, and never be a burden. She had connected her parents' love, and her own sense of worth, to her ability to make herself as small and unobtrusive as possible, and relied on constant discipline and self-control to suppress anything that threatened it, including her own feelings, needs, and desires.

Is it any wonder that when Beth discovered dieting, she quickly became obsessed? Discipline and self-control were already in her wheelhouse, and restricting food made her feel powerful, good, and even more in control of herself. Then as the pounds started to fall away, Beth discovered the joy of being *physically* smaller: even less intrusive, even less of a burden. The smaller she got, the more terrified she became of gaining weight again, having come to associate weight gain with being too much, too needy, too difficult, and too out of control—all very dangerous to someone who believed the only thing that made her lovable was that she wasn't a bother to anyone.

This devastating story highlighted that Beth's food and body issues had been functioning as a way of ensuring her parents' love and protecting her from abandonment, helping her repress and curb what she saw as shameful weaknesses (i.e., having needs and feelings), and helping her hone and display the one talent she was most proud of: the ability to control herself. On top of all that, obsessing over food and body stuff had helped Beth stay distracted and disconnected from all the pain of feeling overlooked, unloved, abandoned, and unworthy of her parents' time and attention, that had nowhere else to go.

Beth's eating disorder and body image issues protected her in so many ways that she was completely reliant on them to get through each day; she was constantly using the thoughts, feelings, and behaviors that accompanied them to cope, regulate, control, numb, or otherwise just . . . survive. Yes, Beth was miserable, but at a certain point being miserable in this way became preferable to the alternative, and almost comfortable.

This was a kind of suffering that she knew how to do; it was something she had practiced for decades. Beth hadn't been able to let go of her body image issues because she still needed them to survive. Even though they made her feel awful, they also made her feel safe.

To keep things simpler, Beth tackled each avatar separately when trying to nail down her hidden body image purpose. With regard to her high achiever side, she decided her body image issues were trying to earn her enough love, acceptance, and external validation that she finally felt good enough as a person, and worthy of love. But as a runner, she acknowledged that her body image issues were also trying to protect her from the pain of abandonment by suppressing and controlling herself into such a small and unbothersome package that people would have no *reason* to abandon her. And her various body control habits and behaviors were helping her cope, self-soothe, and self-regulate—so that she never needed to rely on or burden anyone—but they were also helping to numb, control, repress, and distract her from a lifetime of undealt-with pain.

Food and body image issues had become a sort of multi-tool for Beth, solving a whole bunch of problems. It's why her body image issues were still going strong, even as her relationship with food was improving: she didn't yet have any alternative tools, skills, or solutions to replace her multi-tool!

When I invited Beth to envision a body neutral future, she decided to do it all together as a big bulleted list, rather than dividing it up by avatar or hidden purpose. On a big piece of paper she wrote, "In order for me to no longer need my body image issues . . ." at the top. Then she laid it all out point by point.

- I would need to feel fundamentally good about myself, and worthy of love. I'd need to have a stronger sense of self-worth outside of my body, outside of my discipline or self-control, and outside of my ability to require nothing.

- I would need to believe it's safe for me to take up space, ask for help, and have my own needs, desires, and feelings.

- I would need to either get more of my needs met by my parents *or* find a way of accepting that they're not capable of giving me what I need. (And that that's not my fault!)

- I would need to work on my fear of abandonment so that it doesn't run my whole life, and also so I can stop controlling everything in an effort to keep it from happening all the time. (This will probably get easier the more worthy of love I feel!)

- I would need to get reeducated about body size, health, and weight stigma, and dismantle the anti-fat bias inside myself.

- I would need to overcome the shame I feel about having feelings, needs, urges, and desires . . . and on the flip side, to overcome the superiority I feel about being better than everyone at shrinking, controlling, and repressing those parts of myself. (Note: this is linked to how I see body size, so unlearning fat-phobia will probably help with this.)

- I would need to develop a whole bunch of alternative coping skills and tools for dealing with painful feelings and unmet needs in a healthier way. Basically I'd just need to feel like I could survive and handle the experience of facing and feeling all the unpleasant stuff I currently ignore, avoid, and push away.

- I would probably need to face and work through a lot of the feelings I still have from childhood about my parents, my brother, and myself. This one would probably be best to do with a therapist.

Incredible, right? In one fell swoop, Beth had both come up with the details of her body neutral future, and identified specific micro-goals and action steps for how to get there. Because her list was so specific, she was able to approach each bullet point as its own micro-goal and brainstorm potential action steps for each one. She broke some into even smaller micro-goals, and others straight down into action steps; for some she had immediate ideas, and others she drew a blank. To show you exactly how that looked, I'm including a rough approximation of Beth's early lists, below.

HOW TO FEEL WORTHY OF LOVE

- Figure out what makes me *not* feel worthy of love, and do some shame busting around that if possible.

- Explore what I believe makes another person worthy of love, in an existential/spiritual way—and why I don't include myself in that.

- Connect my self-worth to other aspects of who I am as a person.

  - Name things that make me worthy of love, and focus on them.

  - Ask friends what they think makes me worthy of love, and ask them to remind me of their answers on a regular basis.

  - Post these answers where I can see them every single day.

  - Apply mindfulness and mindset exercises to notice, accept, and redirect my self-critical thoughts away from criticism and toward self-compassion.

  - Identify ways in which I'm not currently living in alignment with my values, and work to shift that.

  - Identify qualities I want to embody, and skills I want to learn, that would help me develop a stronger and more diverse sense of self-worth. (Then start taking action steps toward them!)

    - *I want to be more generous.*

    - *I want to get more educated about, and involved in, social justice.*

    - *I want to prioritize creativity, maybe by taking an art class?*

HOW TO EITHER IMPROVE OR ACCEPT MY RELATIONSHIP WITH MY PARENTS

◆ Identify what I want to express to my parents (like how I feel, and what I want and need from them), and then open that conversation with them!

◆ Improve my skills around communication, self-advocacy, and boundary setting.

  ▸ Read a book.

  ▸ Take a class or workshop.

  ▸ Face my fear of being a burden.

◆ Get better at facing rejection.

  ▸ Start small and practice, to build resilience.

◆ Start asking for the support I need from friends so I can process it with them.

◆ Find a way to separate what I deserve from what they're able to give me.

HOW TO OVERCOME MY FEAR OF ABANDONMENT

◆ Work to identify my abandonment triggers, and come up with new tools for avoiding, tolerating, or handling each one.

◆ Do some fear facing around this?

◆ Cultivate super-secure attachment in my current relationships.

  ▸ Learn more about adult attachment theory!

  ▸ Figure out what I need to feel safe and secure, and ask for it.

  ▸ Fear facing: practice speaking up about my needs and desires in my relationships.

◆ Surround myself with emotionally available and open people, and open up to them more.

◆ Bring this into therapy.

HOW TO OVERCOME SHAME ABOUT
HAVING FEELINGS AND NEEDS

- Get better at identifying, understanding, tolerating, and express-ing my feelings and needs in real time.
    - Ask around for recommendations to learn more about these topics.
    - Do some journaling exercises around my feelings on a daily basis, to bring more self-awareness.
    - Practice mindfulness, and maybe even start a meditation practice, to get better at noticing, accepting, and releasing my feelings.
- Start talking about and owning my feelings and needs more often, to strip them of shame.
- Let go of the belief that my worth comes from my self-sufficiency, and ability to be "good" and "easy."
    - Start telling the people in my life that this is something I'm working on, and ask for both feedback and support as I do.
    - Fear facing around being weak, relying on people, being vulnerable, being a burden, and taking up space.

HOW TO LEARN TO COPE
WITHOUT FOOD OR BODY ISSUES

- Seek out educational resources to learn more about how to do this.
- Identify how each of my compulsive food and body behaviors are serving me, what need they're meeting, and what problem they're solving . . . then find *another* way of handling each situation.
- Learn to let go of control sometimes.
    - Fear facing.
    - Tell the people in my life what I'm working on, and ask for their support.
    - Practice, practice, practice.

- Find other ways of comforting or soothing myself.
  - Figure out what makes me feel comforted or soothed.

- Learn to regulate my nervous system, and increase my window of tolerance (i.e., learn to work *with* my nervous system, to decrease how often and how intensely I get triggered).
  - Learn more about polyvagal theory.
  - Track and use biofeedback, either on my own or with a biofeedback therapist, to better understand my own nervous system.

- Practice slowing my mind down in moments of overwhelm, and calling upon my tools.

HOW TO HEAL AND PROCESS MY OLD SHIT

- Tell my therapist about a few things I've been hiding or avoiding.

- Journal more often.

- Let myself notice those things when they come up, instead of automatically distracting, repressing, avoiding, or numbing them.

- Learn how to connect to my body and my emotions.
  - Seek out educational resources to learn more about how to do this.

With all of this laid out in front of her, Beth picked a few action steps to do immediately: ask her friends to tell her what they like about her, start reading a book on adult attachment theory, and sign up for an art class. Given how complicated her root causes were, and how much work there was to be done between here and there, it should come as no surprise that even though Beth put a lot of time and effort into her action plan, her journey moved slowly. We continued to work together for just over two years, until she felt confident and secure in her ability to carry out the plan on her own, and she was no longer getting triggered by her body image on a regular basis.

At that point, Beth was feeling significantly better about herself as a person, she felt a lot less anxiety and shame about her body, she no longer identified as having an eating disorder, and she only had a few compulsive behaviors left to tackle. She was, however, still struggling to connect to her body, and her arsenal of healthy coping skills still got overwhelmed on a regular basis as she processed a huge amount of rage and grief toward her parents (who had responded to Beth's opening up by criticizing her), and moved through other heavy stuff in therapy.

Put another way, even after two years of working on it, Beth still needed her body image issues. Not as badly as she used to, which is why they were so much less intense and less frequent than they used to be, but because she needed them, they were still there. Luckily, Beth is now able to meet them with gentleness and understanding, instead of panic and despair, and to think of them as nothing more than a misguided attempt to keep her safe. Now, when she finds herself mentally comparing herself with others, spending a lot of time staring at her body in the mirror, bingeing in the middle of the night, or feeling a strong need to download a calorie-counting app, she just notices that. She doesn't fight or reject these thoughts, feelings, or behaviors, and she doesn't treat them like enemies. But she doesn't buy into their song and dance about how her body is the cause of her suffering either. She just acknowledges them with self-compassion, knowing that they get loudest when she's running from something, and goes about trying to identify what she might be running from right then.

Nearly a year after we'd finished working together, I received an email from Beth sharing a huge body neutrality win. She'd been having unusually obsessive body thoughts before a beach vacation with old college friends, but drawing on the tools we've covered in this book, Beth discovered that her body anxiety was trying to cover up the anxiety she felt about not fitting in with these friends again, never having felt like a part of the core group, and then going so many years without seeing each other. This fit into two established hidden body image purposes (coping with discomfort, and preventing abandonment), but it also had its own specific micro-context, so it needed its own specific micro–action plan too.

Beth asked herself what would need to be true for her to no longer need her body-obsessive thoughts in this particular situation. She decided she would either need to feel more confident that her friends liked her and wanted her there, or would need to find a way to face and feel those feelings of vulnerability and self-doubt head-on. This led to a variety of action steps she was able to take before the vacation (opening up to her friends about how she was feeling, increasing how often she meditated and journaled, sitting with and validating her feelings, adding some nervous system regulation tools into her daily mix), and both her obsessive body thoughts and her overall anxiety were significantly decreased.

I recognize that this case study is a little anticlimactic, but that's often how it goes. Beth didn't have some massive breakthrough, she doesn't *love* her body, and she may never get rid of her negative body thoughts, feelings, and behaviors completely. But I think it's important to share a story like this as a reminder that the body neutrality blueprint isn't some instant or magical fix. It takes time, and the amount of time needed is informed by both the severity and the complexity of an individual's root causes. It's also important to remind you that the goal of this process isn't about getting body image issues down to absolute zero, but rather to neutralize their power. That means working to give them less of a reason to show up so that they decrease in frequency and intensity, and also learning to understand, accept, and have compassion for them so that you can work with them rather than fight against them when they do show up.

This is why we worked so hard to nail each piece of the puzzle before putting it all together. We have to find realistic and achievable ways of solving the problems our body image issues have been trying to solve for us, in order to strip them of their power and significance. But once that power and significance are stripped away, body neutrality is the natural end result. For this reason, I can't tell you how *your* specific journey will look, or how long it will take. All I can do is offer you the language and concepts, give you the blueprint, and share some of the most commonly seen action steps for each avatar. The rest will be up to you.

CHAPTER 17

Micro-Goals and Action Steps
for Each Avatar

WHILE YOU'LL HAVE TO DISCOVER the specific details of your body image blueprint for yourself, there are certain micro-goals and action steps that seem to come up for each avatar over and over, and play a huge role in the healing process. Read on to see if any of them apply to you, spark new insight, or give you ideas for your own body neutrality action plan!

THE SELF-OBJECTIFIER

Some Things the Self-Objectifier Often Needs to Learn, Practice, or Cultivate

+ *The Ability to Connect with Their Bodies*

Self-objectfiers tend to spend so much time and energy thinking about how they're being perceived from the outside that they disconnect from (or never fully develop) their internal connection to themselves and their bodies. This means they often can't tell what they're feeling, needing, wanting, or even what their opinion on something is, because the communication channel between their mind and body isn't functioning properly. This makes it very difficult for them to advocate for their own needs, set appropriate boundaries, and trust themselves. It also means they struggle to connect to sensual or sexual pleasure and often feel numb or disembodied during sex, which reinforces the belief that their body exists to give *other people* pleasure and gratification, rather than to experience its *own* pleasure and gratification.

Luckily, reconnecting with the body is a skill that can be learned and cultivated! We can improve our ability to notice, hear, understand, and trust the signals and sensations our body is sending us through an embodied mindfulness practice. Whether you struggle to connect with your five senses, your body's internal cues (like hunger, fullness, needing to pee, etc.), your emotions, or even your intuition, you can strengthen that connection by repeatedly bringing your attention and awareness inward and focusing on it.

Looking for a simple practice to start connecting with your body? Try a body scan. Sit or lie comfortably with your eyes closed, and let your attention and awareness come to the top of your head. What sensations can you notice there externally? Air rustling your hair? Hotness, coldness, or itchiness? How about internally: Can you notice any sensations inside your head? Lightness or darkness? Spaciousness or pressure? Any emotions, imagery, or insight come up as you hold your attention there? Whatever you notice, just stay present and focused on it for a few moments (or more). Then move your attention down to your face and jaw and do the same thing. Repeat until you've gotten all the way down to your toes, having spent time noticing as much as you can about each part of your body, both internally and externally.

There are many embodiment practices like this you can try, including some that center on self-touch, mindful movement, specific signals like hunger and fullness, or emotional awareness, to encourage a mindful awareness of your body's signals and sensations. Consider searching for educational resources to support you (Google can help!), and practice bringing your attention to the signals and sensations in your body however you prefer—just be sure to make whatever you choose a regular practice, doing it daily (or more) over a long period of time, to slowly build that stronger connection to yourself and your body.

+ How to Dismantle the Patriarchy (Including the Objectification and Sexualization of Women) inside Themselves

Self-objectification tends to happen in response to being objectified and sexualized (as is the case for most women in our culture),[1] and this phenomenon, along with the unrealistic beauty and body ideals it leads to, are creations of the patriarchy. For this reason, one of the most powerful body neutrality micro-goals for many self-objectifiers is to learn how to question, challenge, unpack, reject, and dismantle the ways in which we've internalized, and continue to uphold, patriarchal biases, beliefs, and values (including the accepted objectification of women and others). This can be incredibly difficult to do, because the biases, beliefs, and values of patriarchy make up the very fabric of our reality, and like a fish trying to notice water, it's often very difficult for us to see it at first. For that reason, I recommend starting with educational resources that will help you see, conceptualize, and understand the role patriarchy plays in both your habit of self-objectification and your body image issues. You might want to just try a book or class on intersectional feminism, the patriarchy, or the objectification of women (I include several book suggestions for self-objectifiers later in this chapter, as well as in the back of the book), or tackle more specific peripheral concepts like beauty ideals, gender roles, gender identity, compulsory heterosexuality, and compulsory monogamy. Listening to and learning from the perspectives of marginalized and stigmatized folks (i.e., Black, brown, Indigenous, transgender, fat, disabled, queer, kinky, nonmonogamous, neurodivergent, and sex workers) on these topics will offer you the best information, insights, and guidance for setting yourself free from the cramped little box the patriarchy taught you to live in. (Just don't forget to pay these folks for their labor!) Also, adopting a more expansive and liberated worldview like this can be challenging and isolating, so be sure to seek out and connect with other people who are also working to dismantle the patriarchy, to reinforce your new worldview, get support, and hold each other accountable along the way.

✦ Ways of Getting Their Needs Met More Directly—Especially for Attention, Intimacy, and Power

All of the avatars will need to figure out ways of getting their needs met without relying on their bodies (or else find a way of making peace with the fact that they can't), but because the self-objectifier is trying to motivate other people to meet their needs, they often feel disempowered and helpless. They might struggle with feeling needy, clingy, or desperate, and often they don't feel inherently worthy of getting the things they want and need from other people without offering them a "bribe" first (in the form of making the other person feel good). As a result, cultivating the ability to get their own needs met with empowerment and abundance is often a *very* important skill for the self-objectifier. The three most commonly unmet (or inadequately met) needs for the self-objectifier are attention, intimacy, and power. These are the three things women have been taught are most closely linked to attractiveness in our culture, and also the three things that the self-objectifier has a history of going chronically unmet. Getting creative here is often key—a person might practice cultivating intimacy through vulnerable conversation, asking for what they want, hiring a professional cuddler or sex worker, getting a pet, doing eye gazing, joining a sex-positive community, or attending BDSM events, for example, or they might develop their feeling of power through empowered movement or vocal techniques, strength training, learning to speak up for themselves, power posing, or cultivating a community of people who respect and uplift them. The better a self-objectifier becomes at getting their needs met, the more independent, empowered, and confident they feel—and the more they can engage with other people directly and transparently, instead of transactionally.

Some Fears the Self-Objectifier Often Needs to Face

+ *The Excruciating Vulnerability of Loving Someone, and the Innate Risk of Heartbreak They Take by Partnering with Someone*

Whether partnered or single, the self-objectifier often imagines that they could avoid the vulnerability and risk inherent to loving or partnering with someone— if only they were attractive enough, they could guarantee their heart would never be broken. And because this fantasy gives the body an unrealistic and impossible amount of power, it has to be stripped away to make body neutrality possible, which means the self-objectifier has to cultivate their courage and face their deep, massive fear of this vulnerability and risk. They have to find ways of facing, accepting, and tolerating the fact that *nothing* is ever 100 percent guaranteed, and that in allowing themselves to love someone, they may, in fact, get their heart broken. This means learning to tolerate discomfort, take risks, and cultivate resilience in the face of fears like rejection, abandonment, and heartbreak so that they trust themselves to handle those things if (or when) they happen.

+ *Life without Shortcuts or Easy Passes*

The self-objectifier often imagines attractiveness to be like a "get out of jail free" card, offering the attractive person a shortcut to all the good things in life, without needing to risk anything or work at it. Instead of focusing on building up their relationship skills, for example, they might focus on looking hot enough to have a relationship just materialize out of thin air, or instead of working toward their dream job, they might focus on being so desirable that someone offers them their dream job unprompted. As you can imagine, this places a huge and inappropriate amount of power and significance on the body, which is why many self-objectifiers have to face and dismantle this shortcut or "easy pass" fantasy to make body neutrality possible. This means cultivating a more realistic view of the world, as well as facing their fear of putting themselves out there, daring to take risks, and putting in the effort to get what they want. It also means identifying and facing whatever specific fears led to their holding on to this "easy pass" fantasy in the first place, whether that's a fear of failure, success, accountability, rejection, change, or finding out what they're made of.

Some Things the Self-Objectifier Often Feels Shame About

+ Being "Too Much"

The self-objectifier is trying to squish their whole three-dimensional self into a narrow and constricted box of what's "desirable," which is to say they're trying to compress a vast and complex human self into a tiny box marked "sexual object." Because this is an impossible feat, however, it never fully works, and the self-objectifier is left with a ton of shame about the parts of themselves they can't seem to fit into the box. Often this shows up as shame about being "too much" in some way. A woman might feel shame about having her own desires, feelings, needs, or opinions, for example, if she learned that men prefer a woman who has *none* of those things. Someone pretending to be nothing but a perfect lust object might feel shame about the human parts of themselves that blow their cover, like pooping, farting, menstruating, or having body odor or bad breath. All of these things can make the self-objectifier feel like *too much*: too emotional, too needy, too greedy, too human. As a result, they often need to do a whole bunch of shame busting around these parts of themselves in order to accept and reintegrate them and to create a more whole, human, and three-dimensional sense of self. As the self-objectifier strips away layers of shame for the parts of themselves they learned were undesirable or too much, they free themselves to take up space and own their whole vast and complex humanity as a *subject*, rather than an *object*.

+ Being the "Wrong Kind of Person" Sexually or Romantically

In the self-objectifier's mind, there is a sexual and romantic *ideal* they need to embody in order to earn, or be worthy of, sex, intimacy, or partnership. As a result, they tend to feel shame about the ways in which they are "failing" this ideal, and blame those parts of themselves for making it difficult to find a partner, or letting their partner down. Sometimes this is about their appearance (where it might center on the ways they "fail" to meet conventional beauty and body ideals), and sometimes this is about other aspects of themselves, like their personality, sexuality, characteristics, energy, mental health, baggage, or lifestyle. A man might have shame about not feeling "masculine enough," for example, or a person might feel like their attachment style, neediness, intelligence, sexual kinks, or income is a turnoff to others. Finding safe spaces to share, normalize, and connect with other people about these parts of themselves can help the self-objectifier more fully accept and embrace the whole truth of their authentic humanity. This allows them to stop needing to manage how they're perceived all the time, and to have a more realistic sense of their worth as a potential sexual or romantic partner, which leads to the ability to be more discerning in whom they choose, and higher standards for themselves overall.

Some of My Favorite Practices for the Self-Objectifier

+ *Take an Inventory of the Beauty or Body "Rules" You Follow, and then Strip Each One of Its Power*

Write down a list of everything you feel like you "have to do" or "can't do" in order to be attractive. (If you made a body image behaviors list while searching for your hidden body image purpose, that can be a valuable resource here, but also write down any subconscious "rules" you follow, like "I can't get away with a ___ haircut, because my face is ___" or "I have to wear ____ because I have a ___ kind of body.") Then go through your list one by one, implementing a fear-facing practice for each thing you've written down. For example, if you wear makeup every time you leave the house because not wearing makeup would make you feel anxious and insecure, you might challenge yourself to go out without makeup. This doesn't have to happen all at once, though, because fear facing is all about consistent and incremental exposure, until the fear doesn't have any power over you. So you might spend a week just going without mascara until that feels okay, and then another few weeks going without foundation, and continuing that way until going totally barefaced feels possible. Pace yourself however you need to, and be patient. Moving through this list will probably take a long time, and that's okay. Also remember that the goal here isn't to actually stop or change any particular behavior, but rather to just strip it of its power over you. After months of working to get comfortable with your bare face, for example, you might go right on back to wearing makeup because you enjoy it, and that's fine! But after you strip makeup of its power in this way, wearing it would feel like an option rather than an obligation, and that's the goal. Move through your list, taking as long as you need to strip each fear of power, until none of them have power over you anymore.

+ Change Your Approach to Sex

Many self-objectifiers have sex for the validation it offers them, or because they feel like they owe it to someone, rather than because they're turned on. As a result, they often end up having a lot of sex that they don't really want or aren't physiologically ready for. The sex they have doesn't feel particularly pleasureful or satisfying, either, both because their bodies haven't gone through the process of getting sexually aroused first, and because they're focused on what the *other person* wants and likes instead of what they *themselves* want and like. Having a lot of this kind of sex over time can lead to decreased pleasure and orgasm, less overall sexual desire, and numbness of the genitals and erogenous zones.[2] None of this is good for the self-objectifier's relationship with their body, but it especially reinforces their view of themselves as having no innate value or worth outside of giving pleasure, care, or gratification to others. For this reason, many self-objectifiers need to completely overhaul their relationship to sex and pleasure to access body neutrality. Many self-objectifiers are greatly benefitted by the following three practices: setting boundaries around what kind of sex they're willing to participate in, learning about the body's sexual arousal process, and learning to center their own desire and pleasure.

A healing boundary around sex might sound like "I will not have sex until I'm fully mentally turned on *and* my body is fully sexually aroused" or "I'm taking a break from partnered sex until I feel more comfortable focusing on my own sexual arousal and pleasure." The goal is to choose a boundary that both requires you to advocate for yourself in bed, and gives you a break from unpleasurable or others-focused sex, so you can focus on your own desire and pleasure!

When it comes to sexual arousal, I recommend first learning more about the biological sexual arousal process more generally, especially of people with similar genitals and/or gender experience as you, because most of us never learned that stuff! As an ex-self-objectifier myself, I remember being *shocked* to learn that sexual arousal is about more than just "feeling turned on" or wanting sex, and actually includes a whole list of specific biological changes that happen in the body and genitals— including increased body temperature, blood pressure, heart rate, and sensitivity to touch, as well as dramatic changes to the size, shape, texture, and color of the clitoris, vulva, and vagina (very similar to the erection we associate with penises!). If this is news to you, too, consider reading a book or other educational resources (my favorite one for folks with vulvae is *Come As You Are* by Emily Nagoski) to learn more—then start exploring what the sexual arousal process in *your own* body looks and feels like. Examine your genitals in a mirror before, during, and after getting sexually aroused to see visual changes, feel the changes with your fingers, and pay attention to more global changes like increased heart rate, faster breathing, feeling warmer, or flushed skin. Be sure to explore the difference for you between feeling mentally turned on, being willing to say yes to sex, and being fully sexually aroused.

Then, to center and prioritize your desire and pleasure, I recommend starting with a nonsexual pleasure practice at first. Many self-objectifiers find it easier to explore pleasure through their five senses at first, using joy-inducing music, art, scenery, color, scent, taste, or tactile experiences to delight themselves, and then cultivating a mindful awareness of (and connection to) that delight in their bodies. It may also be useful to explore various types of self-touch on the face, body, or genitals, playing with texture, pattern, speed, temperature, and pressure to see what does and doesn't feel good. And discovering what turns you on—by courageously exploring your sexual fantasies, cravings, curiosities, desires, turn-ons, turnoffs, and kinks—will allow your sexual experiences to be more enjoyable and gratifying.

Many self-objectifiers find that stepping away from partnered sex while they're building the skills needed to feel present, embodied, relaxed, and sexually aroused in bed to be incredibly helpful, because it removes the element of wondering what the other person is thinking, feeling, or wanting. A regular self-pleasure practice can help the self-objectifier affirm that they are *worthy* of pleasure, and do not exist to give pleasure to anyone else. Then, if they decide to reintroduce other people to their sex life, they're more likely to feel comfortable advocating for the importance of *their* arousal, pleasure, and orgasm, and more likely to choose sexual partners who center and affirm them.

Book Recommendations for the Self-Objectifier:

Angela Saini, *Inferior: How Science Got Women Wrong and the New Research That's Rewriting the Story* (Boston: Beacon Press, 2017).

Emily Nagoski, *Come As You Are: Revised and Updated; The Surprising New Science That Will Transform Your Sex Life* (New York: Simon & Schuster, 2021).

Lindsay Kite and Lexie Kite, *More Than a Body: Your Body Is an Instrument, Not an Ornament* (Boston: Houghton Mifflin Harcourt, 2020).

Naomi Wolf, *The Beauty Myth: How Images of Beauty Are Used against Women* (New York: Harper Perennial, 2002).

Renee Engeln, *Beauty Sick: How the Cultural Obsession with Appearance Hurts Girls and Women* (New York: Harper, 2018).

THE HIGH ACHIEVER

Some Things the High Achiever Often Needs to Learn, Practice, or Cultivate

+ *A New Understanding of Worthiness and Value, Outside of Social Hierarchies*

Many high achievers learned to understand themselves and their value in a relative way rather than an absolute way, and believe a person's position on the social hierarchies is an accurate reflection of their value, worth, and what they deserve. With so many of these hierarchies having to do with the kind of body a person has, this worldview places a lot of false meaning and significance on a person's body, making body neutrality damn near impossible. That's why the path to body neutrality requires many high achievers to dismantle that entire belief system and cultivate a completely new understanding of value and worthiness outside of the social hierarchies—not only for themselves, but also for everyone else.

Admittedly, unlearning and relearning something that is so deeply woven into our understanding of the world like this is challenging, but it *can* be done. I recommend starting with educational resources that can bring your attention to, and help break apart, your current system of beliefs around what makes a person worthy (or deserving) of what, as well as introducing new concepts and possibilities for how to form a new system of beliefs, in which worthiness isn't relative, but absolute. This is where anti-oppression and social justice work come in! Many high achievers find it's best to start down this path by exposing themselves to (and paying for) the liberation-focused perspectives and teachings of multi-marginalized folks on topics like racism, sexism and misogyny, ableism, ageism, anti-fat bias, and capitalism, in order to start dismantling the myth of individualism, the myth of meritocracy, the just world fallacy, and the whole idea that our value is related to our social status. Let your education lead you to courageous self-inquiry, and your self-inquiry lead to action. Consider where your self-worth comes from and where you learned it's supposed to come from, and then consider what it would look like for it to exist outside of and unrelated to concepts like body size or shape, discipline, hard work, self-control, or accomplishments. How about existing outside of all external validation, social status, social privilege, power, or comparison with others in any way whatsoever?

I also recommend, as with any big shift in worldview, seeking out connections with other people who are also working to divest themselves from these concepts and hierarchies, to help affirm and support your new worldview as well as offer continued growth and learning.

+ *Dismantling the Anti-fat Bias inside Themselves*

In the process of cultivating a new understanding of worthiness and value outside of the social hierarchies, the high achiever will be challenged to dismantle all systems of oppression inside themselves, but weight stigma and anti-fat bias deserve a special mention. Body neutrality includes *weight neutrality*, which tends to go directly against all the fatphobic biases and narratives the high achiever believes in. This is why it's so important for the high achiever to actively unlearn the idea that being thin is an accomplishment, that being fat is bad, and that body size represents *anything* about a person's character, personality, health, or lifestyle habits. This tends to be best done through exposure to anti-diet and fat justice education, communities, and resources, as well as through the learning of skills like intuitive eating,[3] joyful movement, listening to the body, empathy, and compassion.

+ *How to Get Their Needs Met: Self-validation, Self-worth,*
  Happiness, Fulfillment, and Inner Peace

Because the high achiever is often seeking external validation in the hopes that getting enough of it will make them feel how they want to feel, it's important for them to develop the ability to feel how they want to feel in other ways. Often this means they need to learn how to self-validate instead of seeking validation from others, or to cultivate a strong and resilient sense of self-worth so they no longer feel a need to prove their worth to others. Sometimes it means exploring their relationship to happiness and fulfillment, and figuring out ways to build a meaningful and joyful life that satisfies them, instead of trying to "earn" that life by climbing to the top of the social hierarchies or becoming impressive enough. And other times it means learning to reduce or manage their anxiety, and find a sense of inner peace, quiet, or calm so they don't need to stay so busy, distracted, or insecure. (Finding a sense of inner peace, quiet, or calm can be done through mindfulness teachings and practices, meditation, spending more time in nature, learning tools to regulate the nervous system, therapy, medications, or a self-acceptance practice, among other resources and practices.) It might take some creativity, but the goal is to find ways of getting your needs met without relying on your body (or social status) in any way.

Some Fears the High Achiever Often Needs to Face

+ *The Fear of Failure, Imperfection, Making Mistakes, and Being*
  Wrong

The high achiever's self-worth is often so linked to being good, right, perfect, or "on top" that they tend to feel terrified of looking like an idiot, failing, making mistakes, or letting people see their weaknesses. Every moment is pass-fail for them, so they're always trying to prove themselves, which holds them back from getting their needs met, developing a lot of the skills they need to truly thrive, and cultivating a resilient and absolute sense of self-worth. It *also* cultivates their anxiety! In order to reduce their anxiety overall (allowing them to need fewer coping mechanisms and security blankets), as well as to help them develop a sense of self-worth and self-acceptance for their *whole, imperfect* selves, the high achiever often has to face these fears slowly and progressively until they no longer hold any power over the high achiever.

+ *The Fear of Judgment, Especially of Being Seen as Bad, Immoral, Lazy, or Out of Control*

While figuring out how to validate themselves and cultivate an absolute sense of self-worth, many high achievers run into a powerful fear of being judged by other people, particularly when it comes to people thinking they're "bad," immoral, selfish, greedy, or otherwise lacking in respectability or character. The two things they tend to be the most afraid of people thinking about them, though, is that they're either lazy or out of control, because they've spent so long believing those are the two worst and most shameful things a person can be. This fear, combined with the belief that a person's body shape and size are an expression of their character and actions, places a lot of false meaning and significance on the body, and makes body neutrality inaccessible. By facing these fears through gradual exposure (and cultivating a detached tolerance for being judged), avoiding people's judgments will seem less and less important to the high achiever, and they'll be free to do what works best for *them*, without the burden of always making sure other people see them a certain way.

+ *The Big, Wild, Unknown World*

One of the reasons the high achiever is so drawn to body control is that it has a way of shrinking and organizing their world, which is very appealing to someone who finds the massive unknowable chaos of life overwhelming.[4] In order to give up their body control behaviors and obsessions, they'll need to face life in its *true* form: big, wild, uncontrollable, and messy. That means they'll slowly need to give up their protective mechanisms and security blankets, and face their fear of life. As they get comfortable being uncomfortable and increase their tolerance for vulnerability, surrender, and the unknown, the high achiever will no longer need to hide behind the smallness, structure, or orderliness of body control behaviors or body image issues.

Some Things the High Achiever Often Feels Shame About

✦ *Being Human (i.e., Having Imperfections and Weaknesses of Any Kind)*

In the high achiever's mind, perfection is the only acceptable goal, so imperfections of any kind are shameful and must be strictly controlled, hidden, or eradicated. Signs of weakness are also considered shameful, because the high achiever imagines any sign of weakness to represent an alarming level of vulnerability, and an invitation to be attacked, dominated, or oppressed. This makes it extremely important for them to feel "in control," and make themselves appear perfect, which often gets aimed at their bodies. To let go of that pressure and significance, many high achievers have to do some shame busting around anything they perceive as an imperfection or weakness. That includes shame that's focused directly on their perceived physical imperfections, like belly fat, cellulite, or a lack of visible muscle tone—especially important when they believe the imperfection is something they can (and therefore should) be able to change with enough hard work and self-control! It also includes shame that's focused on what they perceive to be *internal* imperfections or signs of weakness, like being bad at something, struggling or being emotional, needing to rely on others, or feeling lazy for wanting to sleep in. The more they strip these sources of shame of their power, the easier it will be for the high achiever to accept themselves, stop managing what people think about them, and access body neutrality.

✦ Being Disobedient, or Going Against Whatever Moral Authority, Structure, or Ideology They've Committed Themselves To

As a moral absolutist, the high achiever tends to be terrified of being "bad," with their measure for what makes them good or bad embedded in an external authority, structure, or ideology, such as religion or diet culture. They tend to report feeling frequent guilt about any ways in which they are bad or disobedient, such as the guilt a Catholic person might feel about having sex before marriage, or the guilt a person on a diet might feel about eating dessert. When we get right down to it, though, it's actually *shame* they're usually feeling, not guilt. The difference is that guilt is about the *action*, while shame is about the *person*. Many high achievers think they feel guilty about the action they've taken, when what they actually feel is shame about being the kind of person who would take it. For this reason, many high achievers need to do a lot of shame busting as they move away from the moral absolutism worldview, moral authorities, structures, and ideologies they've been following and obeying—and take on a sense of morality that is more centered on their *own* values, experiences, and understanding of what makes a person good or bad.

Some of My Favorite Practices for the High Achiever

✦ Choosing Something You're Terrible at (or Brand New to) and Sticking to It

This practice benefits the high achiever in two ways. The first is that it puts them in a position to face their fears and build resilience around making mistakes, being imperfect, failing, and being judged, which has powerful long-term benefits. The second is that it gives them an opportunity to develop a hobby, skill, or activity that interests them, which can be used either to strengthen their sense of identity and self-worth outside of the social hierarchies, or to simply cultivate more joy, pleasure, satisfaction, and fulfillment in their life. So whether it's learning a new musical instrument, taking up an artistic endeavor, learning a new kind of movement skill or sport, joining Toastmasters, or starting a new career path, commit yourself to something that you either know you're terrible at or have to start at the very beginning of. Then just keep showing up in that space no matter how many mistakes you make, and how embarrassed or uncomfortable you feel about failing or being judged!

+ *Committing to Racial Justice, Fat Justice, and Other Anti-oppression Work*

In order to dismantle the social hierarchies inside yourself, you'll need the education, support, encouragement, and exposure that are available through social justice work, particularly racial justice, fat justice, and other anti-oppression work. That means reading the books, taking the classes, joining the community groups, hiring the coaches or teachers, and building the relationships necessary to dismantle the systems of oppression that you've learned, challenge the biases and prejudices you hold, acknowledge your privilege and the ways in which you personally uphold these systems, reckon with what it means to have accidentally caused harm to others and change your harmful habits, learn to hold yourself and others accountable when harm inevitably happens, navigate your *unique* role in anti-oppression work, and commit to always centering the voices and needs of the most marginalized folks. Because this kind of work can be heavy, uncomfortable, and exhausting, it also means finding ways of balancing your commitment to it with your commitment to sustainable self-care, resilience, and self-compassion. (After all, you can't fight for justice if you feel too guilty about your privilege, too afraid of messing up and hurting someone, or too burned out and exhausted to go on.) Seek out the teachings, organizations, and resources created by marginalized people working in the racial justice and anti-oppression space, and pay them for their time and expertise. Then build relationships with people who share a similar type and amount of privilege as you who are also committed to racial and social justice—ideally who are at least a bit further along the path than you are—to process what you're learning, and stay accountable to the work.

Book Recommendations for the High Achiever:

Aubrey Gordon, *What We Don't Talk about When We Talk about Fat* (Boston: Beacon Press, 2020).

Caroline Dooner, *The F*ck It Diet: Eating Should Be Easy* (London: HQ, 2019).

Christine Caldwell and Lucia Bennett Leighton, eds., *Oppression and the Body: Roots, Resistance, and Resolutions* (Berkeley, CA: North Atlantic Books, 2018).

Christy Harrison, *Anti-Diet: Reclaim Your Time, Money, Well-Being and Happiness through Intuitive Eating* (New York: Little, Brown Spark, 2019).

Ibram X. Kendi, *How to Be an Antiracist* (New York: One World, 2019).

Ijeoma Oluo, *So You Want to Talk about Race* (New York: Seal Press, 2018).

Jennifer L. Eberhardt, *Biased: Uncovering the Hidden Prejudice That Shapes What We See, Think, and Do* (New York: Viking, 2019).

Sabrina Strings, *Fearing the Black Body: The Racial Origins of Fat Phobia* (New York: NYU Press, 2019).

THE OUTSIDER

Some Things the Outsider Often Needs to Learn, Practice, or Cultivate

+ *Authentic Self-expression*

The outsider has often spent their entire life prioritizing their need for secure relationships over their need for authentic self-expression, leading to a deeply unmet need to discover and express their true selves.[5]

The first step to doing this is to become better acquainted with their inner authentic self in the first place—a self that may have been completely buried under their idea of who they should be, or need to be, in order to fit in and make people like them. Luckily, by turning their attention inward and working to both understand and connect to their body, emotions, intuition, thought patterns, and desires, the outsider can improve self-awareness and self-trust. Calling upon self-examination tools like meditation, mindfulness, embodiment work, counseling, coaching, journaling, curiosity, art or movement therapy, or self-inquiry practices can all help an outsider get to know their inner selves as well, and some outsiders find it helpful to learn about themselves using personality tests (like the Myers-Briggs Type Indicator, the Big Five Personality Test, the Riso-Hudson Enneagram Type Indicator), astrology, or even more mystical tools like tarot cards. Plus, by cultivating opportunities for self-discovery, the outsider can explore different sides of themselves, and get to know not only who they *are*, but who they're *becoming*. This might mean signing up for new or unusual experiences, meeting new people, going new places, and trying new things—especially things they never would have thought to (or had the courage to) try before, like signing up for a comedy open mic, going to a music festival, or taking a burlesque class!

Whichever path the outsider chooses to get there, once they have a sense of who they are, they can move on to the next step, which is expressing that self to others. This may include learning or improving specific skills, like clear and transparent communication, setting boundaries, advocating for themselves, being vulnerable, getting comfortable with conflict, and trusting/requiring others to clearly communicate as well, so nobody has to rely on subtextual detective work. The outsider may also benefit from cultivating outlets for *creative* self-expression (like art, music, writing, or movement) to practice allowing their internal self into the external world, and many outsiders find it helpful to play with self-expression in the way they look or present themselves. This may include exploring different ways of dressing, different makeup looks or hairstyles, body modifications like piercings and tattoos, new gender expressions, or even new body language; whatever feels interesting or authentic for the individual!

As the outsider cultivates authentic self-expression, they'll be rewarded with more fulfilling relationships; more nourishing connections; less fear of rejection, humiliation, or abandonment; and a feeling of being *truly* seen, heard, known, valued, understood, accepted, and loved—often for the first time. At a certain point, when the outsider feels comfortable both knowing who they are, and expressing that self in the world, this micro-goal will no longer be the priority. But the outsider will probably still find themselves weaving back and forth between self-discovery and self-expression forever, because knowing and expressing your authentic truth is an on-going and lifelong journey.

✦ *How to Turn Their Anger, Shame, Blame, and Disgust* Outward, *Where It Belongs*

Nobody deserves to be bullied, harassed, attacked, violated, discriminated against, or oppressed, and there is no such thing as a body that makes those things happen. There are only people who choose to bully, harass, attack, violate, discriminate, and oppress—and, of course, the society-wide systems of violence and injustice they're upholding as they do so. The outsider blames themselves or their bodies for any bad things that have happened to them; they alchemize their anger and outrage into shame and then aim all those negative feelings inward toward themselves and their bodies. As people pleasers, they've often learned that anger is unacceptable, bad, or dangerous,[6] and that if they make *themselves* the problem, they can avoid risking conflict, retaliation, or the safety of the relationship. For this reason, many outsiders need to cultivate the ability to tap into their own anger: to access it, identify it, validate it, form a positive relationship with it, explore it, and express it in healthy and appropriate ways. By doing this, and stripping away the lies they've been telling themselves in order to keep from getting angry, the real sources of their anger will come into focus.

And as it turns out, the real sources of their anger are *always* outside of themselves! The angrier they get about the people who have hurt them, the injustices they've faced, and the systems of violence and oppression that made them all possible, the less anger they'll have toward themselves. The more they can truly place the blame for what happened to them where it belongs, the less shame they'll feel for having "made it happen." Does this sound like what you need? Try learning more about the relevant systems of injustice at play in your story, doing therapy or healing work around your traumas, improving your emotional awareness and intelligence, practicing forgiveness for yourself and your body, improving self-assertiveness and self-advocacy skills, or taking an active and empowered role in fighting injustice in the world.

+ *The Ability to Speak Up in the Face of Insults, Injustice,*
  Inappropriate Comments, and Inappropriate Behavior

Many outsiders live their lives in a way that's designed to help them avoid judgment, insults, uncomfortable comments, and inappropriate behaviors. Because they don't have the skills to handle those experiences in the moment, they're focused entirely on prevention. This leads to a lot of social anxiety and body image issues, as the outsider is constantly trying to make sure those moments never have a reason to arise. That's why learning to handle those moments with skill, confidence, poise, and conviction is a total game changer for the outsider—it strips them of the need to avoid these experiences, and sets them free to do what they want and have the body they have. If someone insults you, for example, you could respond with something like "wow, that was incredibly rude" or "what a horrible thing to say to someone" or "that hurt my feelings." If someone comments on your body, you could respond with "did you know that comments like that contribute to mental health issues and eating disorders?" or "actually, I'm not accepting comments on my body right now, positive *or* negative" or "that comment made me very uncomfortable." And speaking up when you see or hear racist, sexist, ableist, fatphobic, or transphobic jokes or comments can sound like "wow, that was so inappropriate," or "I don't find racist/sexist jokes funny," or "are you aware of what a harmful thing you just said?" Cultivating this skill mostly just requires practice (e.g., role-playing, trial and error, repetition) and a willingness to feel awkward for a while as you hone it, but it can also be supported through educational resources on self-assertiveness, self-advocacy, and anti-oppression work on how to speak up in the face of injustice. This is also a skill that gets easier as the outsider cultivates authentic self-expression and the ability to turn their anger and blame outward where it belongs, because both of *those* skills help them trust themselves, access their impulses moment to moment, validate their experiences, and stand up for themselves.

Some Fears the Outsider Often Needs to Face

+ *The Fear of Rejection, Conflict, Disappointing People, Being a Burden, Setting Boundaries, and Self-advocacy*

Each of these fears is unique and will require specific fear-facing work to overcome, but they all share a common theme—the outsider is afraid of putting themselves first. They're so used to putting other people's needs, feelings, and experiences first that the thought of putting their *own* needs, feelings, and experiences first is terrifying. They imagine the only thing keeping their relationships relatively secure is the fact that they don't take up space or require anything from the other person, along with the fact that they bend over backward to make the other person happy, so facing each of these fears is really a way of facing their underlying fear of unworthiness and abandonment. They think if they required someone else to do any labor on their behalf (or if they stopped doing so much labor on the other person's behalf), that person would decide the relationship wasn't worth it anymore and disappear. So the outsider has to gradually expose themselves to situations in which they risk rejection, conflict, disappointing people, being a burden, setting boundaries, and advocating for their own needs in order to build up their resilience and capacity in those spaces, strip their fears of power, and finally be able to break free from their people-pleasing patterns. Plus, as an added bonus, this work will help them build a feeling of deeper security, safety, and trust in the relationships that stick around after the outsider stops "bribing" the other person with people-pleasing labor.

+ *Their Anxious Attachment Style*

Many outsiders have an anxious attachment style, which means they may feel overly anxious or clingy in partnership, constantly seeking reassurance in their relationships, and frequently thinking they're about to be abandoned. When this is the case, the outsider may project a lot of their anxiety and insecurity onto their bodies, and therefore need to a find a way of acknowledging, accepting, exploring, and working to heal this part of themselves to make body neutrality accessible. This is often done in therapy, because insecure attachment tends to derive from our earliest childhood experiences,[7] but it can also be supported with self-education, self-awareness, mindfulness, nervous system regulation, and fear facing in relationships. By confronting this part of themselves, the outsider can start to understand and communicate to others what they actually need to feel safe in their relationships, as well as gradually building a tolerance for the uncomfortable feelings that arise when their relationships feel insecure or their abandonment fear gets triggered. With practice and exposure, the outsider can slowly become more comfortable with the moments of space, distance, rejection, and conflict that arise in any healthy and secure relationship, which will allow them the space they need to become their own person.[8]

Some Things the Outsider Often Feels Shame About

+ *The Bad Things That Have Happened to Them*

The outsider blames themselves for the bad things that happen to them, which means they tend to carry a lot of shame for "being the kind of person" who deserved, encouraged, or made something bad happen. This could be true for experiences of random bad luck (like being hit by a drunk driver, or having their home destroyed by a natural disaster), but it's most often true with regard to *other people's treatment of them*. The outsider tends to avoid blaming other people for their harmful behaviors, whether that harm is unintentional, inconsiderate, discriminatory, or violent, and blames themselves instead. Instead of hating the person who abused them, for example, they hate themselves for "making" that abuse happen—for encouraging it, for deserving it, or for letting it happen. None of that is true, of course; a person cannot "deserve" pain, violence, oppression, or trauma. But because of how the outsider processed these experiences, they carry the shame of feeling bad, broken, wrong, unworthy, and undeserving of kindness, respect, acceptance, belonging, or happiness—and their bodies are often scapegoated or blamed. This means there is often a lot of shame busting the outsider will need to do around the stories of bad things happening to them, in order to finally stop blaming themselves, find self-compassion, and heal their relationship with themselves and their bodies. (Reminder: it's important that this shame busting be approached carefully, incrementally, and with appropriate support.)

✦ Having a Body That "Deserves" to Have Bad Things Happen to It

As an offshoot of generally blaming themselves for bad things that happen to them, the outsider often blames *their body* for any negative attention, insults, harassment, exclusion, abuse, discrimination, or violence aimed toward their body. For example, they might blame their thighs for the mean comment someone made about them in high school, blame their fatness for other people's harassment, or blame their body for freezing up instead of running or fighting during a sexual assault. Finding spaces to share these stories and be met with empathy, and connecting to other people who have gone through similar experiences, encourages self-compassion and self-forgiveness, and is often deeply healing for the outsider. Plus, stripping this shame of power makes space for them to aim their anger, disgust, blame, or hatred *outward*, where it actually belongs. This allows the outsider to both forgive their body, and participate in the meaningful fight for justice (if desired).

Some of My Favorite Practices for the Outsider

+ *Disappoint Someone, Get Rejected, or Burden Someone—Every Single Day—for a Month*

If any of the most common outsider fears resonate with you, I suggest choosing one and creating a daily fear-facing practice around it for at least a month—maybe even longer, if you need more time to slowly build up. Start as small as you need to, so that the action you commit to makes you feel uncomfortable, but also feels safe enough to actually get done. And don't worry if that means you have to choose something a bit silly or contrived at first, that's totally normal! If you're terrified of disappointing or upsetting people, it would probably feel way too unsafe to jump right into an emotionally charged scenario, like telling your mom you're not coming home for the holidays, or telling your boss you're no longer available to work weekends. So you might invent a small scenario to practice with first, like role-playing saying no with someone you trust. I do this with clients, sometimes even texting them the first few days with a ridiculous request, like "hey, I need help cleaning my toilet, could you please come over?" and then building up to scenarios they're more likely to come across, like "ugh I just need to vent, do you have the space for that right now?" We both know it's make-believe of course, but after a few days (or weeks) of doing this every day, they're ready to tackle something a *little* more high stakes, whether that means telling their partner they're not in the mood for sex right now or canceling plans with someone—whatever feels uncomfortable, but not overwhelmingly so, to them. The important thing is that you find ways to face your fear, in incrementally higher stakes ways, on a daily basis, for long enough that you're able to strip it of power. Maybe you start by "burdening" someone with tiny requests (like giving you a hug, or picking up toilet paper on their way over), but by the end you're asking for someone to hold space while you process an emotional day, or to help you move. Just start wherever you can, and keep pushing your daily practice to include more and more challenging and vulnerable ways of facing your fear as time goes on.

✛ *Unpack Your Concept of "Everyone"*

The outsider's insecurities and decisions are often informed by the overwhelming feeling that "everyone" or "no one" agrees on something particular, like "everyone prefers thin people to fat people" or "nobody wants to listen to someone complain." When we dig into each specific belief a bit deeper, however, 99 percent of the time, their concept of "everyone" can actually be pinpointed onto five or fewer specific people. By identifying those people and then challenging their credibility as a source on the topic, these kinds of beliefs can be stripped of their power.

Try this exercise: Think of an example from your life in which you feel insecure, ashamed, embarrassed, or wrong, which is based on a belief that "everybody thinks" or "everyone believes" something. For example, if you're ashamed of where you are in your career, you might say, "Everyone thinks I'm just wasting my life," or if you feel insecure about your weight, you might say, "Everyone thinks I'm fat and disgusting." (Note: you can also do this with a "nobody" statement, like "nobody respects me," or "nobody thinks I look good.") Once you've identified the "everyone" belief that's causing you to suffer, identify the people who are standing in for the "everybody" in your mind. Who in your life actually thinks or feels this way, or taught you this? Name the people (up to five) who comprise your sense of "everyone" in this scenario.

Once you have your list, answer the following questions for each:

+ How much do you trust, respect, and value this person's opinion?

+ How much do you even like this person?

+ Would you ever call this person to get advice on your life or body?

+ Is this person really representative of "everyone"? If not, who are they representative of?

To look at an example for this, let's use the belief "everyone thinks I'm too slutty."

The list of people standing in for "everyone" in this belief might look like:

+ My middle school best friend, who later bullied me.

+ My older sister, who lost her virginity at twenty-four years old.

+ That older lady at work who keeps dropping hints about my "revealing clothing."

+ My super-religious neighbors who give me judgmental looks whenever I see them.

And then each person's credibility on this topic would be challenged, like this example for the middle school best friend turned bully:

+ How much do you trust, respect, and value this person's opinion? *Zero.*

+ Do you even like this person? *No, she was so mean and turned into kind of a terrible person.*

+ Would you ever call this person to get advice on your life? *Absolutely never.*

+ Is this person really representative of "everybody"? If not, who are they representative of? *Not at all. She's representative of a mean, hurting fourteen-year-old who was mad at me for getting popular.*

After you've done this for each person on your list, come up with five examples of people who would disagree with your "everyone" statement, whose opinions you trust, respect, and value.

In the "too slutty" example, some trusted and respected sources who disagree with that belief might include *your mom, your partner, your three best friends, and your dog.*

When you're done, freewrite for a few minutes about the experience to consider any insights or discoveries you made.

✛ *Power Posing*

The outsider often has apologetic or disempowered body language, like hunching, hiding, speaking softly or in a pitched-up voice, avoiding eye contact, or trying to shrink themselves so as not to be a burden or draw negative attention. Unfortunately, this kind of body language tends to reinforce their belief that they're unworthy of taking up space and makes them feel more anxious overall. For this reason, I encourage outsiders to explore and practice big and powerful body language! Some research shows that power posing (standing with your body arranged in a big, expansive, and assertive position for several minutes) increases confidence,[9] but consistently practicing this kind of body language over time also seems to help a person feel safer and more confident taking up space in the world, both physically and energetically. If you normally have timid body language, collapsed posture, a quiet or pitched-up voice, or a general desire to shrink yourself down and take up less space, try adopting a daily powerful-physicality practice! This could include any number of ways to practice feeling powerful, like martial arts, lifting weights, the Alexander technique, dance therapy, vocal training, physical therapy, or even primal scream therapy. Do whatever helps *you* feel powerful, and practice taking up space physically, energetically, and vocally! If you're looking for a simple and accessible way to practice this, power posing can't be beat. Try spending a few minutes every day standing with your feet planted firmly, chest tall, shoulders back, eyes up, and arms stretched out wide, breathing deeply and looking around the room like you own the place . . . or do a quick Google search to find other ideas for powerful poses! (Added bonus for shouting, or repeating something as loudly as you can, while doing it!)[10]

Book Recommendations for the Outsider:

Aubrey Gordon, *What We Don't Talk about When We Talk about Fat* (Boston: Beacon Press, 2020).

Amir Levine and Rachel Heller, *Attached: The New Science of Adult Attachment and How It Can Help You Find—and Keep—Love* (New York: TarcherPerigee, 2011).

Marshall B. Rosenberg, *Nonviolent Communication: A Language of Life; Life-Changing Tools for Healthy Relationships* (Encinitas, CA: PuddleDancer Press, 2015).

Sonya Renee Taylor, *The Body Is Not an Apology: The Power of Radical Self-Love*, 2nd ed. (San Francisco: Berrett-Koehler, 2018).

THE RUNNER

Some Things the Runner Often Needs to Learn, Practice, or Cultivate

+ *The Ability to Tune In to, and Connect With, Their Bodies*

The runner is disconnected from their body, but often for different reasons and in different ways than the self-objectifier. Having spent a lifetime trying to repress, numb, avoid, or control their emotions, as well as many of the signals and sensations their body sends them (like hunger, fullness, or a need for comfort)—plus possibly having experienced a dissociative episode during trauma at some point—runners often feel numb and disembodied, almost as if their body were completely separate from and unrelated to them. Being disconnected like this makes it extremely difficult to take good care of their body and make good decisions for themselves, which leads to injury, illness, or other "betrayals" that reinforce the runner's feeling that their body is out to get them and can't be trusted. It also makes the runner feel confused and unsafe a lot, and keeps them from being able to experience much pleasure or joy, making their overall life experience more negative and causing them to rely more heavily on their coping, numbing, distracting, and controlling habits.

For all these reasons, it's important for the runner to rebuild their connection with their body on the path to body neutrality. There are multiple types of mind-body pathways, which is to say multiple channels of awareness and information between the mind and body, that can be improved to accomplish this. (Most of us were born with these channels open, but they can be interrupted or disconnected in such a way that the mind no longer has any awareness of, or connection to, that type of information from the body.) One type is called our *exteroceptive awareness*, which is the ability to identify, access, understand, and appropriately respond to sensations that are triggered externally, like the ones we get from our five senses: taste, touch, sight, hearing, and smell. This awareness can be improved through mindfulness practices (as I mentioned for the self-objectifier), as well as through certain kinds of somatic therapies and practices, like massage, breath work, dance, voice work, sensate focus, neurofeedback, and somatic experiencing. Another channel of mind-body information is our *proprioceptive awareness*, which is the ability to determine where our body parts are in relation to each other without looking at them and track our movement through space. This awareness tends to be particularly impaired when someone has a history of traumatic dissociation, which is why people with unresolved trauma often feel so clumsy, but it can be strengthened through balance work, mindfulness, and mindful movement (like yoga, or lifting weights with an emphasis on noticing and feeling the muscles work). Then there's our *interoceptive awareness*, which is the ability to identify, access, understand, and appropriately respond to the sensations we feel about the internal state of our bodies, like the racing heart, dry mouth, or tingling that indicate fear, or the sensations of being hungry, thirsty, or needing to pee. This mind-body pathway is also what connects us to our emotions, needs, desires, boundaries, sexual arousal, and intuition, which is why it's often so important for the runner to strengthen and improve their interoceptive awareness, using any of the tools mentioned already, as well as practices like intuitive eating, learning to identify and put language to their emotions, journaling, and learning to regulate their nervous system with various types of neuro-feedback.[11]

+ *The Ability to Connect With (and Befriend) Their* Emotions

While this is technically just an offshoot of the ability to tune in to and connect with their body, it's worth mentioning again because of how often runners struggle with emotional awareness, finding it very difficult to recognize, access, identify, tolerate, and respond appropriately to their emotions. That's because the runner is often running from their own emotions—in particular, their uncomfortable or unpleasant emotions—so cultivating a more attuned, positive, and trusting relationship with their emotions can have a huge impact on their ability to stop running. You can cultivate your emotional intelligence and awareness through education, mindfulness or meditation, psychotherapy, discussion, journaling and other self-reflection tools, and by expanding your emotional vocabulary, as well as just trial and error, practice, and repetition. You can also develop a less negative relationship with your emotions by applying the same clear and neutral lens to your emotions that you've been practicing with your body, noticing and stripping away any negative beliefs, interpretations, or false meaning and significance that have been attached to each for you, until you can view your emotions for what they truly are: safe and neutral bits of *information*. It can be especially helpful to learn more about the way emotions work, and why we have them (I recommend reading Lisa Feldman Barrett's *How Emotions Are Made*), on the journey to emotional neutrality, because the runner tends to imagine their feelings are bad or shameful, or have the power to overwhelm or destroy them. But emotions are just biological signals, and each feeling has a beginning and an end; each feeling flows *in* to give us some kind of information that we need, and then flows back *out* once we've adequately acknowledged and responded to it.[12] By learning to differentiate between and tolerate their emotions, the runner will at worst find them far less threatening or overwhelming, and at best discover the respect and appreciation needed to form a friendly alliance.

✦ *The Ability to Remove Their Physical Armor and Physically Relax*

The runner often has no idea how much tension they're holding in their bodies, or that their nervous systems are stuck on high alert. They might know they have tight shoulders, back pain, pelvic floor dysfunction, anxiety, or insomnia without realizing that all those things are related, for example. Unfortunately though, even if someone *does* realize they're stuck in chronic stress and tension, most folks don't know how to address it, outside of trying to calm down with meditation, or calling upon individual (and often expensive) treatments like massage, physical therapy, psychotherapy, or medication.[13] Put another way, many runners need to cultivate the skill of, and capacity for, relaxing their bodies and calming their minds. For this reason, many runners greatly benefit from learning more about the human nervous system and vagus nerve, and using that information to develop tools and skills for intentionally *activating* their parasympathetic nervous system (the one in charge of calming you down, and the rest-and-digest response), and intentionally *deactivating* the sympathetic nervous system (the one in charge of getting you amped up, and the fight, flight, freeze, or fawn response). With practice, this strategy can help the runner maintain homeostasis, a "self-regulating process by which biological systems maintain stability while adjusting to changing external conditions,"[14] more often, and also make it easier for them to release chronic muscle tension.

A runner pursuing this strategy may start by reading a book or article, listening to a podcast, or signing up for a class on the sympathetic and parasympathetic nervous systems or polyvagal theory,[15] and then exploring various tools and techniques for grounding the nervous system, and intentionally getting into a more calm and relaxed state. Some examples include splashing cold water on the face or hands; spending more time in nature; regular meditation; taking deep, slow belly breaths; using certain visualizations or mindfulness practices; humming or singing; cuddling with a trusted loved one or pet, or joining a Dialectical-Behavior Therapy (DBT) skills group. It can also be supported by exploring certain body-centered somatic therapies, which work to address how "a physical body holds on to stress, tension, and trauma,"[16] and can make it easier to release long-held and habitual patterns of tightness and tension. By developing these skills, the runner can often reduce overall anxiety, start feeling safer in their bodies, and discover that they don't need quite as many coping or numbing behaviors as they used to, because there is less to cope with day to day. And by releasing the "armor" of habitual tension, holding, and physical guarding, they may also find it easier to breathe deeply, connect with their bodies, and be more trusting and vulnerable in general.

✛ *More Pleasure, Play, Fun, and Joy*

One of the reasons the runner feels so much resistance to being present in their body is that they associate their bodies with *bad feelings*. Whether due to trauma, anxiety, depression, mental or physical illness, certain disabilities, injury, pain, life circumstances, or just chronically unmet needs, the runner's experience of being a person with a body tends to be skewed dramatically toward the negative. One strategy for the runner to bring themselves back into balance would, of course, be to remove or improve external sources of pain or suffering, like quitting a job they hate, seeking treatment for their mental or physical illness, or leaving an abusive partner. But as it's not always possible to significantly reduce or escape the source of a person's bad feelings, this strategy may not be helpful for everyone. Luckily, there is another strategy that can be employed by all runners, which is to increase sources of *good* feelings, through pleasure, play, fun, and joy! For most runners, this includes both figuring out and prioritizing anything that checks those boxes for them, and also cultivating a mindful presence that allows them to actually take in and connect with those good feelings as they're happening. In your pursuit of pleasure, play, fun, and joy, for example, you might spend more time with people (or in places) that make you happy, take up a new hobby, enroll in a sport or game league, express yourself through art, join a community of like-minded people, or commit to a daily self-pleasure practice—whatever brings you more good feelings! But at the same time, you might need to practice noticing and enjoying those good feelings by slowing down, tuning into the sensations in your body, and cultivating the ability to be present with them, like mindfully savoring your favorite meal, pausing to appreciate your perfume when you put it on, stopping to take in a beautiful sunset, or reveling in the pleasure of seeing live music. The more often you experience and connect with positive feelings in this way, the less you'll associate your body with painful, scary, or bad feelings, and it'll feel safer and easier to tune in to, and be present with, your body.

Some Fears the Runner Often Needs to Face

+ *Their Fear of Intimacy, Letting People In, and Risking Heartbreak*

The runner tends to be afraid of letting anyone get too close, both because that kind of vulnerability is so uncomfortable, and because they don't trust themselves to survive it if they were to let someone in, and then lose them. This makes intimacy terrifying (or even impossible), and often leads the runner to push people away, ghost, create conflict, put up walls, struggle with trust, or develop hyper-independence, in which they decide they can't rely on anyone but themselves, and end up feeling incredibly isolated and lonely.[17] Stripping these fears of their power can be incredibly helpful on the runner's path to body neutrality, but like all fear facing, it must be done gradually and mindfully.

Facing these fears *slowly*—opening up to someone bit by bit—gives you time to check in and make sure the relationship is safe and that vulnerability and trust are being built mutually and appropriately.[18] Learning to be more vulnerable, let people in, and tolerate deeper levels of intimacy takes patience and practice, but it also requires a boatload of courage and a willingness to be scared and do the scary thing anyway, instead of waiting until it's comfortable. By taking risks and letting people in this way (as well as cultivating the skills and tools needed to handle rejection and loss), intimacy and vulnerability will feel less scary and dangerous, and the runner will have an easier time relying on other people for connection, comfort, and support. This opens up a huge new set of resources and possibilities for calming anxiety, regulating the nervous system, having pleasant experiences, and coping with stress in healthy and effective ways.

+ *The Vulnerability of Facing the World without Their Armor*

As the runner learns to release the chronic tension they've been holding in their bodies, and switch off their sympathetic nervous system more often, they face an excruciatingly vulnerable premise: facing the world without armor. The thought of moving through the world unprotected can be unbelievably frightening, especially for a runner who has never done so before, because they've been relying on their armor to feel safe since childhood. Whether it's coping strategies that allow them to never rely on anyone, a constant need to control everything, patterns of distracting or numbing themselves, or chronic tension in the body, the runner has come to rely on their various bits of armor to protect themselves and survive. In some ways, these bits of armor are like security blankets, or imaginary shields, and the prospect of facing life without them can make the runner feel unbearably naked, vulnerable, unsafe, and scared. By facing that fear slowly and incrementally over time, however, the runner has the opportunity to strip it of power, making it possible to finally decrease or release it. If you're used to sucking your stomach in all the time, for example, you might start by trying to increase your awareness of when you're doing it, and then consciously relaxing it when you're home alone, or wearing baggy clothing, until that feels less scary or hard. Then increase the stakes a bit, by practicing relaxing your belly around one or two people you trust, or while wearing more formfitting clothes, and so on, until your belly is soft and relaxed more often than it's not. A lot of emotions or obstacles might come up during this process that require your attention, like discovering you physically can't relax your belly even when you try, or that doing so makes you too panicky to continue. Tending to (and learning to safely tolerate) these emotions, as well as acquiring the resources or support needed to overcome these obstacles, are an important part of this fear-facing practice, because you're training your brain and body to feel safe doing things that have long been categorized as "unsafe." As a runner learns to face the world without their armor, they tend to feel freer, safer, and more confident overall, and have an easier time connecting with both their body and other people.

Some Things the Runner Often Feels Shame About

+ *Their Body Having Betrayed Them, or the Runner Having Betrayed Themselves*

Having so often felt betrayed by their body in some way, the runner tends to holds a lot of resentment and animosity toward their body, or project a lot of shame onto it. Doing some shame busting around those perceived betrayals can help the runner stop seeing their body as their enemy, and move toward healing and wholeness. This can be done by connecting with people who have shared a similar experience, taking in content that normalizes or brings new clarity to what happened, dealing with it in therapy, or sharing your experience with someone you trust. The goal is to strip your shame of power and find a way of acknowledging that your body has actually always been on your side and was trying to protect you (because it was), and possibly even getting to a point where you can forgive your body, apologize for having waged war against it for so long, and move forward as allies. Sometimes, however, the runner feels shame over having betrayed themselves for not listening to their bodies sooner, for example, or for putting themselves in unsafe positions. That shame can negatively affect the runner's self-image, as well as their relationship to their body, and increase their reliance on coping and numbing behaviors. Shame busting around those experiences as well can lead to more self-compassion, self-forgiveness, self-trust, and a decrease in overall anxiety. By stripping their shame and blame of power, the runner becomes able to see themselves—often for the first time—not as two conflicting parts locked in an endless battle for dominance (body versus mind), but as one *whole unified being*.

+ *Feeling Weak, Lacking Willpower, and Being "Out of Control"*

Because *control* makes the runner feel safe, they tend to feel shame about the ways in which they feel "out of control," which generally means the ways in which they either can't get themselves to do something they think they *should* do, or can't *stop* themselves from doing something they think they *shouldn't*. Many of these areas are body related, as the runner believes they should be able to completely dominate and control their bodies, and therefore see any failure to do so as a sign of weakness, a lack of discipline or self-control, or an act of unforgivable self-sabotage. They might feel shame about their inability to stick to a diet, for example, because they think that with enough self-control and willpower they would be able to resist the urge to eat more, or they might feel shame about their failure to do something simple, like send thank-you cards, imagining their behavior to be proof of how weak, lazy, or undisciplined they are. To normalize and shame bust around these kinds of "out-of-control" behaviors, it can be helpful to learn more about the valid physiological and psychological reasons for them, such as the science of why diets fail,[19] or why some people struggle to get seemingly simple tasks done (due to things like difficulty focusing, or mustering up initiative).[20] The truth is that you probably feel out of control because you either have unreasonable and unrealistic expectations for what *can* be controlled, or have been working so hard to control yourself that you're unintentionally creating physiological or psychological backlash (or both!).

Some of My Favorite Practices for the Runner

+ *Mindfulness*

Mindfulness is the practice of bringing one's awareness to the current moment, and it's been proven over and over to reduce stress and anxiety, regulate the nervous system, improve cognitive abilities, increase tolerance for uncomfortable feelings, and boost mood.[21] That's why so many runners benefit from adopting a mindfulness practice and spending some time every day bringing their attention to the present moment. There are so many ways to practice mindfulness that I encourage you to explore whichever path most appeals to you. Some people like to do a traditional seated meditation, closing their eyes and focusing on the breath, for example, or watching their thoughts float by like clouds. Others prefer the various guided meditations available through different apps like Headspace or Calm, or via free content on YouTube. Some find it easiest to practice mindfulness while moving instead of sitting still, or with their eyes open rather than closed, and are therefore drawn to mindful movement practices (like walking meditation, yoga, Tai Chi, or Qigong), or to just spend time bringing mindfulness to daily tasks (like washing the dishes, taking a shower, or eating). Some people are drawn to Buddhism, some to Transcendental Meditation, and some prefer to adopt a more intuitive approach. Some people like to support and cultivate their mindfulness practice via coaching, mentorship, courses, or workshops, while some prefer to do so via podcasts, videos, or books, and others just want to find their own way. There is no right or wrong way to practice mindfulness; just find something that works for you and stick to it.

Note: It has to be said that for some people, trying to be present, sit quietly with their thoughts, or bring their attention to the sensations in their bodies brings up an unproductive or even unsafe amount of discomfort or distress, so mindfulness may not be for everyone.[22] If you decide to move forward with a mindfulness practice, go slowly, pay attention to how it feels (both during and after), and seek out a trauma-informed meditation teacher or therapist if you need extra support.

+ Use the Emotion Wheel to Develop Emotional Granularity

To improve their emotional awareness and emotional intelligence, I encourage many runners to develop their *emotional granularity*. Emotional granularity is the ability to identify, differentiate between, and describe one's feelings with a high degree of specificity and accuracy. Instead of saying they're mad, for example, a person with high emotional granularity might understand themselves to be peevish, exasperated, furious, or resentful. And research shows that people with higher emotional granularity are more resilient and less reactive to stress, feel less overwhelmed when facing challenges, experience less fear and anxiety, have more positive relationships, and require fewer coping behaviors.[23] To start improving your emotional granularity, I recommend learning more about how and why it works (Lisa Feldman Barrett's *How Emotions Are Made* is a great place to start), and then doing a Google search for something called an emotion wheel. Check in with your emotions on a regular basis—maybe a few times per day— to first notice what you're feeling, and then use the wheel to help you practice differentiating between, and describing, your emotions with more specificity and precision.

+ Commit to Choosing How You Want to Suffer

Once we've cleared away the fears, shame, and false meaning and significance obscuring it, we can plainly see the truth: in an ongoing effort to avoid facing or feeling pain, the runner creates a very painful life. There's no denying that pain sucks, but when you refuse to face and feel that pain directly, you have to spend the rest of your life running, hiding, numbing, repressing, distracting, and coping with it. So, sure, you might get to avoid some uncomfortable stuff, but the trade-off usually isn't *less* suffering, it's just *different* suffering. (And frankly, it's a kind of suffering that our minds find especially upsetting: a suffering with no clarity, no solution, no meaning, and no end; the suffering of a pointless, make-believe wild-goose chase.)

If your goal is ultimately to experience less pain and suffering, you need to get honest with yourself and take stock: How is this whole subconscious runner plan working out? Does it actually lead to less pain and suffering for you? If not, what would? And more important—even if living this way does seem to reduce your overall suffering—is this the kind of suffering you want? Seriously. If you're going to suffer either way, is constant running how you want to suffer? Or would you rather occasionally suffer through the thing you've been running from for so long? The first one will always feel a bit frustrating and unsatisfying, because some part of us always knows, deep down, that we're playing a trivial game of pretend and that there's no way to "win." The second one might sound scary as hell, but when we allow ourselves to go there and face it directly, there is something clean about the experience of that pain; there is a feeling of inner calm, clarity, and meaning to it, because we know, deep down, that we're sitting in the truth of the moment.

Facing and embracing this kind of true suffering can take a long time (and include a lot of skill building, fear facing, and shame busting), but it becomes much more tolerable when you've chosen it, and it feels meaningful to you. As Victor Frankl points out in his book *Man's Search for Meaning*, "In some ways suffering ceases to be suffering at the moment it finds a meaning." I invite you right now to just reconsider how you *want* to suffer. Body image suffering both is thrust upon us without our consent and serves absolutely no higher meaning or purpose. By choosing to always meet yourself in the truth of your pain directly, instead of running from it, you can both restore a feeling of power and agency, and connect to the higher meaning and purpose of your suffering (i.e., "I'm suffering the *truth* in order to avoid suffering the *lie*"). Not to mention the fact that pain itself is morally neutral as well, if you're willing to strip away the judgment, significance, and meaning that has been layered onto it for so long. That's why this practice—choosing to always face and feel the truth of your own pain rather than running from it—is one of the most powerful practices for the runner on the path to body neutrality.

Book Recommendations for the Runner:

Bessel van der Kolk, *The Body Keeps the Score: Brain, Mind, and Body in the Healing of Trauma* (New York: Viking, 2014).

Brené Brown, *The Power of Vulnerability: Teachings on Authenticity, Connection, and Courage* (Boulder, CO: Sounds True, 2012).

Deborah Dana, *Anchored: How to Befriend Your Nervous System Using Polyvagal Theory* (Boulder, CO: Sounds True, 2021).

Lisa Feldman Barrett, *How Emotions Are Made: The Secret Life of the Brain* (New York: Mariner Books, 2018).

Resmaa Menakem, *My Grandmother's Hands: Racialized Trauma and the Pathway to Mending Our Hearts and Bodies* (Las Vegas: Central Recovery Press, 2017).

CHAPTER 18

But What about Marginalized Bodies?

A LOT OF THIS BOOK SO FAR HAS FO-cused on how a person can get their needs met and their problems solved more directly once they iden-tify which needs their body image issues are trying to meet, or which problems they're trying to solve. And I stand by the fact that most people have a lot more options for doing this than they think they do, if they're willing to get creative and let go of the way they think it "should look." But the truth is that it's way easier for people in privi-leged bodies to get their needs met and their problems solved than it is for people in marginalized bodies.[1]

Frankly, this topic is just so fucking heartbreaking. Our world is full of violence, discrimination, erasure, bigotry, and prejudice toward peo-ple in certain bodies. Massive systems of oppression and injustice form the very basis of our society.[2] So seeing the world with "clear and neu-tral vision" can actually just . . . really suck. And for people in margin-alized bodies, seeing your body with clear and neutral vision *within* that world can be incredibly painful. When your objective truth is that society is structured to oppress people with bodies like yours, "neutral-ity" can feel anything but neutral.

Absolutely *nothing* about a person's body has the power to "make people" hurt or marginalize them, and body neutrality requires absolute clarity and honesty about that. The blame for harmful behavior *always* lies with the perpetrator of that harm, not your body. Fat bodies don't create anti-fat discrimination or harassment, just like wearing a short skirt doesn't create sexual predators, and Black bodies don't create racism. But while getting angry at the system of violence (and perpetrators of that system) that caused an individual harm might allow them to stop blaming and hating themselves and their bodies, it won't keep them from still facing that violence.

How can we talk about body neutrality in a world that discriminates against and dehumanizes certain people on account of the bodies they happen to live in? Is it even possible to feel neutrally about a body that some people so clearly hate? Can someone ever strip away the meaning and significance they've attached to their body, when that meaning and significance is based on the objective fact that society doesn't consider people with bodies like theirs to be worthy of respect, autonomy, belonging, safety, or even being alive? And how can someone make their body image issues *unnecessary* if they exist to protect them from marginalization, discrimination, and violence?[3]

Whew.

Okay, so here's where I stand on that: Body neutrality is about seeing your body, yourself, and the world exactly as they are, without any additional stories or interpretations layered on top, right? It's about having clear and objective vision. That means we have to admit that while anyone can access body neutrality, body neutrality itself can *only do so much* to improve the quality of life for people in marginalized bodies.

Let's say a transgender woman of color's hidden body image purpose is to "pass" as cisgender to protect her from violence. She hates the many ways in which she is "clockable" as transgender, because they mark her as a target for transphobic violence, and she tries to meet as many Eurocentric beauty ideals as possible in order to avoid racist violence as well. This woman could obviously go through the body neutrality process, but when it comes to envisioning a body neutral future—where she no longer needed her body image issues to protect her—what would that be? Ideally it would be a world in which she was able to make herself safe from transphobic and racist violence without changing the way she looked, but given the world we live in, and the body she has, that might not be possible.

According to the Williams Institute at UCLA School of Law, in the United States 2.3 percent of cisgender women (of all races) are the victims of violent crime; for transgender women, that figure is 8.6 percent (nearly four times more likely). Note that the true figures are likely much higher, because not all crimes are reported, and also because it's a recent phenomenon for gender identity to even be reflected in crime statistics.[4] So we don't know the exact figures for a transgender woman of color, but the heartbreaking reality is that, statistically speaking, this woman is likely to be the target of violence if people clock her as transgender. So she can do the internal work to blame the systems of oppression (and the people who uphold them) for putting her in this position and causing her harm, instead of blaming her body, and that might help ease her body negativity. But the only body neutral futures she could realistically envision would be to choose between *courage* or *self-preservation*, and that's a shit choice. She could bravely show up every day as herself, despite the risks, and cultivate resilience in the face of the oppression and violence she will undoubtedly face that way. Or she can go with *self-preservation*, by staying in the closet, hiding her truth, and shrinking her world to stay safe, or spending all her time and money conforming to standards of femininity and Eurocentric beauty ideals that lower her odds of being targeted.

Maybe she does the work to build courage and resilience, cultivate skills to get more of her needs met, develop a strong support system, and release any shame she feels about being the "wrong" kind of person. She learns to get angry and send her blame and anger outward toward the people and systems causing her harm, instead of inward at herself or her body. She acknowledges that her body is not the source of her suffering, traumas, stigmatization, harassment, or oppression, but rather transphobia, racism, and the patriarchy are. Her body is just a body; it's morally neutral.

Hooray, this woman just found body neutrality! But that doesn't change the fact that she's still going to be living in fear, facing violence, and struggling against injustice. A person's body cannot be the problem, but that doesn't change the fact that *there is still a fucking problem*.

As a side note, this conversation highlights one reason why we should never make assumptions or judgments about the choices other people make with regard to their body or appearance. Inside a system of injustice and oppression, people are just coping however they need to cope, and there is no right or wrong way to do it. All choices a person makes about their own body are morally neutral (not to mention none of our business), and there's nothing morally superior about "looking natural," or refusing to change your appearance to appease society. In fact, sometimes changing your appearance to appease society is the *best* choice a person can make!

This situation sucks. I wish I had a better solution, but all I can offer is the suggestion that we all commit to facing the truth. The *truth* is that we live in a deeply unjust, discriminatory, and violent society in which many people cannot get their needs met or solve their problems because of the kind of body they live in. It's important we acknowledge that people in marginalized bodies might do all this courageous and powerful work only to discover that their body image issues were covering up the deep underlying pain of that truth. And if that doesn't sound like a particularly good deal to you, you're right. Suffering is still suffering, and frankly, believing this is all your fault (and that you could escape your pain by changing your body) might even sound *preferable* to the task of trying to find peace in an unfair and violent world.

That said, hating systems of oppression instead of hating your body *is* an improvement for most people, as is getting angry at the people who caused you harm instead of holding shame about "deserving" that harm. Body neutrality creates space for self-compassion, dignity, self-respect, and the coming back together of all the fractured bits of ourselves we've been taught to scatter so that we can feel whole again.

There is clarity, calm, and power that comes from acknowledging the truth as it is, instead of hiding from it, even if that truth is that we have a huge, unsolvable problem—and in fact, in this case, acknowledging that truth is actually a prerequisite for finding a solution. After all, many people in marginalized bodies want to change their bodies to escape their marginalization, but many people who aren't in marginalized bodies are also terrified of becoming marginalized, which underpins a lot of *their* body image issues. So the more of us who are willing to face this truth, the better, because it means we will finally be acknowledging the *real* problem we're facing as a society, and giving ourselves the opportunity to come together in trying to solve it.

CHAPTER 19

Body Neutrality Success

ODY NEUTRALITY SUCCESS IS, TO BE honest, kind of anticlimactic.

The drama of hating your body is so intense, a daily roller coaster of thoughts and feelings and behaviors, and an endless expenditure of time, energy, attention, and money. It makes sense to imagine body neutrality would be just as interesting and dramatic, but nothing could be further from the truth.

Not only is the process of moving through the body neutrality blueprint slow and gradual for most people, but the end result is that of having *nothing* where once there was *something*, which is both difficult to describe and sort of boring. You know how, when you *really* need to pee, you're completely overwhelmed with the drama of it? Every step you take, every pothole you drive over, every tiny thing that slows down your ability to access a bathroom is a huge deal, because you're completely absorbed by the discomfort you're in, and how to get out of it. But then after you pee, you don't immediately start obsessing over how *good* it feels to have an empty bladder, or how grateful you are for every step you take without pain, do you? You might have a moment of gratitude and relief, but when you're done, you just go back to life as normal, and probably don't think about your bladder again until the next time you have to pee.

That's how it tends to be when a person gets to a state of body neutrality. They're not overwhelmed with gratitude or happiness or even relief, they're just . . . living their lives. It's as though they had been walking around with heavy weights in their pockets for years, and the body neutrality process removed one tiny weight at a time—an insignificant amount each time, hardly even noticeable, and so slowly that they weren't even aware of how much lighter they were getting, until they look back and remember how weighed down they felt six, twelve, or eighteen months ago.

My client Mari told me recently, at the end of six months of coaching, that she didn't think she was getting any better, and that she wasn't any more body neutral than she used to be. When going back through my notes to see how she had described her daily life at the beginning, however, it became clear that a *lot* had changed!

When we first met, Mari was spending twenty to thirty minutes every day criticizing her appearance in the mirror. She was weighing herself three to five times per day, and the number she saw determined how upset or happy she would be all day. She only wore clothing she thought was "flattering," which meant she wore almost exclusively black clothing, she had an anxiety attack around food or exercise if she wasn't able to follow her "plan" for the day (which meant she usually had two or three anxiety attacks per week), and she felt too insecure to be naked around anyone, so she completely avoided dating and sex.

Now, Mari spends about five to ten minutes criticizing her appearance in the mirror every day on average (although some days it's zero!), and the whole experience feels much less painful, because she's totally aware of what she's doing and why. (For example, because she stopped weighing herself and got rid of her scale, some of her anxious body-checking time in the mirror is a way of proving to herself that she's "safe.") She's started buying and wearing more colorful and self-expressive clothing, reports feeling more "herself" than before, and worries far less about whether or not an item of clothing is "slimming." And while she still sets a plan for herself around food and exercise, the intense and time-consuming anxiety attacks have been downgraded to a sort of irritable mood when she goes off plan and happen with far less frequency, because her food and exercise plan is more realistic and flexible now. Plus, Mari started exploring sex and dating, and it's going well!

As we went through this comparison, Mari kept saying things like "ooh, that's right!" and "oh my god I forgot I used to do that!" and "whoa, it's been a while since I've even thought about that." This is very typical for folks who go through the blueprint, because they're completely unaware that so many little weights are being removed from their pockets throughout the journey. After only six months of this work with her, I know Mari will continue to get closer and closer to body neutrality as she moves through her action plan, gets more of her needs met, builds up her collection of skills and resources, and strips her shame and fear of power. In fact, if she's anything like my other clients, a year or so from now Mari will be marveling at the way she used to body check, dress, care about her weight, and make a food and body plan at all, because all those things will have slowly faded into memory too.

This is how the process goes. When I look back at my life before body neutrality, I did all kinds of things I find bewildering now. I weighed myself daily (sometimes multiple times per day), counted macros, got my body fat percentage measured every few months, posed, pinched, and body checked in mirrors or my phone all day, and thought about how I looked *constantly*. I wore makeup, dressed in accordance with conventional beauty and body "rules," sucked in my belly, and obsessed over my "flaws." And while all these habits are in my rearview mirror now, it's not like I go around feeling euphoric and blissful all the time. It's just that now I get to spend all that time, attention, and energy on things that are more *real* and that feel more meaningful, rewarding, and interesting to me. Instead of thinking about my weight, I can think about my gender identity and sexuality. Instead of cultivating a perfect body, I'm cultivating the ability to be kind, generous, and present. Instead of working toward body goals, I work toward bucket list and career goals. Instead of spending time and energy trying to improve my appearance, I spend it trying to improve the world.

The biggest difference is that when I feel pain now, that pain is real; untouched by projections, distractions, moral judgment, cover-ups, or false meaning. There is a tangible, vulnerable directness to my pain now. Instead of feeling fat or ugly, if I'm feeling unloved now, I just feel . . . *unloved.* If I'm feeling lonely, I just feel *lonely,* and if I'm feeling angry, I just feel *angry.* It's still unpleasant, but there is a sort of peace to knowing I'm dealing with the *truth,* because that means there is nothing else lurking behind it that will jump out and hurt me.

Also, because I have such a deep understanding of my hidden body image purpose, I can now use my occasional bouts of body dysmorphia or preoccupation as a sort of *warning sign;* the "canary in the coal mine" of my mental health. I've gotten so used to having clear and neutral vision that when I look in the mirror and see something totally different, I immediately know something is up. About eight months into the global pandemic, for example, I had about a week of body dysmorphia in which I looked *horrible* to myself—bloated, old, pale, and bizarrely wide. I asked my partner if I looked different to them, and they said no, so I checked in with myself. *What is going on with me emotionally? What needs are going unmet? What might my brain be protecting or distracting me from noticing right now?*

Because I already knew my body image patterns, it only took me about half an hour to realize that I was not doing okay emotionally, that I was dealing with a shit ton of anxiety and depression, and that I needed support immediately. I talked to my partner and my mom about how dark things had gotten inside my heart and mind, and started looking into telehealth options for counseling and medication. The next day, I looked normal to myself in the mirror. Why? Because once I started tackling the problem directly, I no longer needed my dysmorphia to distract, alarm, or alert me that something was wrong.

Similarly, a few months before my thirty-fifth birthday, I found myself "feeling old," meaning, I was spending a lot of time looking at my new silver hair and wrinkles, and wondering if I should "do something about them." When I caught these kinds of thoughts popping up for several days in a row, I realized something was up, and returned to my body neutrality basics. *What purpose does "feeling old" serve for me right now? What am I really feeling, needing, or avoiding this time?*

Over the next few days I did some processing, and realized that turning thirty-five was bringing up a ton of anxiety about time passing too quickly, specifically around the pending loss of my parents, and about heading toward the end of my reproductive years and needing to make peace with whether or not I want kids. Whew! Not light or easy stuff to deal with, but *real*. And as soon as I named it, I forgot all about looking or feeling "old." Why? Because once I started dealing with the real issues head-on, I didn't need to be distracted from them. *This* is long-term body neutrality success.

In my experience, it takes a year or two of moving through the body neutrality blueprint for a person to identify their biggest and most deeply rooted problems, build the skills and solutions to make those body image issues obsolete, and remove the main sources of false or excess meaning and significance from their body. Depending on how many reasons *your* body image issues have to exist, this might take more or less time, but this first part of the process is about getting to a place where, even if you still have issues to tackle and layers to peel back, you feel stable and neutral more often than not.

Once you arrive at this "mostly neutral" place, you can start viewing your body image issues as little invitations from your brain to dip back into this work and see what's going on. My client Raven, for example, is a Black nonbinary self-objectifier in their thirties whose body anxiety and obsession had faded for the most part, as they got their need for attention, intimacy, partnership, self-expression, and autonomy met in their daily life. After a while, though, they started to get curious about the random couple of bad body image days that cropped up every so often out of nowhere. Time to dive back in and apply the blueprint to this specific situation!

I asked Raven what was going on for them emotionally when their old body insecurities flared up. What were they feeling, and what emotional needs were going unmet? What were they craving or wanting? What were they afraid of or avoiding? We searched for a new hidden body image purpose by exploring what problem their body image issues might be trying to solve for them under these particular circumstances.

Raven discovered that every example they could think of where their body insecurities had flared up again had been a day in which they felt *pissed* about something. Once was when they had been blamed for something at work that hadn't been their fault, once was when their parents had visited and criticized their life choices, and a few times they had been misgendered or disrespected in various ways. When I asked Raven how they felt about the emotion of anger, they said they generally thought of it as a "bad" emotion you shouldn't express to other people because it's impolite, but even *more* so because they were often misgendered as a woman, and "people don't like angry Black femmes." Mystery solved!

Every time Raven felt angry, they turned all that angry energy inward toward their body, to avoid coming off to others as threatening or unlikable. In other words, this particular experience of body image issues existed to solve the problem of not feeling safe expressing their anger toward others. And when thinking about what it would take to no longer require body image issues under these circumstances (and how to get there), we had to consider the fact that anti-Black biases did *indeed* make Raven's anger unsafe to express under certain circumstances. Several pathways and action steps emerged from there: Raven started naming their anger when it showed up, writing about it in their journal, or sharing it with me, their therapist, their partner, or a few friends. This helped strip some of the shame and fear away from Raven's experience of feeling angry, and made their anger feel much more valid, respected, and witnessed. They decided they could safely express anger to their parents, but not at work, so they started a dialogue with their parents about not wanting to be criticized, but kept their feelings to themselves in the office. When people misgendered them, they also started speaking up. "Actually I use they/them pronouns," they would say, or "wow, that was a rude comment," or "I don't think that joke was funny."

Slowly, as Raven became comfortable naming, feeling, and having their anger witnessed, as well as advocating for themself more often, this particular type of body image flare-up stopped happening. They reported feeling less trapped and more empowered, as the same moments that used to bring up body insecurities now just brought them face to face with the truth of their own anger, and the injustice of needing to hide it.

This is one of the things I want to make clear about the body neutrality blueprint: yes, it's a system for addressing your individual body image suffering right now, but it's also a system for understanding yourself, and getting to your truth, *forever.*

I can't tell you how many clients have reflected that they used the same exact steps of the blueprint to tackle behaviors, thoughts, and feelings that had nothing whatsoever to do with body image, with great results. Many runners will explore their various numbing habits through the lens of "what problem is this trying to solve for me," "what is this helping protect me from," and "what am I hoping I'll get, feel, or avoid from this?" They've used the insights from that exploration to come up with action plans to make everything from drinking, smoking weed, Netflix marathons, doom scrolling, playing video games, and online shopping, to workaholic tendencies and even compulsive sexual behavior powerless and unnecessary. I've had clients report figuring out what fears, shame, or unmet emotional needs were being hidden underneath their self-sabotaging behaviors, their judgments of others, their insecurities in other areas of life, and even their depression. Many times I've even heard stories of people using this model to explore their racist, sexist, or ableist biases and bigotry, and dismantling other blocks to what is, essentially, "human neutrality."

Being able to clear away the false meaning, significance, stories, and interpretations obscuring the truth from us is powerful, and this process can be applied *anywhere the truth is hidden*. Stripping away meaning, significance, and interpretation can be anti-oppression work, because all systems of oppression are based on lies, and being able to see with clear and neutral vision instead is liberation. Consider the following questions to see where else it might apply.

+ Where might your clear and neutral vision be currently obscured by layers of false meaning or significance when it comes to friendship or partnership? How about parenting, family structure, or monogamy? Sex? Rest? Money? Religion? Politics?

+ Which of your habits, patterns, thoughts, feelings, behaviors, or insecurities still carry negative meaning or interpretation in your mind? What would be different for you if they didn't?

+ What would be different in the world if everyone explored their own "bad habits" and coping strategies with curiosity and compassion (instead of judgment), and then strove to *make them unnecessary* (instead of trying to stop them with willpower)?

+ What would be different in the world if everyone explored their own biases around race and ethnicity, gender, age, ability, weight, and appearance this way, until they could see everyone *else* with clear and neutral vision too?

This is where I want to leave you: with an invitation to do this work to overcome your own personal body image suffering, and also to do it in service of building the world you want to live in—a world where body image issues don't make *sense*, both because neutrality has replaced hierarchy as the societal default, and because we are all so skilled at dealing with the truth that there is simply no longer a need for them.

Acknowledgments

Thank you to everyone who helped make this book possible. To Amy, my editor, and the whole team at Penguin Life, for believing so emphatically in this book. To Laura, my agent, for warmly helping me navigate the world of publishing. To Gretchen, for insisting that I write it. To Rachel, for drawing the avatars out of me. And to Harv and Annie, for investing in me before I knew I was worth investing in.

Thank you, too, to everyone who was in the trenches with me as I wrote it. To my mom, for all the love, support, hugs, and dinners. To Celia for always being there when I needed her. To my brother Ben for workouts that helped me survive, and my brother Jason for reminding me to play. To my dad for his long-distance support, and to Erica, Benny, and Jade for bearing witness. To my partner Drew for tending to me day in and day out: for loving me, for holding me when I cried, for feeding me when I needed to eat, and for making it safe for me to put the book first. And finally, to my cat Walden, for just being the sweetest boy.

Appendix:
Recommended Reading

BODY LIBERATION BOOK LIST, BY CATEGORY

Racial Justice

An Indigenous Peoples' History of the United States, by Roxanne
    Dunbar-Ortiz
Between the World and Me, by Ta-Nehisi Coates
How to Be an Antiracist, by Ibram X. Kendi
I'm Still Here: Black Dignity in a World Made for Whiteness, by Austin
    Channing Brown
*Me and White Supremacy: Combat Racism, Change the World, and
    Become a Good Ancestor*, by Layla F. Saad
Minor Feelings: An Asian American Reckoning, by Cathy Park Hong
*My Grandmother's Hands: Racialized Trauma and the Pathway to
    Mending Our Hearts and Bodies*, by Resmaa Menakem
*Racism without Racists: Color-Blind Racism and the Persistence of Racial
    Inequality in America*, by Eduardo Bonilla-Silva
So You Want to Talk about Race, by Ijeoma Oluo

Tears We Cannot Stop: A Sermon to White America, by Michael Eric Dyson

The New Jim Crow: Mass Incarceration in the Age of Colorblindness, by Michelle Alexander

We Want to Do More Than Survive: Abolitionist Teaching and the Pursuit of Educational Freedom, by Bettina L. Love

We Were Eight Years in Power: An American Tragedy, by Ta-Nehisi Coates

White Rage: The Unspoken Truth of Our Racial Divide, by Carol Anderson

Why Are All the Black Kids Sitting Together in the Cafeteria?: And Other Conversations About Race, by Beverly Daniel Tatum

Why I'm No Longer Talking to White People about Race, by Reni Eddo-Lodge

Fat Justice

Fattily Ever After: A Black Fat Girl's Guide to Living Life Unapologetically, by Stephanie Yeboah

Fearing the Black Body: The Racial Origins of Fat Phobia, by Sabrina Strings

Heavy: An American Memoir, by Kiese Laymon

Hunger: A Memoir of (My) Body, by Roxane Gay

Landwhale: On Turning Insults Into Nicknames, Why Body Image Is Hard, and How Diets Can Kiss My Ass, by Jes Baker

The Body Is Not an Apology: The Power of Radical Self-Love, by Sonya Renee Taylor

The Other F Word: A Celebration of the Fat & Fierce, edited by Angie Manfredi

Thick: And Other Essays, by Tressie McMillan Cottom

What We Don't Talk about When We Talk about Fat, by Aubrey Gordon

What's Wrong with Fat?, by Abigail Saguy

You Have the Right to Remain Fat, by Virgie Tovar

Feminism and Beauty Ideals

Ain't I a Woman: Black Women and Feminism, by bell hooks

Americanah: A Novel, by Chimamanda Ngozi Adichie

Appetites: Why Women Want, by Caroline Knapp

Bad Feminist: Essays, by Roxane Gay

Beauty Sick: How the Cultural Obsession with Appearance Hurts Girls and Women, by Renee Engeln

Down Girl: The Logic of Misogyny, by Kate Manne

Fed Up: Emotional Labor, Women, and the Way Forward, by Gemma Hartly

Feminism Is for Everybody: Passionate Politics, by bell hooks

Hood Feminism: Notes from the Women That a Movement Forgot, by Mikki Kendall

More Than a Body: Your Body Is an Instrument, Not an Ornament, by Lexie Kite and Lindsay Kite

Not That Bad: Dispatches from Rape Culture, by Roxane Gay

Pleasure Activism: The Politics of Feeling Good, by Adrienne Maree Brown

The Beauty Myth: How Images of Beauty Are Used Against Women, by Naomi Wolf

Sex and Gender

Amateur: A Reckoning with Gender, Identity, and Masculinity, by Thomas Page McBee

Come As You Are: The Surprising New Science That Will Transform Your Sex Life, by Emily Nagoski

Girls & Sex: Navigating the Complicated New Landscape, by Peggy Orenstein

Life Isn't Binary: On Being Both, Beyond, and In-Between, by Meg-John Barker and Alex Iantaffi

Love's Not Color Blind: Race and Representation in Polyamorous and Other Alternative Communities, by Kevin A. Patterson

Mating in Captivity: Unlocking Erotic Intelligence, by Esther Perel

Pure: Inside the Evangelical Movement That Shamed a Generation of Young Women and How I Broke Free, by Linda Kay Klein

Sensual Self: Prompts and Practices for Getting in Touch with Your Body; A Guided Journal, by Ev'Yan Whitney

Sex at Dawn: How We Mate, Why We Stray, and What it Means for Modern Relationships, by Cacilda Jetha and Christopher Ryan

The Ethical Slut: A Practical Guide to Polyamory, Open Relationships, and Other Freedoms in Sex and Love, by Dossie Easton and Janet W. Hardy

The Purity Myth: How America's Obsession with Virginity Is Hurting Young Women, by Jessica Valenti

The Transgender Issue: Trans Justice Is Justice for All, by Shon Faye

Anti-Diet

Anti-Diet: Reclaim Your Time, Money, Well-Being, and Happiness Through Intuitive Eating, by Christy Harrison

Intuitive Eating: A Revolutionary Anti-Diet Approach, by Evelyn Tribole and Elyse Resch

The F*ck It Diet: Eating Should Be Easy, by Caroline Dooner

Important, but Harder to Categorize

A Disability History of the United States, by Kim E. Nielsen

Caste: The Origin of Our Discontents, by Isabel Wilkerson

Clean and White: A History of Environmental Racism in the United States, by Carl A. Zimring

Decolonizing Wealth: Indigenous Wisdom to Heal Divides and Restore Balance, by Edgar Villanueva

Oppression and the Body: Roots, Resistance, and Resolutions, by Christine Caldwell and Lucia Bennett Leighton

Appendix:
Frequently Asked Questions

Over the years, I've found there to be a handful of very common situations, problems, and obstacles that people run into along the path to body neutrality, which leads them to the question: "How should I handle it when . . . ?" And while I believe there is never one right way to handle these moments, I want to provide you with a few options, ideas, and examples to help you feel better prepared, should you run into them too.

How do I get my family/friends/partner to be more supportive of body neutrality? They're still deep in diet and wellness culture and see what I'm doing as "unhealthy," stupid, weak, or even dangerous.

It's so hard to evolve within our established relationships, because people come to expect (and even rely upon) certain aspects of the relationship to feel secure. If you and your best friend have spent years bonding over hating your bodies, dieting, or trash-talking other people's looks, they might feel threatened when you turn your back on those behaviors.

I say this only because a lot of the emotionally loaded pushback people get for adopting a new worldview isn't so much the result of the new worldview itself as it is the result of defensiveness and insecurity in the people who now feel judged, criticized, shamed, or left behind. If people in your life seem to have an inappropriately big or emotional response to what you're doing, they may be experiencing something similar.

How do you handle this? Totally up to you. You might find that some relationships just don't feel good anymore, because they were too dependent on your old values, beliefs, or behaviors around food, health, weight, and body stuff. It's completely valid to want to distance yourself from those relationships, either to protect your mental health and body image, or just because those relationships no longer hold any value or appeal for you. I give you full permission to reconsider your relationships, set new boundaries, and safeguard your time and energy for people who nourish, support, and fulfill you, as well as those who naturally align with your new system of values and beliefs.

That said, people are often tempted to write off a relationship before giving the other person a chance to make things better, because those kinds of conversations tend to be scary, hard, and uncomfortable. But if you've never told your friend that you're working on body neutrality and would like to get away from body bashing or diet talk, then they never have a chance to rise to the occasion. Personally, I recommend facing the discomfort of such a conversation, and giving people a chance whenever possible. If they start to get on board, and show up with more respect and understanding, great! If not, you can always shift gears to boundary setting, or distancing yourself from the relationship—but at least you gave them the opportunity first.

Want to open a dialogue with someone who is currently pooh-poohing body neutrality? First consider what outcome you're looking for from the conversation. Do you want them to genuinely understand and support what you're doing? Get educated about the dangers of diet culture and weight stigma? Be nicer to you about it? See how their behaviors are hurting you? Stop dieting and hating their own body? Each of these outcomes would dictate a different approach and conversation, so be sure to get clear before moving forward!

Once you know exactly what outcome you're looking for, consider whether you can safely talk to them about it from a vulnerable place, perhaps explaining how you were or are struggling with body image and how this approach to food, weight, and appearance is helping you. Also consider whether you can say it in such a way that *doesn't* sound judgmental or critical, or as if you're looking down on them from a moral high horse. I know these two considerations are a tall order, but most people aren't particularly motivated to learn a whole new approach to life (especially one that flies in the face of everything they've ever known or believed) just because someone told them they *should*, or because someone thinks their perspective is bad, wrong, or dangerous. So if your goal is genuinely to get the person to learn about, invest in, and connect to the value of body neutrality, you're not gonna do it by criticizing their beliefs or sending them an article about why they're wrong.

With all of this in mind, I find it's best to be very honest and direct about what you're asking for, while also connecting it to a real and vulnerable place in you—and bonus points if you can include some reassurance about your relationship too. Also, the kind of transformation you're hoping for probably won't happen within one conversation, because dismantling and rebuilding a whole worldview like this takes exposure, processing time, self-inquiry, and support. Because it will probably play out over *many* conversations, you can consider the first conversation to be a place where you're just opening a dialogue, planting seeds, and inviting them to show up for you. Here are a few ways that might look:

- Hey, Mom, have I ever talked to you about my struggle with body image issues? I know it's weird for you that I stopped dieting, and that you worry about my health. But I've been battling some serious food and body image issues for a long time, and I'm just trying to break free from them. I'd like to tell you more about how badly those issues were affecting me if you're interested, and I'd also be curious to hear more about your relationship to your own body. Where do you think *you* learned that it was important to be thin?

♦ Hey, friend, I've been reading this book called *Body Neutral*, and it's blowing my mind about why people actually struggle with body image issues. I'm dying to hear your thoughts about it, because we've always had such similar struggles around body image. Can I lend it to you so we can talk about it together?

♦ Hey, partner, I so admire your dedication to health and fitness, and you know I've always strived to be like that too. But I'm not sure if I've been completely honest with you about *why* I was so into it, or how unhealthy my approach was. It came from a very dark place, where I felt like I needed to be perfect or else nobody would ever love me, and I'm finally working to heal that now. So it might look on the surface like I don't care about my health anymore, but it's exactly the opposite—body neutrality is one of the most important things I've ever done for my health! It's okay if you don't understand, but I want you to know that criticizing my new approach, or making fun of it, makes me feel like you think I'm stupid, and that *you're* the one who doesn't care about my health. Either way it's hurtful. How can I support you in getting on board with this? Would an article or book recommendation to learn more about body neutrality help?

♦ Hey, sibling, I know body neutrality isn't your jam, and that's fine. But would you be willing to have a conversation about your specific issues with it? I want to understand your concerns better, because I love and respect you, but I also want an opportunity to help you understand that I'm being safe and healthy.

If the first conversation leads to the outcome you wanted (or just more conversations), that's fantastic. If the person refuses to consider your request or engage about their beliefs and behaviors in a respectful way, however, or if you don't have the time and energy available to support them as they transform, you can always just start setting boundaries or distancing yourself from them.

I'm trying to release the negative associations I have with my body and appearance, but it's hard when other people reinforce them all the time. How do I respond when someone criticizes, makes a negative comment about, or offers unsolicited advice about my body or appearance?

My answer to this totally depends on the relationship itself, as well as the outcome you want. As mentioned above, you may want to invite certain people into a more honest and ongoing dialogue unpacking the biases, beliefs, and assumptions leading to such a comment, how their comment makes you feel, how it causes harm to others, and why it's not actually true. But often these kinds of comments happen so fast, or with people you're not about to spend time or energy educating, that it can be hard to know how to respond.

Personally in these moments, I like to feign naive confusion, or sort of bright-eyed curiosity, and ask the commenter to explain what they meant, what the joke was, or where they got that information. This immediately alters the power dynamic, and puts all the discomfort and awkwardness of their comment right back on them, without me needing to educate anyone. I know this approach won't be everyone's cup of tea, but I still wanted to offer you some examples, and encourage you to try it:

- You walk into a party, and someone sees you and says, "Whoa, *someone* hasn't been hitting the gym lately!" in a sort-of joke about your weight. You respond with a big smile, bright eyes, and a sort of expectant pause, like you know they're probably being *hilarious* but you just can't quite figure out the joke yet. Still smiling encouragingly, you say, "Wait . . . what do you mean?" They now have to stand there, in front of the other people nearby, and either name the joke explicitly (to which you might just shrug and shake your head like you're still not getting it), or backpedal like crazy. This moment immediately inverts the power dynamic. They believed they could make that comment without consequences, because they're in a position of power, and you're not, so *of course* you will automatically agree to hold and absorb the consequences of the comment for them. By asking them to explain the joke, you are refusing to "play your part," and suddenly they realize they have no protection from the consequences of their behavior. In that moment, on the spot like that, and without getting the laugh they expected, most people will feel very awkward and uncomfortable and choose to backpedal with something like "what? Oh, nothing, never mind."

♦ You're chatting with coworkers, and someone says, "You should try the keto diet, I've been doing it for a few months and I've already lost ten pounds!" You cock your head and ask, with an air of complete confusion, "Why should *I* try it, though?" (If you're feeling a bit bolder or snarkier, you could say, with the same air of confusion, "Why would I try a diet, when I'm already at my goal weight?" That hands the awkwardness and discomfort back to them in a *big* way.)

If this strategy isn't for you, don't worry. There are five other strategies that can work well in these situations—you'll just have to try them out, find your own style, and consider what each individual situation calls for. One strategy to responding is to risk a bit of vulnerability with a response that invites a human connection: "That comment really hurt my feelings." Two is to be direct or even blunt, saying something true without putting yourself in the picture: "That comment was not appropriate." Three is to challenge the other person to see where they've erred, for example by asking, "Where did you learn it was okay to make comments like that?" Four is to educate or inform the other person in some way: "I'm sure you didn't realize, but comments like that lead to eating disorders and other fatal mental health issues." And the last way to respond is to just set a boundary, with something like "please don't say that kind of thing to me." Here are a bunch more examples of each:

BEING VULNERABLE.

- "Wow, that comment makes me *so* uncomfortable."
- "Ouch."
- "I have severe body image issues, and comments like that sometimes take weeks to get past."
- "Are you trying to hurt my feelings?"
- "I don't like it when you say things like that."
- "Lately I've been learning about how damaging comments like that are to my mental health, do you think it would be possible to refrain from making them?"

BEING DIRECT.

- "What a rude comment."
- "That kind of joke is harmful."
- "Nobody likes unsolicited advice."
- "Would you feel comfortable if I criticized *your* body?"
- "That was a shitty thing to say."

- "Thank you, but a person's health is between them and their doctor."

- "That's a *very* weird thing to volunteer out of nowhere."

- "I think you and I have very different ideas about how I should look."

- "I wasn't asking for, nor am I interested in, your opinion on my appearance."

- If they offer unsolicited advice: "No, I don't think I will," or "I disagree."

CHALLENGE.

- "Does it bother you at all to know you're making people uncomfortable with comments like that?"

- "How do you know I don't have an eating disorder?"

- "Actually I'm good with how I look, but it sounds like *you* have some food or body image issues you need to deal with."

- "Are you aware that comments like that uphold sexist and racist beauty ideals?"

- "You have such an old-school approach to bodies . . . nobody thinks that stuff anymore."

- With a bit more snark, but along the same lines, a self-identified southern belle once told me she responded with: "bless your heart, for not caring if you hurt people's feelings."

- And you can always confuse people with responses like "why would I do that when I love how I look?" or "but I'm *already* at my goal weight!" (Note: these are valid responses even when they're not true, because you don't owe your truth to people who are insulting your body.)

CHOOSING TO EDUCATE.

- "Did you know that eating disorders are the most deadly of all mental illnesses? Yeah, up to 20 percent of them end in death. And comments like that contribute to their developing."

- "Do you know how harmful that joke would be to someone with an eating disorder or body image issues?"

- "Thoughtless comments like that can put people in the hospital, just so you know."

- "Are you implying I would be more worthy of love and respect if I were thinner? If so, where do you think that belief came from?"

- "It sounds like you're playing into an essentialist view of gender, as well as conventional beauty ideals. Why do you think that feels so important to you?"

- "It sounds like you care a lot about people following certain rules when it comes to beauty and body ideals. What are you afraid would happen if someone broke them?"

SETTING A BOUNDARY.

- "Please don't make jokes like that around me."

- "Because I'm sure you wouldn't like people making rude comments like that to *you*, I ask that you not make them to *me*."

- "I've decided not to tolerate insults about how I look anymore. Will that be a problem for you?"

- "In order for this relationship to continue, I'm going to need you to stop commenting on my body."

> ▸ "I'm not okay with having my appearance criticized. If you continue to do so, I'll have to rethink how much time we spend together."

> ▸ "Actually I'm not available for unsolicited advice right now."

> ▸ "If we can't find something else to talk about, I probably won't stay very long."

> ▸ "I know you mean well, but I'm actually not interested in hearing your opinion on how I look."

I'm working to disconnect my appearance from my identity and self-worth, so I don't *really* want to hear other people's opinions on how I look, good or bad. How do I respond when someone *compliments* my body or appearance, though? Obviously, they mean well.

People make comments all the time that they *think* are compliments, but actually just reinforce and uphold sexist, racist, ableist, ageist, and anti-fat beauty and body ideals, like "oh my god you look *great*, have you lost weight?!" or gushing over how incredible a Black celebrity looks when she straightens and lightens her hair. These kinds of "compliments" are actually examples of something called a *microaggression*, which is a comment or action that indirectly, subtly, or unintentionally expresses discrimination or prejudice toward a member of a marginalized group. Microaggressions are harmful to folks in marginalized bodies (I once had a queer Black client describe them as "death by a thousand paper-cuts"), but they're also harmful to anyone practicing body neutrality.

So how do you respond? The above five strategies can still work: inviting the person into a more vulnerable conversation, being blunt or direct, challenging them, taking the opportunity to educate, or just setting a boundary. The only difference is that, because the person thinks they're complimenting you or being nice, you *might* want to respond with a softer or gentler touch. (Although you are absolutely not obligated to!) Here are some examples:

BEING VULNERABLE.

- "I love that you think I'm beautiful, but lately I've been trying to disentangle my appearance from my identity and sense of self-worth, so comments like that feel kind of confusing and uncomfortable to me."

- "You know, I used to love comments like that because they made me feel temporarily confident about how I looked. But then I discovered they actually made me feel worse about myself overall, because they reinforce the feeling that people only value me for my looks."

- "When you say things like that, I feel like the only nice things you can think of to say to me are about how I look. I know it's not intentional, but it makes me feel like you don't actually see or value me as a person."

- "When people compliment my appearance, I feel objectified."

BEING DIRECT.

- "Compliments like that aren't really compliments, because they uphold sexist, racist, and fatphobic beauty ideals."

- "I'm actually not interested in whether or not people find me attractive or think I look good."

- "I don't consider comments like that to be compliments. After all, if we don't want 'fat' to be an insult, then we can't consider 'thin' to be a compliment."

- "I prefer not to be complimented in ways that cause harm to other people."

▸ "Giving someone your unsolicited opinion of their appearance is a form of objectification."

CHALLENGING.

▸ "What makes you think I care whether or not you approve of my appearance?"

▸ "Why do you think you compliment my appearance so often, but never my intelligence, sense of humor, kindness, courage, or passion?"

▸ "I'm so tired of talking about appearances, can't we compliment each other on something more meaningful?"

▸ "What makes you think I consider it a compliment to say that my body is smaller?"

▸ "Talking about how people look is so boring, can we go a bit deeper?"

▸ "If you're interested in me, it had better be for something more interesting or important than how I look."

▸ Disarm someone who compliments your appearance by responding with something like "yes, I know," or "I agree," or "you're right." This is jarring because we're *supposed to* respond with gratitude, disagreement, or self-deprecation (especially women), and will force the commenter to think about what just happened.

EDUCATING.

▸ "Have you ever noticed you have a habit of complimenting my appearance every time we see each other? Why do you think that is?"

- "Men seem to feel like it's okay to tell a woman when he finds her attractive, but more often than not it's actually just sexist, objectifying, and creepy."

- "Recently I discovered that when I have the urge to compliment someone's appearance, there's actually something truer and more vulnerable underneath that I'm shying away from saying, like how I might tell someone they look amazing when I actually just want to tell them how *happy* it makes me to see their face again. Do you think you do the same thing?"

- "You know, seemingly positive compliments like that actually send a pretty dark message."

SETTING A BOUNDARY.

- "This might sound strange to you, but I have a no-compliments-on-my-appearance policy. Is that something you can honor?"

- "I can tell you're just trying to be nice, but I actually don't want to hear *any* comments on my appearance anymore, even if they're positive ones."

- "Thank you, I know you meant that in a kind way. But I've been learning more about how compliments on my appearance aren't very good for my mental health or body image issues. Would you be willing to try finding other ways to compliment me?"

- "I'd prefer if you found something to comment on *other than* my appearance, please."

- "If you want to talk to me, please keep your thoughts about how I look to yourself."

How do I respond when someone comments on my *weight* (either good or bad)?

Everything already stated above still applies when responding to these kinds of comments, but I also want to offer some more specific responses.

Here are some examples for how to handle *negative* comments, criticisms, or unsolicited advice about your weight:

- "What makes you think I consider weight gain to be a bad thing?"

- "Thank you! I *love* having a bigger body!" (Or "I actually feel most beautiful when I gain weight." Again, this doesn't have to be true to use it. It's just a way of flipping the expected power dynamic, and you don't owe your truth to people insulting you.)

- "You know, when I was in a smaller body, I was unhealthy and miserable. But you didn't seem to worry about my health or happiness then. Why do you think that is?"

- "The assumption that smaller bodies are healthier than bigger bodies is actually a false bias that causes a lot of harm to people in larger bodies. It's called weight stigma, and if you want to learn more, I can send you an article."

- "It's very rude to comment on someone's weight."

- "What on earth makes you think you're qualified to comment on my health, diet, or body size?"

- "Are you aware that over 95 percent of intentional weight loss attempts fail, and over half of them lead to more weight gain in the end? Would you go around and give the unsolicited advice to cancer patients that they should try a treatment with only a 5 percent success rate, and a more than 50 percent chance it'll make them worse?"

- ◆ "Comments like that are why so many people have eating disorders and body image issues."
- ◆ "Wow, it sounds like you have some seriously fatphobic beliefs you might want to consider exploring."
- ◆ "Please don't comment on the size of my body."
- ◆ "My body size isn't any of your business."

And here are some examples for how to respond to seemingly *positive* comments about your weight (usually praising weight loss):

- ◆ "Thanks, I have an eating disorder." (Or "thanks, I have a chronic disease that causes me to lose weight," "thanks, I lose weight when I'm depressed," or "thanks, my medications keep me from being able to maintain a healthy weight." True or untrue, responding this way makes the commenter hold the full awkwardness of what they've done.)
- ◆ "So you didn't think I looked good before?"
- ◆ "What makes you think I consider weight loss a good thing?"
- ◆ "Now that you've said that, how do you think I'll feel around you if I gain weight again?"
- ◆ "Compliments like that make it clear how you feel about people in bigger bodies."
- ◆ "I don't consider weight loss a compliment."
- ◆ "I don't consider thinness an achievement."
- ◆ "What makes you assume I lost weight in a healthy way?"
- ◆ "Where do you think you learned to associate thinness with health and happiness?"
- ◆ "I feel like you're making a *lot* of assumptions about me based on my body size. Can we talk about what you're assuming, and what's actually true instead?"
- ◆ "Comments like that are fatphobic and harmful to everyone."

> ◆ "I'm actually not interested in hearing what people think about my body size."

I've recently become aware of how anti-fat bias is false, dangerous, and _everywhere_. What should I say when I hear comments that uphold thin privilege and fat oppression? I want to make people more aware, but I don't want to be rude.

It's very common to hear people making comments on their own (or a third party's) body that contribute to weight stigma. This can include people talking about their new diet plan, weight loss, or how they "need to lose weight," as well as making fat jokes, offering unsolicited weight loss advice to another person, or just associating fat bodies with laziness, lack of health, unintelligence, or unattractiveness. In such situations, you can still respond with the above five categories I mentioned earlier (be vulnerable, be direct, challenge, educate, or set a boundary), but it's also worth considering who is being harmed in this situation, and what it would look like to stand on the side of justice for them.

For example, if your grandma is constantly criticizing your cousin for being fat, and you're _not_ fat, your body size might position you to have a bigger impact on Grandma's beliefs and behavior than your cousin ever could. Stepping in might look like setting a boundary on your cousin's behalf, like saying, "Hey, Grandma, it's very rude to talk about people's weight, can you please find something else to talk about?," _or_ it might look like inviting Grandma into an ongoing transformative dialogue about her beliefs and behaviors, as mentioned in the first question.

You might not always (or ever) have the resources available to stand up for justice in this way every time, and some situations just aren't worth investing that labor into. That's valid, and folks in marginalized bodies _especially_ do not owe the world this kind of labor. But personally, for folks with a lot of body privilege, I consider it to be something of a responsibility to use that privilege to protect people with less privilege, and fight for justice. And because the most effective way to get people inside our circle of influence to change their minds is to challenge them from a place of love and respect, expose them to new ideas and information, be patient, and show up for ongoing and hard conversations, that might be where you want to invest your energy.

If this applies to you, try using a seed-planting conversation opener like I described in the first question, and invite the person to engage on the topic of weight and body size with as much curiosity and as little judgment as possible. Here are a few examples:

+ "I notice you make a lot of negative comments on your body size. Do you want to share any more about your relationship to your body?"

+ "I know you're a very kindhearted person and would never hurt anyone on purpose. That's why it's so weird to me when you talk about people's weight. That kind of anti-fat bias just doesn't seem in alignment with your values." (I love this one, because it holds the person accountable to *their own values*, rather than trying to push a new value onto them.)

+ "I know you're an incredibly accepting and open-minded person, which is why I feel safe coming to you with a concern I have. I've noticed you comment on people's weight in some ways that seem inappropriate or even harmful. Would you be open to talking to me about that?"

+ "You're such an intelligent and deep person, so it's strange to hear you place such an emphasis on people's body size. Why do you think that might be?"

+ "Have you ever heard of the term 'weight stigma'? It's something I've been learning a lot about lately, and I think you in particular might find it interesting."

+ "Comments like that always strike me as kind of weird, because it implies a person is automatically harder working, healthier, and happier in a thinner body. But that's not always the case, right? Where do you think *you* learned that kind of thing?"

♦ "When you talk about your diet, or how much you want to lose weight, I feel a bit uncomfortable, because you're placing such a high value on thinness and how you look in general. And if you feel that about yourself, how must you feel about *me*?" (Especially useful if the person talking about their own weight loss is smaller than you.)

♦ "I hear you make such negative comments about your body, and I worry about you. You deserve better than a life spent beating yourself up and trying to lose weight. Have you ever thought about getting support for your body image issues?"

♦ "You know, I used to make comments like that, too, back when I felt the worst about my *own* body size. If there's ever anything you want to talk to me about when it comes to body image stuff, I'm here to listen."

Of course, you'll also hear weight stigma being upheld outside your circle of influence, too, like if a stranger on the street calls out, "Lose weight, fatty!" to another stranger, meeting a new person at a party who is talking about how badly they need to go on a diet, or hearing the woman next to you in the coffee shop fat-shaming her daughter. In these moments, consider who is being harmed, and what it would look like to be an ally to them, protect them, or stand up for justice on their behalf. This will be different in every situation, of course. If you see a fat-shaming billboard, you might call your local representative to get it taken down. If your neighbor complains about how fat his kids are, you might offer him a simple resource on weight stigma that you "just think he might find interesting." If a friend of a friend makes a fat joke, you might respond with "I didn't think that joke was very funny" or inform your friend about the incident. If your boss is considering an office-wide weight loss challenge, you might speak up about how harmful that is, gather a bunch of signatures to stop it, or submit a complaint to HR. And if you see a fat person being harassed in public, you might ask whether they're okay, find out if they want any company or help, report it to management, or even confront the harasser.

There is no one right answer here, and sometimes it won't even be appropriate, available, or safe to respond. So you'll have to feel out each situation individually, and choose to invest your time, energy, and labor into dismantling body oppression wherever (and however) you feel is best for you.

I know I'm not supposed to compliment people on their appearance, because it reinforces the idea that their appearance matters, but what should I say instead? Sometimes people want to be complimented like that!

Such a great question! My biggest piece of advice when it comes to giving compliments is to focus on sharing *impact* rather than sharing *opinion*.

Far too many compliments are an expression of the person's opinion as if it were *fact*. These compliments tend to involve some kind of hierarchical ranking system of assessment and often objectify the other person. Opinion-sharing compliments generally sound like this:

- You look amazing.
- I think you're beautiful.
- You're so sexy.
- You look incredible since you lost weight.
- Your butt looks great in that.
- You're the hottest person in the room.
- I love your body in that outfit.
- You have amazing eyes.

Each of these "compliments" functions to remind the receiver that their appearance has just been (and is constantly being) ranked and assessed. This reinforces and upholds some false and dangerous ideas: their body exists to be enjoyed or consumed by others, they owe other people a pleasant experience of looking at them, other people's opinions on their appearance should matter to them, and how they look is intrinsically linked to their value and worth as a person. While opinion-sharing compliments are very common, they have the potential to cause harm, and they don't usually have much of an effect on the person being complimented, because an opinion can always just be disagreed with. (Which explains why so many compliments seem to just bounce right off folks struggling with body image issues—someone says, "You're beautiful," and your mind just immediately says, "Nope, they're wrong.")

In an *impact-sharing* compliment, you let the person know *how their presence affects you*. There is no opinion involved with this (because you're just sharing your personal experience), so the person can't really disagree. This causes the compliment to feel more true and meaningful and to have a bigger impact on the person being complimented. Here are some impact-sharing compliments you can use to replace opinion-sharing compliments on a person's appearance:

+ I'm so happy to see you!
+ I've missed your face so much.
+ I want you.
+ Your whole vibe right now feels like happiness to me.
+ Getting to be near you is making me so happy right now.
+ Knowing someone like you desires me makes me feel incredible.
+ I could stare into your eyes forever.
+ Seeing you is making me feel giddy!
+ I'm so into you.

- Being around you feels like sunlight.

- Everything about you is turning me on right now.

- Seeing how you express yourself through clothes always brings me joy.

Of course, you can also go even deeper, and share ways in which you're affected by their *internal* qualities and characteristics, or how they show up in relationship with you. This gets you ever further away from their appearance and affirms who they are as a whole person. Here are some ideas:

- I love the way you show up for me.

- Your thoughtfulness makes me feel so cared for.

- I think I'm a better version of myself after hanging out with you.

- Your playfulness has encouraged me to take life less seriously.

- My life is better because you're in it.

- I feel so lucky that I have you to bounce ideas around with.

- Your passion inspires me.

- The way you think turns me on.

- Joking around and laughing with you always makes me feel so much better.

- Your willingness to be vulnerable has made me feel safe enough to do the same.

As far as how you want to handle it when someone is *fishing* for a compliment on their appearance, it's up to you. If you're in the habit of regularly complimenting a specific friend or partner's appearance, you might want to let them know in advance that you're trying to stop, and ask them what other kinds of compliments would feel good. And if someone clearly wants to be praised for their weight loss efforts, you might find a way to comment instead on an internal quality that led to it, like "I'm so impressed with the way you've been putting yourself first lately," or "it makes me so happy to see you be proud of yourself." Personally, I also like to deepen the conversation in these moments by asking questions like "what story are you telling yourself about this weight loss?" or "what meaning are you attaching to having a smaller body?"

Lastly, I just want to encourage you to be gentle with yourself as you try to break the habit of commenting on or complimenting people's appearance. It can be difficult at first, but it gets easier with practice. Even now, for example, I still sometimes have to bite my tongue to not comment on how my little siblings look. Why? Two reasons. One is that they're five and seven, so their faces and bodies are constantly growing and changing, and my brain finds that process notable and interesting. The other is that *they're the cutest little goblins on the planet and I just freak out with pleasure whenever I see their perfect little faces.* I don't judge myself for having the impulse to blurt this stuff out, but I do consciously choose not to. They'll hear that stuff from other people anyway, and *I'd* rather they feel seen and valued by me for *who they are as people*, so I focus on sharing impact and affirming internal qualities instead.

I'm working to be weight and body neutral for my mental health, but I also want to take care of my physical health. Is it possible to do both?

Oh my goodness, *absolutely.* In my experience, body neutrality actually makes it a lot easier to be healthy, because you're not attaching moral judgment or false meaning to your body's signals (or to your own behaviors), and you're not getting derailed by subconscious coping strategies. Plus, it's also a lot easier to take care of yourself when you believe you deserve to be healthy and feel good.

The key is improving your health while practicing body neutrality to focus on the health-promoting *behaviors* rather than your weight or appearance. For example, you might decide to eat more nutrient-dense foods to improve your health. And that's great, but it has nothing whatsoever to do with your weight. Eating more nutrient-dense foods could possibly lead to weight gain *or* weight loss (or no weight change at all!), but none of that is relevant to the goal of improving your health. No matter what happens to your weight, eating more nutrient-dense foods *will* have a positive impact on your health.

Likewise, you might decide to exercise, meditate, drink more water, stretch, quit smoking, or work on your balance, to improve your health. Each of these health-promoting behaviors is likely to make you healthier, so whether or not they impact your weight is irrelevant. Being thinner doesn't automatically mean being healthier, but implementing more health-promoting behaviors *does*. So there's no reason to consider weight at *all* when trying to get healthier. (Plus, focusing on weight loss has a *negative* impact on a person's health outcomes overall—read the book *Anti-Diet* by Christy Harrison to learn more about why that is.)

Without weight standing in as a (false) symbol of health success, you'll have to pay attention to *more important and accurate* ways of measuring health outcomes. You'll know your new behaviors are having a positive impact on your health, for example, if you find yourself sleeping better, feeling less stressed, experiencing less pain, feeling more energized, noticing an increase in libido, seeing an improvement in your digestion, or finding yourself in a better mood more often. And if you want even *more* feedback about your progress, get a checkup with a doctor before starting or test your resting heart rate—then check back in with *those* bits of data. You'll know your health is improving if your blood pressure or cholesterol improve, you're more insulin sensitive, or you have a lower resting heart rate.

That said, if you've spent a long time with a disordered relationship to food, exercise, or your body, you may need to take a fairly significant amount of time putting your mental and emotional health first, even if that means hitting pause on various health-promoting behaviors for a while. I know it seems counterintuitive, but it's something I see play out for the majority of my clients, and it's all part of a long-term strategy for overall better health. (Bear in mind that chronic stress has an explicitly negative impact on physical health . . . and that includes the stress and distress of food and body image issues.)

The truth is that it's often impossible to heal your relationship with your body while *also* engaging in the same "healthy habits" you used to do from a place of shame, anxiety, insecurity, or self-loathing. While learning to eat and exercise intuitively, for example, most people can't *also* be following a restrictive diet or structured exercise plan.

So while body neutrality is super compatible with a desire to get healthy, I encourage you to consider how you're defining "physical health," and to keep a long-term mindset. For example, the best thing many people can do for their physical health is to stop exercising for a year or two while they rewire their brain to believe they're worthy and deserving of good things, no matter what size their body is, how fit they are, and whether or not they've "earned" it. Even though exercise is "healthy," and even if they miss it terribly when they stop, taking a break from exercise is sometimes the only way for a person to face and heal the underlying stuff that exercise has been hiding, disguising, or repressing. Don't misunderstand me though, the end goal isn't for everyone to get rid of exercise for good, and this strategy isn't in the best interest of everyone's long term health. (Be sure to check with yourself and your doctor before making changes to your exercise routine!) I'm just sharing this as an example of how focusing on long-term health can sometimes require seemingly "unhealthy" choices in the short-term. Plus, the purpose of taking a break from exercise is to strip away the false or excess meaning and significance a person has been assigning to exercise, so that they can access something we might call "exercise neutrality." After that, they can move however they like!

The same goes with eating. People who have spent many years dieting and assigning labels like "good" and "bad" to different foods or eating behaviors often need to go through a significant period of eating all the foods they'd been restricting, and breaking all their eating rules. (You can learn more about this process through the books *The F*ck It*

Diet by Caroline Dooner, *Anti-Diet* by Christy Harrison, and *Intuitive Eating* by Elyse Resch and Evelyn Tribole.) Just like with the exercise example above, this process may seem "physically unhealthy" to someone focused on the short-term health effects of nutrition, but this is about holistic health in the long-term. (That said, this strategy can be unhealthy or even dangerous for some people in both the short- and long-term, so again, be sure to check with yourself and your doctor before making any dietary changes!) This is just another example of how your perception of what's "healthy" and "unhealthy" tends to change, whether you're detail-focused, or thinking big picture.

Health is more subjective and context-dependent than people realize! A dry salad might seem healthier than a cheeseburger, for example, if you're focused on minimizing calories or maximizing fiber or hydration, but a cheeseburger might be the healthier option if it's the only meal you'll get to eat today, you're low in iron, or you only want the salad because eating a burger sends you into a panic-and-shame spiral. A free-for-all phase around food helps a lot of people strip away the false or excess meaning, significance, and morality they've been assigning to food and eating, and teaches their brain and body to feel safe and secure around food again, which ultimately reduces stress, and improves their health. Admittedly, some people do feel like crap physically while they go through this phase—eating Pop-Tarts every day can do that—but with time and practice, this strategy helps a lot of people break free, psychologically and physiologically, from the inappropriate amount of power that food and eating have over them, *forever*.

Why do you call people "fat"? It feels rude, or like an insult. Why don't you say "obese" or "overweight"?

I use the word "fat" because it's descriptive, and because it's the term most often used by the fat justice and liberation communities. (Check out the book *The Other F Word*, edited by Angie Manfredi, to learn more.) If an individual prefers a different term, I'll use their preferred term with them, of course. But when speaking to a broad audience, I try to use the language that is *most* representative of how fat people want to be identified. Many fat communities have reclaimed the word "fat" as a neutral (or even friendly!) descriptor for their bodies, rather than an insult, kind of like how LGBTQIA+ folks have reclaimed the word "queer." And because I'm all about stripping away false significance and power from concepts and language, I'm especially here for it. In my view, using the word as a neutral descriptor promotes body size and weight neutrality.

And as far as person-first language goes, I do say things like "folks in larger bodies," or "individuals living in a marginalized body," and I recognize some people vastly prefer this to "fat." But I can't make everyone happy, and "fat" seems to currently be the best word for it.

As for why I don't use the words "obese" and "overweight," that's simple. Those terms have roots in, and associations with, the scientifically inaccurate—not to mention wildly oppressive and violent—system of categorizing people's body size called the body mass index.

BMI uses a person's height divided by their weight to categorize their weight into labels like "underweight," "healthy weight," "overweight," and "obese," as a way of supposedly determining their risk for certain diseases. I want to position myself as far away from it as possible for the following reasons:

- **It's inappropriate.** BMI was created in the 1830s by a mathematician (with no medical training or interest) to measure population, not individuals. The creator himself even said it was never intended to measure the fatness of any given individual, and it certainly wasn't intended to measure anything about an individual's health!

- **It's inaccurate.** BMI doesn't account for different factors like race, ethnicity, age, gender, body shape, body density, or muscle mass. This means whole demographics end up regularly miscategorized (like how lean and muscular folks get categorized as "overweight" or "obese") and that BMI is an entirely inaccurate way of determining an individual's health risks.

- **It's racist.** BMI was based exclusively on French and Scottish participants, which means it's absurdly inaccurate to use for non-European white folks, *and* it continues to uphold the racism and white supremacy of two hundred years ago.

- **It's arbitrary.** In 1998, the National Institutes of Health arbitrarily lowered the threshold for the categories, suddenly making millions of Americans "overweight" or "obese" overnight. The only people who benefited from this alteration were the pharmaceutical, medical, and weight loss industries.

- **It's dangerous.** BMI encourages weight stigma, and weight stigma causes many doctors to treat their fat patients with less respect and empathy, leading to less thorough testing, more inaccurate diagnoses and medical neglect, and higher fatalities. Plus, being exposed to weight stigma has a negative impact on the health outcomes and life expectancy for people in bigger bodies in general. So using BMI in medical settings isn't just ignorant, pointless, and outdated—it's also outright harmful, bigoted, violent, and dangerous.

Check out the books *Fearing the Black Body* by Sabrina Strings or *Anti-Diet* by Christy Harrison to learn more about BMI.

Notes

CHAPTER 2: Body Positivity

1. Elizabeth Gulino, "Body Positivity Doesn't Mean What You Think It Does," *Refinery29*, updated March 25, 2021, 9:42 a.m., refinery29.com/en-us/2021/03/10370504/body-positivity-neutrality-movement-history.

2. Shayahi Nathan, "Beauty and the Biased: How Algorithms Perpetuate Body Dysmorphia," Medusa, October 9, 2020, medusacreatives.com/2020/10/09/beauty-and-the-biased-how-algorithms-perpetuate-body-dysmorphia.

3. Charlotte Betts, "Perceptions of the Self: How Social Media Leads to Body Dissatisfaction," Medium, July 28, 2020, medium.com/@charlotteebetts/perceptions-of-the-self-how-social-media-leads-to-body-dissatisfaction-7ce918be978. See also Nealie Tan Ngo, "What Historical Ideals of Women's Shapes Teach Us About Women's Self-Perception and Body Decisions Today," *AMA Journal of Ethics* 21, no. 10 (October 2019): E879–901, doi.org/10.1001/amajethics.2019.879.

4. Roberto A. Ferdman, "Why Diets Don't Actually Work, According to a Researcher Who Has Studied Them for Decades," *Washington Post*, May 4, 2015, washingtonpost.com/news/wonk/wp/2015/05/04/why-diets-dont-actually-work-according-to-a-researcher-who-has-studied-them-for-decades; Traci Mann, *Secrets from the Eating Lab: The Science of Weight Loss, the Myth of Willpower, and Why You Should Never Diet Again* (New York: Harper Wave, 2015).

5. Nick Trefethen, letter to *The Economist*, January 5, 2013, people.maths.ox.ac.uk/trefethen/bmi.html; Christian Nordqvist, "Why BMI Is Inaccurate and Misleading," *Medical News Today*, updated January 19, 2022, medicalnewstoday.com/articles/265215; and Adele Jackson-Gibson, "The Racist and Problematic History of the Body Mass Index," *Good Housekeeping*, February

23, 2021, goodhousekeeping.com/health/diet-nutrition/a35047103/bmi-racist -history.

6. Lindsay Kite, "Body Positivity or Body Obsession? Learning to See More and Be More," filmed September 9, 2017, at TEDxSaltLakeCity, TED video, 16:47, November 6, 2017, ted.com/talks/lindsay_kite_body_positivity_or _body_obsession_learning_to_see_more_and_be_more. See also Lindsay Kite and Lexie Kite, *More Than a Body: Your Body Is an Instrument, Not an Ornament* (Boston: Houghton Mifflin Harcourt, 2020).

7. Jon Greenberg, "10 Examples That Prove White Privilege Protects White People in Every Aspect Imaginable," Everyday Feminism, November 26, 2015, everydayfeminism.com/2015/11/lessons-white-privilege-poc; and "White Men See White Privilege More Clearly If They Have Experienced Social Disadvantages," Duke University's Fuqua School of Business, February 21, 2022, fuqua.duke.edu/duke-fuqua-insights/ashleigh-shelby-rosette -white-men-see-white-privilege-more-clearly-if-they-have.

8. Amanda Mull, "Americans Can't Escape Long-Disproven Body Stereotypes," *The Atlantic*, November 6, 2018, theatlantic.com/health/archive /2018/11/body-stereotypes-personality-debunked-eugenics/575041.

9. Sarah Parker Harris, Rob Gould, and Courtney Mullin, "Experience of Discrimination and the ADA," ADA National Network Knowledge Translation Center, 2019, adata.org/research_brief/experience-discrimination -and-ada; Rebecca M. Puhl and Chelsea A. Heuer, "The Stigma of Obesity: A Review and Update," *Obesity* 17, no. 5 (2009): 941–964, https://www.doi .org/10.1038/oby.2008.636; and Adele Jackson-Gibson, "What Is Thin Privilege?," *Good Housekeeping*, April 15, 2021, goodhousekeeping.com /health/diet-nutrition/a35047908/what-is-thin-privilege.

10. Williams Institute at UCLA School of Law, "Transgender People over Four Times More Likely Than Cisgender People to Be Victims of Violent Crime," March 23, 2021, williamsinstitute.law.ucla.edu/press/ncvs-trans -press-release. Note that the data came from the 2017 and 2018 National Crime Victimization Survey, the first comprehensive and nationally representative criminal victimization data to include information on the gender identity and sex assigned at birth of respondents.

11. Susan Green, "Violence against Black Women—Many Types, Far-Reaching Effects," Institute for Women's Policy Research, July 13, 2017, iwpr.org /iwpr-issues/race-ethnicity-gender-and-economy/violence-against-black -women-many-types-far-reaching-effects; Asha DuMonthier, Chandra Childers, and Jessica Milli, executive summary, "The Status of Black Women in the United States," Institute for Women's Policy Research, June 7, 2017, iwpr.org/iwpr-issues/race-ethnicity-gender-and-economy/the-status -of-black-women-in-the-united-states.

12. University of Alberta, "Perception: Skinny People Aren't Lazy but Overweight People Are," *Science Daily*, April 22, 2010, www.sciencedaily.com /releases/2010/04/100420152839.htm.

13. Christine Hope, "Caucasian Female Body Hair and American Culture," *Journal of American Culture* 5, no. 1 (Spring 1982): 93–99, doi.org/10.1111/j.1542-734X.1982.0501_93.x; Phil Edwards, "How the Beauty Industry Convinced Women to Shave Their Legs," *Vox*, May 22, 2015, vox.com/2015/5/22/8640457/leg-shaving-history.

14. Ngo, "What Historical Ideals of Women's Shapes Teach Us."

CHAPTER 3: What *Is* Body Neutrality?

1. *Encyclopedia Britannica Online*, s.v. "Four Noble Truths," by Donald S. Lopez, accessed April 20, 2022, https://www.britannica.com/topic/Four-Noble-Truths.

2. Bessel van der Kolk, *The Body Keeps the Score: Brain, Mind, and Body in the Healing of Trauma* (New York: Viking, 2014), 210–11; Jon Kabat-Zinn, *Full Catastrophe Living: Using the Wisdom of Your Body and Mind to Face Stress, Pain, and Illness* (New York: Dell, 1990).

3. Van der Kolk, *The Body Keeps the Score*.

4. Anne Hollander, "When Fat Was in Fashion," *New York Times*, October 23, 1977, nytimes.com/1977/10/23/archives/when-fat-was-in-fashion-abundant-flesh-was-a-thing-of-beauty-to.html.

5. Katelyn Burns, "The Internet Made Trans People Visible. It Also Left Them More Vulnerable," *Vox*, December 27, 2019, vox.com/identities/2019/12/27/21028342/trans-visibility-backlash-internet-2010.

CHAPTER 4: The One Big, Crucial Lie

1. Kendra Cherry, "How Confirmation Bias Works," Verywell Mind, updated July 30, 2021, verywellmind.com/what-is-a-confirmation-bias-2795024.

2. Terry Marks-Tarlow, "I Am an Avatar of Myself: Fantasy, Trauma, and Self-Deception," *American Journal of Play* 9, no. 2 (Winter 2017): 189, files.eric.ed.gov/fulltext/EJ1141578.pdf.

CHAPTER 5: Why Am I Lying to Myself?

1. Terry Marks-Tarlow, "I Am an Avatar of Myself: Fantasy, Trauma, and Self-Deception," *American Journal of Play* 9, no. 2 (Winter 2017): 190–95.

2. Lindsay Kite, "Body Positivity or Body Obsession? Learning to See More and Be More," filmed September 9, 2017, at TEDxSaltLakeCity, TED video, 16:47, November 6, 2017, ted.com/talks/lindsay_kite_body_positivity_or_body_obsession_learning_to_see_more_and_be_more. See also Lindsay Kite and Lexie Kite, *More Than a Body: Your Body Is an Instrument, Not an Ornament* (Boston: Houghton Mifflin Harcourt, 2020).

CHAPTER 8: The Self-Objectifier

1. Tanjare' McKay, "Female Self-Objectification: Causes, Consequences and Prevention," *McNair Scholars Research Journal* 6, no. 7 (2013): commons .emich.edu/cgi/viewcontent.cgi?article=1065&context=mcnair.

2. Lindsay Kite and Lexie Kite, *More Than a Body: Your Body Is an Instrument, Not an Ornament* (Boston: Houghton Mifflin Harcourt, 2020), 3.

3. Evangelia (Lina) Papadaki, "Feminist Perspectives on Objectification," Stanford Encyclopedia of Philosophy, December 16, 2019, plato.stanford .edu/entries/feminism-objectification.

4. Papadaki, "Feminist Perspectives on Objectification."

5. Liliana Almeida, "What Is Body Checking?," Verywell Mind, updated March 22, 2022, verywellmind.com/reduce-body-checking-with-two-easy -steps-1138366.

6. Paul D. Trapnell, Cindy M. Meston, and Boris B. Gorzalka, "Spectatoring and the Relationship between Body Image and Sexual Experience: Self-Focus or Self-Valence?," *Journal of Sex Research* 34, no. 3 (Summer 1997): 267–78, doi.org/10.1080/00224499709551893.

7. Emily Nagoski, "What Does 'Spectatoring' Mean When Referring to Sex?," Sharecare, accessed May 10, 2022, sharecare.com/health/erectile -dysfunction-causes/what-spectatoring-mean-sex. See also Emily Nagoski, *The Good in Bed Guide to Female Orgasms* (Good in Bed Guides, 2011), https://b-ok.cc/book/783203/20704e; and Emily Nagoski, *Come as You Are: Revised and Updated: The Surprising New Science That Will Transform Your Sex Life* (New York: Simon & Schuster, 2021), 249.

8. Stephanie Pappas, "Our Brains See Men as Whole and Women as Parts," *Scientific American*, July 25, 2012, scientificamerican.com/article/our-brains -see-men-as-whole-as-women-as-parts.

9. Valerie Curtis, Mícheál de Barra, and Robert Aunger, "Disgust as an Adaptive System for Disease Avoidance Behaviour," *Philosophical Transactions of the Royal Society B* 366, no. 1563 (2011): 389–401, doi.org/10.1098/rstb.2010.0117.

10. Tom W. Smith, "Public Attitudes toward Homosexuality," NORC/University of Chicago, September 2011, www.norc.org/PDFs/2011%20GSS %20Reports/GSS_Public%20Attitudes%20Toward%20Homosexuality _Sept2011.pdf.

11. "Moral Stance towards Gay or Lesbian Relations in the United States 2021," Statista Research Department, August 12, 2021, statista.com/statis tics/225968/americans-moral-stance-towards-gay-or-lesbian-relations.

12. Charlie Kurth, "Disgust Can Be Morally Valuable," *Scientific American*, May 9, 2021, scientificamerican.com/article/disgust-can-be-morally-valuable.

13. Peter J. de Jong, Mark van Overveld, and Charmaine Borg, "Giving In to Arousal or Staying Stuck in Disgust? Disgust-Based Mechanisms in Sex and Sexual Dysfunction," in "Annual Review of Sex Research," ed. Jacques van Lankveld, special issue, *Journal of Sex Research* 50, nos. 3–4 (March 12,

2013): 247–62, doi.org/10.1080/00224499.2012.746280; and Diana S. Fleischman et al. "Disgust versus Lust: Exploring the Interactions of Disgust and Fear with Sexual Arousal in Women," *PloS One* 10, no. 6 (June 24, 2015): e0118151, doi.org/10.1371/journal.pone.0118151. See also Debra Lieberman and Carlton Patrick, *Objection: Disgust, Morality, and the Law* (Oxford: Oxford University Press, 2018).

14. Christy Harrison, *Anti-Diet: Reclaim Your Time, Money, Well-Being, and Happiness through Intuitive Eating* (New York: Little, Brown Spark, 2019).

15. Marissa E. Wagner Oehlhof et al., "Self-Objectification and Ideal Body Shape for Men and Women," *Body Image* 6, no. 4 (September 2009): 308–10, doi.org/10.1016/j.bodyim.2009.05.002.

16. Sarah Vanbuskirk, "What Is the Male Gaze?," Verywell Mind, updated September 11, 2021, verywellmind.com/what-is-the-male-gaze-5118422; and Pappas, "Our Brains See Men as Whole and Women as Parts."

17. Shawn Meghan Burn, "The Psychology of Sexual Harassment," *Teaching of Psychology* 46, no. 1 (January 2019), doi.org/10.1177/0098628318816183; Vanbuskirk, "What Is the Male Gaze?"; Sharon G. Smith et al., *The National Intimate Partner and Sexual Violence Survey: 2010–2012 State Report* (Atlanta, GA: National Center for Injury Prevention and Control, Centers for Disease Control and Prevention, 2017); Lili Loofbourow, "The Female Price of Male Pleasure," *The Week*, January 25, 2018, https://theweek.com/articles/749978/female-price-male-pleasure; and "Domestic Violence," National Coalition against Domestic Violence, 2020, assets.speakcdn.com/assets/2497/domestic_violence-2020080709350855.pdf?159681107999.

18. Julian Real, "'Unpacking the Male Privilege Jockstrap': The 100 Male Privileges Checklist," *A Radical Profeminist* (blog), December 1, 2009, radicalprofeminist.blogspot.com/2009/12/100-male-privileges-checklist.html; Barry Deutsch (items 1–42), *Expository Magazine* 2, no. 2 (October 2, 2008); Peggy McIntosh, "White Privilege: Unpacking the Invisible Knapsack," 1990.

19. Michelle R. Hebl, Eden B. King, and Jean Lin, "The Swimsuit Becomes Us All: Ethnicity, Gender, and Vulnerability to Self-Objectification," *Personality and Social Psychology Bulletin* 30, no. 10 (October 2004): 1322–31, doi.org/10.1177/0146167204264052.

20. Wsoemarg, "Do You Even Lift? Muscle Fetish and Masculinity," W. Soemargo (blog), May 4, 2016, soemargo.wordpress.com/2016/05/04/do-you-even-lift-muscle-fetish-and-masculinity.

21. Jonathan Rauch, "Short Guys Finish Last," Jonathan Rauch website, originally published in *The Economist*, December 23, 1995, jonathanrauch.com/jrauch_articles/height_discrimination_short_guys_finish_last; M. Dittmann, "Standing Tall Pays Off, Study Finds," *Monitor on Psychology* 35, no. 7 (July/August 2004): 14, apa.org/monitor/julaug04/standing; fem4him2please, "The Truth about Penis Size (A Woman's Perspective)," September 9, 2000, http://www.misterpoll.com/polls/5407/results.

22. Sean Jameson, "Does Size Matter? 91.7% of Women Say It Does [1,387 Woman Study]," Bad Girls Bible, April 5, 2022, badgirlsbible.com/does -size-matter; "Size Does Matter," accessed May 10, 2022, datavizproject .com/data-type/pictorial-stacked-chart/yes-penis-size-does-matter.

23. Jason Okundaye, "The Fetishisation of Black Masculinity," *GQ*, October 13, 2020, gq-magazine.co.uk/lifestyle/article/fetishisation-black-masculinity.

24. Eddie Kim, "The Myth of the Small Asian Cock," MEL, [2019] accessed April 24, 2022, melmagazine.com/en-us/story/the-myth-of-the-small-asian -cock; and "The Myth of an Asian Penis," *TheUNPUZZLED* (blog), July 20, 2020, https://medium.com/the-noodle-shop/the-myth-of-an-asian-penis -9af59d248e7c.

25. Janice Gassam Asare, "What Is Fetishization and How Does It Contribute to Racism?," *Forbes*, February 7, 2021, forbes.com/sites/janicegassam/2021/02 /07/what-is-fetishization-and-how-does-it-contribute-to-racism/?sh =47de4d866e39; Rachel Ramirez, "The History of Fetishizing Asian Women," *Vox*, March 19, 2021, vox.com/22338807/asian-fetish-racism-atlanta-shooting.

26. Beth Azar, "Oxytocin's Other Side," *Monitor on Psychology* 42, no. 3 (March 2011): 40, apa.org/monitor/2011/03/oxytocin.

27. Heather Jones, "What to Know about Anxious Attachment and Tips to Cope," Verywell Health, November 29, 2021, verywellhealth.com/anxious -attachment-5204408#toc-strategies-for-coping.

28. Rita Watson, "Oxytocin: The Love and Trust Hormone Can Be Deceptive," *Psychology Today*, October 14, 2013, psychologytoday.com/us/blog/love -and-gratitude/201310/oxytocin-the-love-and-trust-hormone -can-be-deceptive; Azar, "Oxytocin's Other Side," 40; Hallie Gould, "This Is What Happens to Your Brain When You Have Sex," TheThirty, February 2, 2022, thethirty.whowhatwear.com/what-happens-during-sex; and Marjan Khajehei and Elmira Behroozpour, "Endorphins, Oxytocin, Sexuality and Romantic Relationships: An Understudied Area," *World Journal of Obstetrics and Gynecology* 7, no. 2 (October 2018): 17–23, doi.org/10.5317/wjog.v7.i2.17.

29. Zawn Villines, "Sex, Lies, and Visual Stimulation: Debunking the Myths about Men," GoodTherapy, February 17, 2013, goodtherapy.org/blog/sex -lies-men-myths-0217137; and Kelly Gonsalves, "Men Aren't 'More Visual' or More Easily Turned On Than Women Are, Study Finds," mindbodygreen, July 15, 2019, mindbodygreen.com/articles/men-not-more-visual-or-easily -aroused-than-women-research-shows.

30. James Giles, *The Nature of Sexual Desire* (Westport, CT: Praeger, 2004); Nikolaos D. Kiskiras, "Sexual Desire(s) and the Desire for Intimacy: An Au-toethnographic Exploration" (PhD diss., Duquesne University, 2016), dsc .duq.edu/etd/99; and Ingrid Wickelgren, "Decoding Sexual Desire: Why You're into It—or Not," *Streams of Consciousness* (blog), *Scientific American*, October 11, 2011, blogs.scientificamerican.com/streams-of-consciousness /decoding-sexual-desire-why-youre-into-itor-not.

CHAPTER 9: The High Achiever

1. "Size Diversity & Health at Every Size," National Eating Disorders Association, accessed May 10, 2022, nationaleatingdisorders.org/size-diversity -health-every-size; and "Body Size Diversity and Acceptance," University of Illinois at Urbana-Champaign Counseling Center, 1999, accessed May 10, 2022, ndsu.edu/fileadmin/counseling/Body_Size_Diversity___Accep tance.pdf.

2. Tomas Chamorro-Premuzic, "Attractive People Get Unfair Advantages at Work. AI Can Help," *Harvard Business Review*, October 31, 2019, hbr.org /2019/10/attractive-people-get-unfair-advantages-at-work-ai-can-help; and Deborah L. Rhode, "Hooters Hires Based on Looks. So Do Many Companies. And There's No Law Against It," *New Republic*, August 30, 2014, new republic.com/article/118683/why-we-need-law-protect-against -appearance-discrimination.

3. Charlotte Ruhl, "Implicit or Unconscious Bias," *Simply Psychology*, July 1, 2020, simplypsychology.org/implicit-bias.html. See also Jennifer L. Eberhardt, *Biased: Uncovering the Hidden Prejudice That Shapes What We See, Think, and Do* (New York: Viking, 2019).

4. Benjamin Elisha Sawe, "What Is Moral Absolutism?," WorldAtlas, May 15, 2018, worldatlas.com/articles/what-is-moral-absolutism.html.

5. "What," Just World Fallacy, justworldfallacy.com/what. See also Melvin J. Lerner, *The Belief in a Just World: A Fundamental Delusion* (New York: Plenum Press, 1980).

6. Arash Javanbakht and Linda Saab, "What Happens in the Brain When We Feel Fear," *Smithsonian*, October 27, 2017, smithsonianmag.com/science -nature/what-happens-brain-feel-fear-180966992.

7. Emily Addison, "High Achievers and Mental Health: What Is the Link?," Everymind at Work, July 12, 2021, everymindatwork.com/high-achievers -and-mental-health.

8. Hilary Jane Grosskopf, "Pairs of Unlikely Compliments: Compassion and Competition," Medium, July 4, 2017, medium.com/awake-leadership -solutions/pairs-of-unlikely-compliments-compassion-and-competition -9997e77ff720.

9. William J. Burns, "The United States Needs a New Foreign Policy," Carnegie Endowment for International Peace, July 14, 2020, https://carnegieen dowment.org/2020/07/14/united-states-needs-new-foreign-policy -pub-82295.

10. "Size Diversity & Health at Every Size," National Eating Disorders Association; and "Body Size Diversity and Acceptance," University of Illinois at Urbana-Champaign Counseling Center.

11. Sirena Bergman, "Society Insists That Laziness Makes Us Fat—Now Science Proves This Is Baseless Bigotry," *Independent*, January 25, 2019, independent

.co.uk/voices/fat-overweight-dna-study-thin-people-women-tess-holliday
-donald-trump-a8746166.html.

12. York University, "When Does Clean Eating Become an Unhealthy Obsession?," ScienceDaily, May 14, 2019, sciencedaily.com/releases/2019/05/190
514115822.htm.

13. Merriam-Webster, s.v. "apophenia (n.)," accessed April 24, 2022, merriam
-webster.com/dictionary/apophenia.

14.. Michael Bar-Eli, Simcha Avugos, and Markus Raab, "Twenty Years of 'Hot
Hand' Research: Review and Critique," *Psychology of Sport and Exercise* 7,
no. 6 (November 2006): 525–53, doi.org/10.1016/j.psychsport.2006.03.001.

CHAPTER 10: The Outsider

1. Beverly Amsel, "Terrified People Pleasers: Why Can't I Love and Be
Loved?," GoodTherapy, December 21, 2016, goodtherapy.org/blog/terri
fied-people-pleasers-why-cant-i-love-be-loved-1221164.

2. Gareth Cook, "Why We Are Wired to Connect," *Scientific American*, October
22, 2013, scientificamerican.com/article/why-we-are-wired-to-connect.

3. Cindy Lamothe, "Conflict Avoidance Doesn't Do You Any Favors,"
Healthline, March 30, 2020, https://www.healthline.com/health/conflict
-avoidance.

4. Kendra Cherry, "The Different Types of Attachment Styles," Verywell
Mind, updated June 3, 2020, verywellmind.com/attachment-styles-2795344.

5. Sayli Agashe, Sunil Kumar, and Rishabh Rai, "Exploring the Relationship
between Social Ties and Resilience from Evolutionary Framework," *Frontiers in Human Dynamics* (August 5, 2021): doi.org/10.3389/fhumd.2021
.683755.

6. Mariska E. Kret et al., "Perception of Face and Body Expressions Using
Electromyography, Pupillometry and Gaze Measures," *Frontiers in Psychology* 4, no. 28 (February 8, 2013): doi.org/10.3389/fpsyg.2013.00028.

7. Olivia Remes, "Loneliness Is Contagious—and Here's How to Beat It," *The
Conversation*, July 13, 2018, theconversation.com/loneliness-is-contagious
-and-heres-how-to-beat-it-94376; and John Amodeo, "Are You Wondering
Why You're Lonely?," *Psychology Today*, April 1, 2018, psychologytoday
.com/us/blog/intimacy-path-toward-spirituality/201804/are-you
-wondering-why-youre-lonely.

8. Robin Stern, "I've Counseled Hundreds of Victims of Gaslighting. Here's
How to Spot If You're Being Gaslighted," *Vox*, updated January 3, 2019,
vox.com/first-person/2018/12/19/18140830/gaslighting-relationships
-politics-explained.

9. Alex Eichler, "'Askers' vs. 'Guessers,'" *The Atlantic*, May 12, 2010, the
atlantic.com/national/archive/2010/05/askers-vs-guessers/340891.

10. Brené Brown, "The Power of Vulnerability," filmed June 2010 at TEDx-
Houston, TED video, 20:03, ted.com/talks/brene_brown_the_power_of

_vulnerability; see also Brené Brown, *Daring Greatly: How the Courage to Be Vulnerable Transforms the Way We Live, Love, Parent, and Lead* (New York: Avery, 2012).

11. Willie Garrett, "Marginalized Populations," Minnesota Psychological Association, April 1, 2016, mnpsych.org/index.php?option=com_dailyplan etblog&view=entry&category=division%20news&id=71:marginalized -populations.

12. Peg Streep, "Tackling Self-Blame and Self-Criticism: 5 Strategies to Try," *Psychology Today*, January 10, 2018, psychologytoday.com/us/blog/tech -support/201801/tackling-self-blame-and-self-criticism-5-strategies-try; and Darius Cikanavicius, "6 Ways Childhood Abuse and Neglect Leads to Self-Blame in Adulthood," PsychCentral, July 2, 2018, https://psychcen tral.com/blog/psychology-self/2018/07/abuse-neglect-blame#1.

13. "A Guide to Finding Yourself," PsychAlive [2017], accessed May 11, 2022, psychalive.org/finding-yourself; and "Know Yourself—Socrates and How to Develop Self-Knowledge," The School of Life, accessed May 11, 2022, theschooloflife.com/article/know-yourself.

14. Harper West, "Factor 5: Attachment—Why Attachment Is So Important," Harper West website, accessed May 11, 2022, harperwest.co/self-acceptance /five-factors/5-attachment.

15. Maya Al-Khoujaa et al., "Self-Expression Can Be Authentic or Inauthentic, with Differential Outcomes for Well-Being: Development of the Authentic and Inauthentic Expression Scale (AIES)," *Journal of Research in Personality* 97 (April 2022): doi.org/10.1016/j.jrp.2022.104191.

16. Marlena Tillhon, "The Power of Speaking Our Truth in Intimate Relationships," Medium, June 15, 2018, https://marlenatillhon.medium.com/the -power-of-speaking-our-truth-in-intimate-relationships-81eb87bcff7.

CHAPTER 11: The Runner

1. Fred Rothbaum, John R. Weisz, and Samuel S. Snyder, "Changing the World and Changing the Self: A Two-Process Model of Perceived Control," *Journal of Personality and Social Psychology* 42, no. 1 (January 1982): 5–37, doi.org/10.1037/0022-3514.42.1.5

2. Ruth Cohn, "Trauma & Neglect," accessed May 10, 2022, Ruth Cohn website, ruthcohnmft.com/trauma-neglect; see also [Priya Watson,] "What Is Developmental Trauma / ACEs?," Childhood Trauma Toolkit, accessed April 29, 2022, porticonetwork.ca/web/childhood-trauma-toolkit/devel opmental-trauma/what-is-developmental-trauma.

3. Zhongqiu Li, Yang Yang, Xue Zhang, and Zhuo Lyu, "Impact of Future Work Self on Employee Workplace Wellbeing: A Self-Determination Perspective," *Frontiers in Psychology* (July 15, 2021): doi.org/10.3389 /fpsyg.2021.656874; and Naina Dhingra et al., "Help Your Employees Find Purpose—or Watch Them Leave," McKinsey & Company, April 5, 2021,

mckinsey.com/business-functions/people-and-organizational-performance/our-insights/help-your-employees-find-purpose-or-watch-them-leave.

4. Saul McLeod, "Maslow's Hierarchy of Needs," Simply Psychology, updated April 4, 2022, simplypsychology.org/maslow.html.
5. Bessel van der Kolk, *The Body Keeps the Score: Brain, Mind, and Body in the Healing of Trauma* (New York: Viking, 2014), 205.
6. Meagan Mullen, "Is It Binge Eating Disorder (BED) or Are You Stuck in a Vicious Cycle?," Multi-Service Eating Disorders Association, accessed May 11, 2022, medainc.org/bed-or-binge-restrict-cycle; Naveed Saleh, "9 Adverse Health Effects of Too Much Exercise," MDLinx, updated August 17, 2020, mdlinx.com/article/9-adverse-health-effects-of-too-much-exercise/70VZzE7JPAtHBOXq4O8Ltw; and "Burnout Prevention and Treatment," HelpGuide.org, accessed May 11, 2022, helpguide.org/articles/stress/burnout-prevention-and-recovery.htm.
7. Erin Olivo, "Here's Why You Struggle to Stay Present," mindbodygreen, August 27, 2020, mindbodygreen.com/0-16126/heres-why-you-struggle-to-stay-present.html.
8. Dianne Grande, "The Neuroscience of Feeling Safe and Connected," *Psychology Today*, September 24, 2018, psychologytoday.com/us/blog/in-it-together/201809/the-neuroscience-feeling-safe-and-connected.
9. Kristine Klussman, "Numbing vs. Relaxing: Are You Disconnecting from Life?" Kristine Klussman PhD website, accessed May 11, 2022, kristineklussman.com/numbing-vs-relaxing.
10. Michael Clark [pseud.], "Emotional Numbing: Why Avoiding Uncomfortable Feelings Gets Us Nowhere," Ananias Foundation, April 10, 2020, ananiasfoundation.org/emotional-numbing.
11. Van der Kolk, *The Body Keeps the Score,* 210.
12. Brené Brown, *The Gifts of Imperfection: Let Go of Who You Think You're Supposed to Be and Embrace Who You Are* (Center City, MN: Hazelden, 2010).
13. Van der Kolk, *The Body Keeps the Score.*
14. Stacey Colino, "When You Can't Put Your Feelings into Words: The Emotional Ignorance of Alexithymia," *U.S. News & World Report*, March 28, 2018, health.usnews.com/wellness/mind/articles/2018-03-28/when-you-cant-put-your-feelings-into-words-the-emotional-ignorance-of-alexithymia; René J. Muller, "When a Patient Has No Story to Tell: Alexithymia," *Psychiatric Times* 17, no. 7 (July 1, 2000): psychiatrictimes.com/view/when-patient-has-no-story-tell-alexithymia.
15. "Dissociation and Dissociative Disorders," Mind, March 2019, mind.org.uk/information-support/types-of-mental-health-problems/dissociation-and-dissociative-disorders/about-dissociation.
16. Peter A. Levine with Ann Frederick, *Waking the Tiger: Healing Trauma* (Berkeley, CA: North Atlantic, 1997), 16–21; see also Robert M. Sapolsky,

Why Zebras Don't Get Ulcers: The Acclaimed Guide to Stress, Stress-Related Diseases, and Coping, 3rd ed. (New York: Henry Holt, 2004).

17. Asaf Rolef Ben-Shahar, *Touching the Relational Edge: Body Psychotherapy* (London: Routledge, 2018); see also Sheila L. Ferguson (jealousyjane), "Trauma & Body Armoring: Why We Are So Tense?," Steemit, December 18, 2017, steemit.com/health/@jealousyjane/trauma-and-body-armoring -why-we-are-so-tense.

18. Rolef Ben-Shahar, *Touching the Relational Edge;* see also Ferguson, "Trauma & Body Armoring."

19. Julianne Ishler, "How to Release 'Emotional Baggage' and the Tension That Goes with It," Healthline, September 16, 2021, healthline.com/health /mind-body/how-to-release-emotional-baggage-and-the-tension-that -goes-with-it.

20. "Stress Effects on the Body," American Psychological Association, November 1, 2018, apa.org/topics/stress/body.

CHAPTER 13: Identifying Your Hidden Body Image Purpose

1. Margaret Neale, "How Your Appearance Is Affecting Your Behavior," HuffPost, updated September 28, 2014, huffpost.com/entry/how-your -appearance-is-affecting_b_5628517; and Tonya K. Frevert and Lisa Slattery Walker, "Physical Attractiveness and Social Status," *Sociology Compass* 8, no. 3 (March 2014): 313–23, doi.org/10.1111/soc4.12132.

2. Nancy Etcoff et al., "Beyond Stereotypes: Rebuilding the Foundation of Beauty," Dove Beauty, January 21, 2016, https://fliphtml5.com/trmf/mxyo.

CHAPTER 14: Creating a Vision for a Body Neutral Future

1. Courtney E. Ackerman, "Coping Mechanisms: Dealing with Life's Disappointments in a Healthy Way," PositivePsychology.com, updated March 29, 2022, positivepsychology.com/coping; and Amy Morin, "Healthy Coping Skills for Uncomfortable Emotions: Emotion-Focused and Problem-Focused Strategies," Verywell Mind, updated November 29, 2021, verywellmind .com/forty-healthy-coping-skills-4586742.

CHAPTER 15: Creating a Body Neutrality Action Plan

1. Megan Call, "Neuroplasticity: How to Use Your Brain's Malleability to Improve Your Well-Being," Accelerate, University of Utah Health, August 8, 2019, accelerate.uofuhealth.utah.edu/resilience/neuroplasticity-how-to -use-your-brain-s-malleability-to-improve-your-well-being.

2. American Psychological Association, "What Is Exposure Therapy?," PTSD Clinical Practice Guideline, July 2017, apa.org/ptsd-guideline/patients-and -families/exposure-therapy; APA Div. 12 (Society of Clinical Psychology).

3. Brené Brown, "Shame vs. Guilt," Brené Brown website, January 15, 2013, brenebrown.com/articles/2013/01/15/shame-v-guilt; see also Brené Brown,

"Listening to Shame," filmed March 2012 at TED2012, Long Beach, CA, Ted video, 20:22, ted.com/talks/brene_brown_listening_to_shame.

4. Brené Brown, *Daring Greatly: How the Courage to Be Vulnerable Transforms the Way We Live, Love, Parent, and Lead* (New York: Avery, 2012), 68.

CHAPTER 17: Micro-Goals and Action Steps for Each Avatar

1. Kathrin Karsay, Johannes Knoll, and Jörg Matthes, "Sexualizing Media Use and Self-Objectification," *Psychology of Women Quarterly* 42, no. 1 (March 1, 2018): 9–28, doi.org/10.1177/0361684317743019; Chiara Rollero and Norma De Piccoli, "Self-Objectification and Personal Values. An Exploratory Study," *Frontiers in Psychology*, (June 23, 2017), doi.org/10.3389 /fpsyg.2017.01055.

2. Emily Nagoski, *Come As You Are: Revised and Updated; The Surprising New Science That Will Transform Your Sex Life* (New York: Simon & Schuster, 2021).

3. Christy Harrison, *Anti-Diet: Reclaim Your Time, Money, Well-Being and Happiness through Intuitive Eating* (New York: Little, Brown Spark, 2019).

4. Catherine Goldberg, "This Is Mine: The Only 7 Things You Can Control in Life," Greatist, updated August 31, 2020, greatist.com/grow/what-you -can-control-for-happiness-success.

5. Courtney E. Ackerman, "What Is Self-Expression and How to Foster It?," PositivePsychology.com, updated March 28, 2022, positivepsychology.com /self-expression; and Judith E. Glaser, "Self-Expression: The Neuroscience of Co-creation," Psychology Today, February 15, 2016, psychologytoday .com/us/blog/conversational-intelligence/201602/self-expression.

6. Melissa Mesku, "The Problem with Being a People Pleaser," Medium, March 7, 2015, medium.com/the-ascent/the-problem-with-being-a-people -pleaser-6a9714c6c8a1.

7. Kerry Jamieson, "ACEs and Attachment: Why Connection Means Everything," Center for Child Counseling, July 15, 2021, centerforchildcounsel ing.org/aces-and-attachment-why-connection-means-everything.

8. Heather Jones, "What to Know about Anxious Attachment and Tips to Cope," Verywell Health, November 29, 2021, verywellhealth.com/anx ious-attachment-5204408#toc-strategies-for-coping.

9. Kim Elsesser, "The Debate on Power Posing Continues: Here's Where We Stand," *Forbes*, October 2, 2020, forbes.com/sites/kimelsesser/2020/10 /02/the-debate-on-power-posing-continues-heres-where-we-stand/?sh =260f1281202e.

10. Tal Shafir, Rachelle P. Tsachor, and Kathleen B. Welch, "Emotion Regulation through Movement: Unique Sets of Movement Characteristics Are Associated with and Enhance Basic Emotions," *Frontiers in Psychology* (January 11, 2016): doi.org/10.3389/fpsyg.2015.02030.

11. Cynthia J. Price and Carole Hooven, "Interoceptive Awareness Skills for Emotional Regulation: Theory and Approach of Mindful Awareness in

Body-Oriented Therapy (MABT)," *Frontiers in Psychology* 28 (May 28, 2018): doi.org/10.3389/fpsyg.2018.00798.

12. Mark Manson, "Happiness Is a Problem That Can Be Solved," Quartz, April 26, 2017, excerpt from *The Subtle Art of Not Giving a F*ck: A Counterintuitive Approach to Living a Good Life* (New York: HarperOne, 2016).

13. Kyli Rodriguez-Cayro, "The Way You Sit While You Answer Emails Can Have a Surprising Effect on Your Body," Bustle, April 18, 2018, bustle.com /p/9-ways-posture-affects-your-health-that-might-surprise-you-8793625; Harvard Health Publishing, "3 Surprising Risks of Poor Posture," Harvard Medical School, February 15, 2021, health.harvard.edu/staying-healthy /3-surprising-risks-of-poor-posture; and James Roland, "Want to Kick Your Slouching Habit? Try These 8 Strategies," Healthline, September 12, 2019, healthline.com/health/slouching.

14. George E. Billman, "Homeostasis: The Underappreciated and Far Too Often Ignored Central Organizing Principle of Physiology," *Frontiers in Physiology* (March 10, 2020): doi.org/10.3389/fphys.2020.00200.

15. Arianne Missimer, "How to Map Your Own Nervous System: The Polyvagal Theory," The Movement Paradigm, March 22, 2020, themovement paradigm.com/how-to-map-your-own-nervous-sytem-the-polyvagal -theory.

16. Ariane Resnick, "What Is Somatic Therapy?," Verywell Mind, updated July 29, 2021, verywellmind.com/what-is-somatic-therapy-5190064.

17. Ann Pietrangelo, "Defining and Overcoming a Fear of Intimacy," Healthline, January 10, 2019, healthline.com/health/fear-of-intimacy#treatment.

18. Bessel van der Kolk, *The Body Keeps the Score: Brain, Mind, and Body in the Healing of Trauma* (New York: Viking, 2014), 96, quoting in part Antonio Damasio, *The Feeling of What Happens: Body and Emotion in the Making of Consciousness* (New York: Harcourt Brace, 1999), 28.

19. Roberto A. Ferdman, "Why Diets Don't Actually Work, According to a Researcher Who Has Studied Them for Decades," *Washington Post*, May 4, 2015, washingtonpost.com/news/wonk/wp/2015/05/04/why-diets-dont -actually-work-according-to-a-researcher-who-has-studied-them-for -decades; Traci Mann, *Secrets from the Eating Lab: The Science of Weight Loss, the Myth of Willpower, and Why You Should Never Diet Again* (New York: Harper Wave, 2015).

20. Jack Wilkinson, "Difficulty Concentrating," Buoy Health, updated September 17, 2020, https://www.buoyhealth.com/learn/difficulty-concentrating; see also Sarah Fielding, "How the 'Impossible Task' Affects Anxiety—and What You Can Do about It," Healthline, updated July 2, 2019, healthline .com/health/mental-health/impossible-task-anxiety#The-line-between -normal-laziness-and-the-impossible-task.

21. "The Science of Mindfulness," Mindful, September 7, 2020, mindful.org /the-science-of-mindfulness.

22. Jeremy Adam Smith et al., "The State of Mindfulness Science," *Greater Good Magazine*, December 5, 2017, greatergood.berkeley.edu/article/item /the_state_of_mindfulness_science.

23. Eric Barker, "New Neuroscience Reveals Three Secrets That Will Make You Emotionally Intelligent," Observer, September 1, 2017, observer.com /2017/09/new-neuroscience-reveals-three-secrets-that-will-make-you -emotionally-intelligent-happiness-relationships; and Lisa Feldman Barrett, *How Emotions Are Made: The Secret Life of the Brain* (New York: Mariner Books, 2018).

CHAPTER 18: But What about Marginalized Bodies?

1. Kathleen Ebbitt, "Why It's Important to Think about Privilege—and Why It's Hard," Global Citizen, February 27, 2015, globalcitizen.org/en /content/why-its-important-to-think-about-privilege-and-why.

2. "Social Identities and Systems of Oppression," National Museum of African American History & Culture, Smithsonian Institution, nmaahc.si.edu /learn/talking-about-race/topics/social-identities-and-systems-oppression; and Nathaniel Granger, "Marginalization: The Pendulum Swings Both Ways," Unbound, Saybrook University, April 5, 2013, saybrook.edu/un bound/marginalization.

3. Nicole Hawkins, "Battling Our Bodies: Understanding and Overcoming Negative Body Images," Center for Change, updated August 2014, center forchange.com/battling-bodies-understanding-overcoming-negative -body-images; Margo Maine, *Body Wars: Making Peace with Women's Bodies; An Activist's Guide* (Carlsbad, CA: Gürze Books, 2011).

4. Williams Institute at UCLA School of Law, "Transgender People over Four Times More Likely Than Cisgender People to Be Victims of Violent Crime," March 23, 2021, williamsinstitute.law.ucla.edu/press/ncvs-trans -press-release. In addition, according to the advocacy group Forge, "multiple studies indicate that over 50% of transgender people have experienced sexual violence at some point in their lives." Compare this figure—one in two—with the commonly reported rates of sexual abuse to cisgender individuals: one in three girls, or one in six boys. "Transgender Rates of Violence," Victim Service Providers' Fact Sheet #6, Forge Forward, October 2012, forge-forward.org/wp-content/uploads/2020/08/FAQ-10-2012-rates -of-violence.pdf.

Bibliography

Barrett, Lisa Feldman. *How Emotions Are Made: The Secret Life of the Brain*. New York: Mariner Books, 2018.

Ben-Shahar, Asaf Rolef. *Touching the Relational Edge: Body Psychotherapy*. London: Routledge, 2018.

Betts, Charlotte. "Perceptions of the Self: How Social Media Leads to Body Dissatisfaction." Medium, July 28, 2020. medium.com/@charlotteebetts /perceptions-of-the-self-how-social-media-leads-to-body-dissatisfaction -7ce918be978.

Brown, Brené. *The Power of Vulnerability: Teachings on Authenticity, Connection, and Courage*. Sounds True, 2012.

Damasio, Antonio. *The Feeling of What Happens: Body and Emotion in the Making of Consciousness*. New York: Harcourt Brace, 1999.

Dana, Deb. *Anchored: How to Befriend Your Nervous System Using Polyvagal Theory*. Boulder, CO: Sounds True, 2021.

Daswani, Nico. "We Should Care More for Each Other—It's Good for Our Health." World Economic Forum Annual Meeting, January 21, 2019. weforum.org/agenda/2019/01/we-should-care-more-for-each-other-after-all -its-in-our-own-interest.

Dooner, Caroline. *The F*ck It Diet: Eating Should Be Easy*. London: HQ, 2019.

Eberhardt, Jennifer L. *Biased: Uncovering the Hidden Prejudice That Shapes What We See, Think, and Do*. New York: Viking, 2019.

Engeln, Renee. *Beauty Sick: How the Cultural Obsession with Appearance Hurts Girls and Women*. New York: Harper, 2018.

Ferdman, Roberto A. "Why Diets Don't Actually Work, According to a Researcher Who Has Studied Them for Decades." *Washington Post*, May 4, 2015. washingtonpost.com/news/wonk/wp/2015/05/04/why-diets-dont-actually-work -according-to-a-researcher-who-has-studied-them-for-decades.

Fox, Kate. "Mirror, Mirror: A Summary of Research Findings on Body Image." SIRC (Social Issues Research Centre), 1997. sirc.org/publik/mirror.html.

Gordon, Aubrey. *What We Don't Talk about When We Talk about Fat.* Boston: Beacon Press, 2020.

Gulino, Elizabeth. "Body Positivity Doesn't Mean What You Think It Does." *Refinery29*, updated March 25, 2021, 9:42 a.m. refinery29.com/en-us/2021/03/10370504/body-positivity-neutrality-movementhistory.

Harrison, Christy. *Anti-Diet: Reclaim Your Time, Money, Well-Being, and Happiness through Intuitive Eating.* New York: Little, Brown Spark, 2019.

Hollander, Anne. "When Fat Was in Fashion." *New York Times*, October 23, 1977. nytimes.com/1977/10/23/archives/when-fat-was-in-fashion-abundant-flesh-was-a-thing-of-beauty-to.html.

Ishler, Julianne. "How to Release 'Emotional Baggage' and the Tension That Goes with It." Healthline, September 16, 2021. healthline.com/health/mind-body/how-to-release-emotional-baggage-and-the-tension-that-goes-with-it.

Jackson-Gibson, Adele. "The Racist and Problematic History of the Body Mass Index." *Good Housekeeping*, February 23, 2021. goodhousekeeping.com/health/diet-nutrition/a35047103/bmi-racist-history.

Jackson-Gibson, Adele. "What Is Thin Privilege?" *Good Housekeeping*, April 15, 2021. goodhousekeeping.com/health/diet-nutrition/a35047908/what-is-thin-privilege.

Jarrett, Christian. "A Biological Mechanism That Protects against Rape?" *British Psychological Society Research Digest*, January 11, 2011, digest.bps.org.uk/2011/01/11/a-biological-mechanism-that-protects-against-rape.

Kabat-Zinn, Jon. *Full Catastrophe Living: Using the Wisdom of Your Body and Mind to Face Stress, Pain, and Illness.* New York: Dell, 1990.

Kite, Lindsay. "Body Positivity or Body Obsession? Learning to See More & Be More." Filmed September 9, 2017, at TEDxSaltLakeCity. TED video, 16:47, November 6, 2017. ted.com/talks/lindsay_kite_body_positivity_or_body_obsession_learning_to_see_more_and_be_more.

Kite, Lindsay, and Lexie Kite. *More Than a Body: Your Body Is an Instrument, Not an Ornament.* Boston: Houghton Mifflin Harcourt, 2020.

Levine, Amir, and Rachel Heller. *Attached: The New Science of Adult Attachment and How It Can Help You Find—and Keep—Love.* New York: TarcherPerigee, 2011.

Levine, Peter A. *Waking the Tiger: Healing Trauma.* With Ann Frederick. Berkeley, CA: North Atlantic, 1997.

Lewis, Marc. "Why We're Hardwired to Hate Uncertainty." *The Guardian*, April 4, 2016. theguardian.com/commentisfree/2016/apr/04/uncertainty-stressful-research-neuroscience.

Maine, Margo. *Body Wars: Making Peace with Women's Bodies; An Activist's Guide.* Carlsbad, CA: Gürze Books, 2011.

Mann, Traci. *Secrets from the Eating Lab: The Science of Weight Loss, the Myth of Willpower, and Why You Should Never Diet Again.* New York: Harper Wave, 2015.

Mannino, Brynn. "TODAY/AOL 'Ideal to Real' Body Image Survey." AOL, February 24, 2014. aol.com/article/2014/02/24/loveyourselfie/20836450.

Menakem, Resmaa. *My Grandmother's Hands: Racialized Trauma and the Pathway to Mending Our Hearts and Bodies.* Las Vegas: Central Recovery Press, 2017.

Nagoski, Emily. *Come As You Are: Revised and Updated; The Surprising New Science That Will Transform Your Sex Life.* New York: Simon & Schuster, 2021.

Nathan, Shayahi. "Beauty and the Biased: How Algorithms Perpetuate Body Dysmorphia." Medusa, October 9, 2020. medusacreatives.com/2020/10/09/beauty-and-the-biased-how-algorithms-perpetuate-bodydysmorphia.

Rhode, Deborah L. "Hooters Hires Based on Looks. So Do Many Companies. And There's No Law Against It." *New Republic*, August 30, 2014. newrepublic.com/article/118683/why-we-need-law-protect-against-appearance-discrimination.

Rosenberg, Marshall B. *Nonviolent Communication: A Language of Life; Life-Changing Tools for Healthy Relationships.* Encinitas, CA: PuddleDancer Press, 2015.

Ryder, Gina, and Taneasha White. "How Intergenerational Trauma Impacts Families." Psych Central, April 15, 2022, https://psychcentral.com/lib/how-intergenerational-trauma-impacts-families.

Saini, Angela. *Inferior: How Science Got Women Wrong and the New Research That's Rewriting the Story.* Boston: Beacon, 2017.

Sapolsky, Robert M. *Why Zebras Don't Get Ulcers: The Acclaimed Guide to Stress, Stress-Related Diseases, and Coping.* 3rd ed. New York: Henry Holt, 2004.

Tan Ngo, Nealie. "What Historical Ideals of Women's Shapes Teach Us About Women's Self-Perception and Body Decisions Today." *AMA Journal of Ethics*, October 2019, E879–901. https://www.doi.org/10.1001/amajethics.2019.879.

Taylor, Sonya Renee. *The Body Is Not an Apology, Second Edition: The Power of Radical Self-Love.* San Francisco: Berrett-Koehler, 2021.

van der Kolk, Bessel. *The Body Keeps the Score: Brain, Mind, and Body in the Healing of Trauma.* New York: Viking, 2014.

Wolf, Naomi. *The Beauty Myth: How Images of Beauty Are Used against Women.* New York: Harper Perennial, 2002.

YaleNews. "Yale Study Shows Weight Bias Is as Prevalent as Racial Discrimination." *YaleNews*, March 27, 2008. news.yale.edu/2008/03/27/yale-study-shows-weight-bias-prevalent-racial-discrimination.